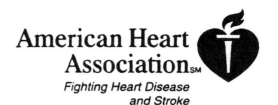

American Heart
Association℠

*Fighting Heart Disease
and Stroke*

Monograph Series

COMPLIANCE IN HEALTHCARE
AND RESEARCH

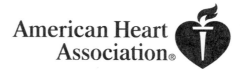

American Heart Association®

Fighting Heart Disease and Stroke

Monograph Series

COMPLIANCE IN HEALTHCARE AND RESEARCH

Edited by

Lora E. Burke, PhD, MPH, RN

Associate Professor
University of Pittsburgh School of Nursing
Pittsburgh, PA

and

Ira S. Ockene, MD

Professor of Medicine
Division of Cardiovascular Medicine, Department of Medicine
University of Massachusetts Medical School
Worcester, MA

Futura Publishing Company, Inc.
Armonk, NY

Library of Congress Cataloging-in-Publication Data

Compliance in healthcare and research / edited by Lora E. Burke,
  Ira S. Ockene.
  p. cm.
  Includes bibliographical references and index.
  ISBN 0–87993–474–3 (hardcover : alk. paper)
  1. Patient compliance. 2. Cooperativeness. 3. Behavior
modification. 4. Medical personnel and patient. 5. Compliance. I.
Burke, Lora E. II. Ockene, Ira S.

  R727.43 .C66 2001
  615.5—dc21fw00–051414

Copyright © 2001
Futura Publishing Company, Inc.
135 Bedford Road
Armonk, New York 10504

ISBN #:0–87993–474–3

Contributors

Deborah J. Aaron, PhD, MSIS   Assistant Professor, Department of Epidemiology, University of Pittsburgh, Pittsburgh, PA

Joan M. Amatruda, RN   Yale-New Haven Hospital Center for Outcomes Research and Evaluation, New Haven, CT

Tom Baranowski, PhD   Professor of Behavioral Nutrition, Children's Nutrition Research Center, Department of Pediatrics, Baylor College of Medicine, Houston, TX

Janice C. Baranowski, MPH, RD, LD   Project Director of Behavioral Nutrition, Department of Behavioral Science, University of Texas M.D. Anderson Cancer Center, Houston Texas

Deborah J. Bowen, PhD   Fred Hutchinson Cancer Research Center, Seattle, WA

Milo L. Brekke, PhD   Brekke Associates, Minneapolis, MN

Hans R. Brunner, MD   Professor, Division of Hypertension and Vascular Medicine, CHUV, Lausanne, Switzerland

Lora E. Burke, PhD, MPH, RN   Associate Professor, University of Pittsburgh School of Nursing, Pittsburgh, PA

Michel Burnier, MD   Professor Associate, Division of Hypertension and Vascular Medicine, CHUV, Lausanne, Switzerland

Karen Cullen, DrPH, RD, LD   Assistant Professor of Behavioral Nutrition, Department of Behavioral Science, University of Texas M.D. Anderson Cancer Center, Houston, Texas

Susan M. Czajkowski, PhD   Behavioral Medicine Scientific Research Group, Division of Epidemiology and Clinical Applications, National Heart, Lung, and Blood Institute, National Institutes of Health, Bethesda, MD

Ed Davis, MD   Professor, University of North Carolina Department of Biostatistics, School of Public Health, Chapel Hill, NC

Mohsen Davoudi, MD   Yale-New Haven Hospital Center for Outcomes Research and Evaluation, New Haven, CT

Jacqueline Dunbar-Jacob, PhD, RN, FAAN   Professor of Nursing, Epidemiology and Occupational Therapy, Chair, Department of Health and Community Systems, University of Pittsburgh School of Nursing, Pittsburgh, PA

Cara B. Ebbeling, PhD   Senior Research Fellow, Division of Endocrinology, Children's Hospital, Boston, MA

Deborah Echement, BA   Associate Director of Data Management, Epidemiology Data Center, University of Pittsburgh, Pittsburgh, PA

R. Brian Haynes, MD, PhD   Professor of Clinical Epidemiology and Medicine, McMaster University, Faculty of Health Sciences, Hamilton, Ontario, Canada

James R. Hebert, ScD   Professor and Chair, Department of Epidemiology and Biostatistics, University of South Carolina, School of Public Health, Columbia, SC

Almut Helmes, MS   Fred Hutchinson Cancer Research Center, Seattle, WA

Laurie A. Kopin, MS, ANP   Senior Nurse Manager, Cardiac Rehabilitation Center, University of Rochester School of Medicine, Rochester, NY

Thomas E. Kottke, MD, MSPH   Mayo Clinic and Foundation, Rochester, MN

Harlan M. Krumholz, MD   Paul Beeson Faculty Scholar, Section of Cardiovascular Medicine, Department of Medicine and the Section of Chronic Disease Epidemiology, Department of Epidemiology and Public Health, Yale University School of Medicine, Yale-New Haven Hospital Center for Outcomes Research and Evaluation, New Haven, CT, Qualidigm, Middletown, CT

Shiriki K. Kumanyika, PhD, MPH, RD   Professor (designate) of Epidemiology, Associate Dean for Health Promotion & Disease Prevention, Center for Clinical Epidemiology and Biostatistics, University of Pennsylvania School of Medicine, Philadelphia, PA

Ronald E. LaPorte, PhD   Professor, Department of Epidemiology, University of Pittsburgh, Pittsburgh, PA

Erika Lease, BA   Fred Hutchinson Cancer Research Center, Seattle, WA

Thomas H. Lee, MD   Medical Director, Partners Community Healthcare, Inc., Associate Professor of Medicine, Brigham and Women's Hospital, Harvard Medical School, Boston, MA

Yunsheng Ma, MD, MPH   Research Associate, Division of Preventive and Behavioral Medicine, Department of Medicine, University of Massachusetts Medical School, Worcester, MA

Jeffrey P. Martin, MBA   Associate Director of Computing, Epidemiology Data Center, University of Pittsburgh, Pittsburgh, PA

Charles E. Matthews, PhD   Assistant Professor, Department of Epidemiology and Biostatistics, University of South Carolina, School of Public Health, Columbia, SC

Kimberly A. Morris, PhD   Instructor of Pediatrics, Cystic Fibrosis Center, Children's Hospital of Pittsburgh, Department of Pediatrics, University of Pittsburgh, Pittsburgh, PA

Patricia A. Nixon, PhD   Associate Professor of Pediatrics, Cystic Fibrosis Center, Children's Hospital of Pittsburgh, Department of Pediatrics, University of Pittsburgh, Pittsburgh, PA

Ira S. Ockene, MD   Professor of Medicine, Division of Cardiovascular Medicine, Department of Medicine, University of Massachusetts Medical School, Worcester, MA

Judith K. Ockene, PhD, MEd   Professor of Medicine and Chair, Division of Preventive and Behavioral Medicine, University of Massachusetts Medical School, Worcester, MA

Neil B. Oldridge, PhD   Professor of Physical Therapy and Medicine, Indiana University Center for Aging Research, Regenstrief Institute for Health Care, Indiana University, Indianapolis, IN.

Thomas A. Pearson, MD, PhD   Professor and Chair, Department of Community and Preventive Medicine, University of Rochester School of Medicine, Rochester, NY

Michael G. Perri, PhD   Professor, Department of Clinical and Health Psychology, University of Florida Health Science Center, Gainesville, FL

Cynthia Rand, PhD   Associate Professor, Asthma and Allergy Center, Johns Hopkins University School of Medicine, Baltimore, MD

Sarah A. Roumanis, RN   Yale-New Haven Hospital Center for Outcomes Research and Evaluation, New Haven, CT

Elizabeth A. Schlenk, PhD, RN   Assistant Professor, University of Pittsburgh School of Nursing, Pittsburgh, PA

Eleanor Schron, MS, RN   Clinical Trials Scientific Research Group, Division of Epidemiology and Clinical Applications, National Heart, Lung, and Blood Institute, National Institutes of Health, Bethesda, MD

Susan Sereika, PhD   Associate Professor, University of Pittsburgh School of Nursing and Graduate School of Public Health, Pittsburgh, PA

Leif I. Solberg, MD   HealthPartners Research Foundation, Minneapolis, MN

John Urquhart, MD, FRCP(Edin)   Professor of Pharmaco-epidemiology, Maastricht University, Maastricht, Netherlands

Contents

PART IV.   Measurement of Compliance

PART V.   Issues in Special Populations

PART VI.   Issues Across Settings

PART VII.   Special Topics

PART VIII.   Future Directions

Section I

Introduction

Improving Patient Adherence:
State of the Art, With a Special Focus on Medication Taking For Cardiovascular Disorders

R. Brian Haynes, MD, PhD

Introduction

Many more medical disorders can now be managed with self-administered treatments than ever before. Of most importance is the advance of effective treatments for chronic disorders. People can live longer and better if they take these treatments, but almost all treatments are palliative and exact a price. Because they do not cure the disorder, patients must follow the treatments for as long as the disorder persists, often for the rest of their lives. The treatments can cause adverse effects and also are often expensive for the patient and inconvenient to take. Furthermore, the prescription often includes "lifestyle changes" including weight reduction, stopping smoking, and increasing exercise. While all of these nondrug treatments have merit, each of them places a heavy behavioral demand on the patient—an additional adherence burden.[1] Although sometimes we might wonder why patients do not follow our prescriptions, there is not much mystery here.

During the past 25 years, randomized controlled trials have validated several interventions to help patients to follow their treatment regimens,[2] the main subject of this paper. Unfortunately, most of these methods don't work very well or are labor-intensive and expensive to implement. Worse still, most practitioners and scientists who discover the adherence limitations of their treatments begin from scratch in de-

This chapter is an update and expansion of an earlier article,[79] and is published with permission of Marcel Dekker Inc.

From: Burke LE, Ockene IS (eds). *Compliance in Healthcare and Research.* Armonk, NY: Futura Publishing Company, Inc.; © 2001.

veloping ways to improve adherence, oblivious to the research of others in similar circumstances, albeit for different treatments. In addition to the fragmentation of adherence research, it is not imaginative, and is largely impractical for application in usual clinical settings. Thus, much of the effort to date to develop innovations that will improve adherence is wasted, while the problems of adherence persist. To make matters worse, little of what is known and practical about improving adherence is applied in usual clinical practice. Indeed, because the "state of the art" for improving adherence is relatively static while new treatments abound, the gap is widening between what we could achieve with full application of current best care, and what we are achieving.

This chapter will provide a general narrative review of selected knowledge concerning patient adherence, with more detailed results from systematic reviews of evidence from randomized controlled trials of interventions to improve adherence with medications in which both adherence and at least one clinical outcome have been measured in at least 80% of the patients that were enrolled in the study.[2] While adherence with nondrug treatments will not be reviewed systematically, general comments will be made based on more comprehensive reviews.[3-5] Finally, some practical considerations will be discussed and a preliminary research agenda proposed.

The Nature and Determinants of Nonadherence

Definition

Compliance has been defined as the extent to which a person's behavior (in terms of taking medication, following a diet, modifying habits or attending clinics) coincides with medical or health advice.[6] Some people object to the term "compliance" because they believe it implies subservience on the part of the patient, or constitutes blaming the patient for noncompliance. Some prefer "adherence" or "concordance" to compliance.[7] Perhaps "acceptance" would be the best term of all, but it is not widely used. I will use the terms adherence and compliance interchangeably in this chapter with the explanation that I am using them without prejudice.

Types of Nonadherence and Their Magnitude

Nonadherence can undermine the effectiveness of care at many steps in the process.[8] Following community screening for high blood pressure, for example, from 35% to 49% of those whose blood pressures are elevated may fail to follow through with a referral for follow-up assessment.[9-10] Once assessed and prescribed therapy, over a third of patients may drop out of care entirely and are particularly prone to do so in the few months following their initial diagnosis.[11,12] While in care, patients frequently do not take all of their medication, the average consumption rate being reported as about 50%.[13,14] Adherence with instructions to lose weight or stop smoking is less still, with long-term rates of less than 10% for substantial weight loss and smoking cessation in most situations.[15,16]

The rates of nonadherence in most reports imply that few patients receive much benefit from therapy. However, most of the studies from which the figures are derived were relatively short-term. A study with longer follow-up periods has found that, for hypertension for example, many of those who left care eventually returned, and most patients in care eventually got enough treatment to bring their blood pressures under control.[17] One way of thinking about this is that the short-term disadvantages of following chronic disease therapy substantially out-weigh the short-term benefits and patients require persistent reminding of the long-term benefits to swing this unfavorable balance in a positive direction.

Key Determinants of Adherence

Literally hundreds of studies have attempted to "crack the adherence nut," discovering the causes of low adherence and the determinants of high adherence. If understanding the causes of chronic diseases is complicated, it is not difficult to imagine that understanding nonadherence is more so. Studies of sociodemographic factors, such as age, gender, socioeconomic status, intelligence, marital status and so on, have not provided consistent findings, and neither have any consistent psychological features of nonadherence been discovered. Indeed, we are virtually all nonadherent with medical treatments at one time or another. Thus, there is no "stereotypical" nonadherer. This has obvious implications for detecting nonadherence (see "Measurement" section below). There are two exceptions to this generalism: first, difficult social circumstances such as marital discord, social isolation,[18,19] and unemployment,[1] adversely affect adherence. Second, patients with mental disorders, particularly those with paranoid or depressive features, tend to be less adherent.[1]

Key care process factors that affect adherence that we can often do something about include the time between screening and follow-up appointments,[20-22] the amount of waiting time at clinic visits,[23-24] the complexity of the regimen,[25-29] adverse effects from therapy,[1,30] and the cost of therapy.[20,24,25] These factors affect individual patients differently, so that the clinician needs to become aware of each patient's situation, with particular attention to barriers to adherence that can be modified.

Measurement of Adherence

In Practice

Clinicians are notoriously poor judges of the adherence of their patients, and it is essential to use methods of measuring adherence that have been validated.[31] As it happens, most accurate measures of adherence are not very easy to apply and most easy measures are not accurate. Fortunately, however, most important adherence problems can be detected by three simple maneuvers, used in sequence:

1. Watch for patients who fail to attend appointments. Nonattendance is evidence of the most severe form of nonadherence: dropping out of treatment. Also, patients who are irregular attendees are less likely to be following their prescribed regimen.[32-34]
2. Watch for nonresponders. The match between treatment and response is inexact in individual patients.[35] However, for patients whose condition fails to respond to increments in medication, nonadherence is the most frequent explanation, as long as the treatment is known to be efficacious when taken. This method can be augmented for some medications by observing their effects on other body processes, for example, slowing of heart rate with beta-blockers, or lowering of serum potassium and elevation of uric acid for diuretics. However, these effects may be no better correlated with medication consumption than measures of the clinical disorder itself.[5]
3. Ask nonresponders about their adherence. A meta-analysis of studies of measures of adherence has shown that the simple clinical measure of asking the patient has a sensitivity of 55% with a specificity of 87%.[36] That is, about half of nonadherers will confirm this on direct questioning, and few patients who are taking most of their medication will indicate that they are not. A nonthreatening approach is best, such as, "Many people have difficulty taking all the medications we prescribe. During the past week, have you missed *any* tablets?" In my experience, many patients will

indicate that they have taken virtually all their medication but "may have missed one or two pills on Saturday night" when they were visiting outside the home. Qualifying statements such as these are associated with an average adherence rate of less than 50%![35]

In Research

Other ways of assessing adherence are impractical in most clinical settings but are possible—and often necessary—in research settings. Careful pill counts can be useful on one occasion but these require a home visit, a very careful inventory of the pills, an accounting of when the pills were dispensed and whether pills from a previous prescription were added to the container, and questioning the patient about whether they share their pills with others, or have some of their supplies in other locations, such as the car, office, or cottage.[35] Some initial deception is required in setting up the visit (eg, indicating that the main purpose of the visit is to measure the blood pressure in the home) or the result is no more likely to be accurate than asking the patient directly. Also, after the first occasion, the patient will usually know what's up and may modify their pill count to reflect what they want the assessor to know. The deception raises ethical issues that are discussed further below, but the ethical concerns can often be dealt with satisfactorily by asking the patient at the time of the visit if their pills can be counted, making clear the reason for the count and that it is entirely up to them whether the count is done. Counting pills that patients bring to clinic visits gives rates of 90% to 100%, making a mockery of the procedure,[37] although it is remarkable how many drug trials blithely report such figures.

Monitoring pharmacy records for refills of medication is a useful variant of counting pills in settings where there is a single-source pharmacy for patients.[38–40] The validity of monitoring depends on the assumption that what is taken from the pharmacy actually ends up passing through the lips of the patient in the intended way, which is not always the case. Nevertheless, it can provide an inexpensive indirect method of monitoring adherence if trouble is taken to correlate pharmacy records with prescriptions, including changes in dosing and medications.

Drug assays are available routinely for some drugs such as digitalis and in some settings for some beta-blockers[41,42] but these assays can be expensive and the measurements can be misleading if the medication has a short serum half-life as the patient may have taken their pills only just before the time of determination or may have missed just that

---

Table 1

Methods of Measuring Adherence

In clinical practice
- attendance at appointments
- clinical response to medications
- patient self-report

In research
- pill counts at home visits
- monitoring prescription refills
- drug assays in body fluids
- tracers
- "memory" pill containers

---

dose. Urinary measures, for example, of diuretics, provide no more information than simply asking the patient.[35] A variant on these methods is to add a tracer to the medication, such as riboflavin[43] or a homeopathic dose of digoxin[44] or phenobarbital[45] and measure this, but there are obvious logistical and regulatory problems of doing so. An additional disadvantage to these direct measures of adherence is that they can be applied only to specific medications, compared with pill counts, prescription monitoring, memory-cap pill containers and self-reports which apply to any medication the patient is prescribed.

Finally, a number of special pill containers have been created with computerized memory chips[37,46] in their caps that can provide valuable information about the timing of dosing and gaps in dosing—as long as the patient removes and replaces the lid with each dosing. Their use in drug trials has revealed patterns of drug taking that include long and irregular periods between doses, including "holidays" of several days, even while patient diaries indicate much more regular consumption.[47] Unfortunately, these "medication event monitors" add cost to care (which might be offset by improved outcomes), require computer downloading of the monitor memories, and ultimately depend on the patient's cooperation. (See Table 1.)

The Ethics of Attempting to Improve Adherence

Several circumstances exist in which encouraging high adherence is of dubious merit, so that it is important to consider each patient's situation before intervening to improve adherence. First, the diagnosis must be clearly established before adherence becomes an issue. Second, the treatment being prescribed must be of known efficacy for the pa-

Table 2

Ethical Issues in Using Adherence-Enhancing Strategies

1. The diagnosis of hypertension must be established.
2. The benefits of treating the condition must outweigh the adverse effects for the individual patient.
3. The method of improving adherence must be of known efficacy.
4. The patient must be willing.

tient's specific condition and their circumstances (including the severity of the condition and the nature and tolerability of adverse effects the patient may suffer). Third, the method of improving adherence must be of established effectiveness. If for no reason other than efficiency, the maneuvers used to increase adherence should have been documented to work in properly designed studies. Unfortunately, many practitioners feel that they have done their job in promoting adherence when they have instructed the patient on the need for, and details of, the regimen,[48] even though simple instruction has no lasting effect on adherence. Many studies have shown that instruction alone does not improve long-term adherence and, while clear instructions are necessary to promote adherence, they are not sufficient for long-term regimens, such as those required for most cardiovascular disorders.[49] Finally, the patient must be a willing partner in the process of improving adherence. The patient has a right to refuse treatment and this right must be respected. Attempts to coerce or intimidate the patient to adhere (for example, by emphasizing that they will have a stroke or heart attack if they do not comply) have not been shown to work any better than positive reinforcement and supportive reminders, but they do cause some patients with high anxiety levels to withdraw from care. Thus, such tactics might be considered unethical and potentially dangerous. (See Table 2.)

Improving Adherence

Compared with the relatively straightforward research that has established the efficacy of many treatments, research into methods of improving adherence is often difficult and complex. Most of the interventions that have been tested to improve adherence are not easily packaged or standardized (the term "disembodied technology" might be used to describe them), and the theoretical underpinnings of these strategies are not always apparent. These interventions will be considered at two levels, first reviewing the randomized controlled trials of attempts to improve adherence to medical treatments, based on a systematic review,[2] and then describing a theory-based practical formulation of the empirical studies.

Empirical Research

There have been many studies of attempts to improve patient adherence with medical therapies.[2-5] To be reasonably certain of the validity of the findings, I believe that these studies should be randomized controlled trials with follow-up of at least 80% of the participants, and that the studies measure both adherence and clinical outcomes. The reason for the latter requirement is that effective adherence interventions are usually costly; if they are not potent enough to improve at least intermediate clinical outcomes (such as cholesterol levels, blood pressure, blood sugar, heart failure, or angina severity) then the findings are really only of academic interest. All of the trials reviewed here meet all of these criteria.

Several studies have shown no benefits for adherence or clinical outcomes of interventions as diverse as self-monitoring of blood pressure, home visits, worksite care, programmed teaching, counseling by a nurse, or health educator, peer group discussions, tangible rewards, or unit dose-reminder packaging.[14,50-54] Fortunately, even more studies, summarized in Table 3, show that adherence and clinical outcomes can be improved by a number of interventions, often including those that were not successful in the studies just cited. This is not as mysterious as it might seem; no single maneuver works very well, but the combination of complementary strategies is often beneficial[5] and all the studies of successful strategies for longer-term treatments included two or more maneuvers. We will return to the theoretical underpinnings and a practical formulation after a description of the effective strategies.

In 1976, Haynes and colleagues[13] reported that adherence could be improved and blood pressure lowered among nonadherent patients with uncontrolled hypertension by a complex intervention with a nonhealth professional research assistant helping patients at their worksite to plan their medication taking in concert with usual daily activities ("cueing" or "tailoring"); teaching them to monitor their own blood pressures and adherence at home; and rewarding patients for higher adherence and blood pressure improvements by praising their efforts, allowing them to earn credits towards purchasing their blood pressure monitoring equipment, and reducing the frequency of their follow-up visits. The research assistant was not allowed to change medications

Table 3

Randomized Trials of Interventions to Improve Adherence with Therapy for Cardiovascular and Related Disorders§

Authors	Condition	Intervention
Sackett et al.	Hypertension	Instruction vs. worksite care vs. both vs. neither (usual care)†
Haynes et al.	Hypertension	Self-monitoring, cueing of medications, frequent follow-up visits at the worksite, rewards administered by a researh assistant vs. usual care by primary care physicians
Logan et al.	Hypertension	Worksite nurse with specialty clinic physician backup, self-monitoring, cueing, recalls, frequent visits, rewards vs. usual care by primary care physicians
Johnson et al.	Hypertension	Self-monitoring vs. home visits vs. both vs. neither†
Bass et al.	Hypertension	Cueing of medications, recalls for missed appointments, frequent visits vs. usual care by primary care physicians
Takala et al.	Hypertension	Written instruction, monitoring cards, recalls vs. usual care
Levine et al.	Hypertension	Counseling, social support, group discussions vs. usual care
Nessman et al.	Hypertension	Self-monitoring, group discussion, self-management vs. usual care
Swain et al.	Hypertension	Instruction, contingency contracts vs. usual care
Friedman et al.	Hypertension	Telephone-linked computer system (TLC)-an interactive computer system that conversed with patients in their homes between office visits to their physicians vs. regular medical care
Baird et al.	Hypertension	Controlled release metoprolol once-a-day vs. regular metoprolol twice-a-day*
Becker et al.	Hypertension	Special "reminder" pill packaging vs. regular pill containers†
Brown et al.	Hyperlipidemia	Controlled release niacin twice a day vs. regular niacin 4 times a day
Bailey et al.	Asthma	Standardized information pamphlets, a skill-oriented self-help workbook, a one-to-one counseling session, support group and telephone calls from a health educator, with physician's emphasis of skills at regular clinic visits vs. pamphlets alone
Cote et al.	Asthma	Extensive asthma education program plus written self-managed action plan based on PEF or based on asthma symptom monitoring vs. basic information provided plus verbal action plan could be given by physician†

§ All studies showed significant improvements in both adherence and clinical outcomes unless otherwise noted

* Significant effect on adherence but not on clinical outcome

† No significant effect on adherence or clinical outcome.

but could notify the patient's physician if adherence appeared to be high without blood pressure being controlled. This "kitchen sink" approach resulted in a statistically significant, absolute 21% increase in adherence compared with control patients who received usual care from their physicians. Blood pressures improved significantly within the intervention group ($P<0.001$) but the difference compared with the control group was not significant ($P = 0.12$).

Logan and colleagues[55] used the same adherence procedures, also administered at the worksite, but in this study they were administered by nurses who also made changes in medications in consultation with the study physician. Control patients were simply referred to their family physicians for continuing care. Again there was a significant improvement in adherence in comparison with control patients, but this time there was also a statistically significant improvement in blood pressure control in favor of the intervention group patients. Although this intervention was quite elaborate, a full economic analysis showed that it was cost-effective in comparison with usual community care by primary care physicians.[56]

A study of Bass and colleagues[57] changed the venue to family physicians' offices, with practice nurses working in an extended role with the physician, screening patients for hypertension and helping hypertensive patients to achieve high adherence through instruction, cueing, recalling patients who missed appointments, and seeing some patients on extra visits. There was a modest improvement in adherence among intervention group patients compared with patients in control practices, and a small, statistically significant difference in systolic but not diastolic blood pressure at the end of the four-year follow-up in the trial.

Brown et al.[58] showed improved adherence and cholesterol lowering with a polygel niacin formulation given twice a day, compared with a regular niacin preparation given four times a day, among patients with coronary heart disease who were on a complex regimen to lower cholesterol. Although the study by Baird et al.[59] did not show an improvement in blood pressure with once versus twice per day metoprolol, a small improvement in adherence was shown.

Several other investigations have used similarly elaborate approaches, with additional innovations, including social support and group discussions for patients with hypertension,[53,60] and contingency contracts in which patients agreed to do specific tasks (eg, showing up at clinic on time) for simple rewards (eg, being seen on time!).[61] Of interest, in the latter study, few patients contracted to take their pills more often. Nevertheless, the drop-out rate was substantially reduced and blood pressures were lowered. One of these studies[53] also showed reduced mortality among patients receiving the adherence enhancement program, compared with controls, when the patients were followed over a five year period.[62] In a recent innovative study, Friedman et al.[63] showed increased adherence and blood pressure control with an automated telephone support program that "conversed" with patients once a week, allowed them to record their blood pressures and pill adherence, and reminded them of appointments and the importance of adherence.

Almost all trials of what proved to be successful adherence strategies used very complicated interventions, too complex to use in most practice settings, but the studies of failed adherence strategies showed that simple, single strategies are ineffective.[14,50,51,53,54] Is there a middle ground? A Finnish study by Takala and colleagues[64] was perhaps the first to demonstrate the success of a complex but practical approach. Patients in a community health center were given simple written information and instructions about their high blood pressure and its treatment, treatment cards on which their blood pressures and medications were recorded and amended at follow-up visits, and telephone recalls if they missed appointments. The dropout rate over one year was reduced from 19% in the control group to 4% in the intervention group, and significantly more intervention group patients had improvements in their blood pressures. Keeping patients in care is of paramount importance and recalling nonattenders is likely the most important single intervention, although the weight of evidence would suggest that recalls would have limited effectiveness if they were the only adherence maneuver.

The descriptions of adherence interventions in reports of individual studies can leave the reader in a state of confusion about what works and what does not, particularly as the studies have come from researchers of a number of different scientific disciplines including psychology, sociology, health education, and clinical epidemiology, each with their own jargon. Some theories of adherence behavior can clarify this situation and lead to practical generalizations.

Theories of Adherence and Their Practical Application

As described by Leventhal and Cameron,[65] theories from psychology can provide a basis for classifying adherence strategies and understanding why certain strategies work while others do not. A full discussion of the current theories is beyond the scope of this paper; a simple framework classifies adherence interventions into three broad categories: cognitive, behavioral, and social support.[49] Cognitive factors include what the patient knows about the disease and its treatment. Behavioral factors include the reminders and rewards a patient receives to comply with appointments and prescribed therapy. Social support is a more nebulous concept, but includes the emotional support and encouragement that the patient receives from their family, friends and health professionals to help them cope with their disorder and its treatment. It is important to bear in mind that no single intervention has been shown to maintain long-term adherence; one must combine strategies from two or more of these three categories to achieve success.

Practical Cognitive Strategies

The cognitive aspect of most importance to adherence is what the patient understands about the details of following the regimen. The schedule of pill taking, what to do if pills are missed or delayed, what common side effects may occur, what serious side effects should be watched for, and what to do when the first prescription is running out, are all far more important than information about the nature of the disease and the mechanics of how the treatment works. (This is not to say that information about the nature of disease and treatment should not be made available to patients if they wish it, but that such information will not help improve long-term adherence and may compete with the vital information the patient needs to follow the regimen.) Information should be provided in the form of clear, simple instructions about the schedule of medication and its duration. To ensure that the necessary information has been understood, key instructions should be provided both verbally and in written form, asking the patient to verify that they understand the instructions. Common misconceptions should be anticipated and avoided, including that the medication can be stopped when the prescription runs out or the condition comes under control, that different medications cannot be taken together at the same time of day, and that symptoms are guides to when to take the medication.

At the heart of simple instructions is a simple regimen. Medications that can be given once a day are best.[59,66,67] For patients who require more than one medication, all should be prescribed to be taken at the same time if this is consistent with therapeutic activity. (Patients often make their own regimens unnecessarily complicated by spreading their pills over the day.) If clinically sensible, combination medications may help. Mixing nondrug and drug treatments may be appropriate therapeutically but can be confusing for the patient. Nondrug treatments, such as weight control, salt restriction, or regular exercise are often harder for patients to follow and probably should be reserved for highly motivated patients or introduced after the condition is brought under control with medication, as a possible means of reducing medication.[1]

Behavioral Strategies

Behavioral interventions are the most important ingredients of any adherence improvement program,[49] the two main forms being cues (reminders) and rewards (reinforcements). Reminders of various sorts are important to keep the patient on track. Reminders about upcoming appointments can reduce nonattendance and, if patients miss appointments, they should be contacted as soon as possible.[64,68] Medication should be prescribed in concert with constant features of the patient's daily schedule so that events such as brushing one's teeth act as cues to take a pill that has been prescribed at that time of day.[13] Pill organizers (available at all pharmacies) also help to remind patients to take their pills and enable them to see if they have done so.

To reward adherence, the practitioner's recognition of, and praise for, the patient's efforts to comply at each visit provide potent reinforcement. The importance of adherence should be stressed at each visit (this need take only a few seconds). Some patients need to be seen more frequently than others to ensure adequate adherence. On follow-up, if control of the condition seems to have slipped, rather than attempting to adjust medication, the practitioner should ask the patient to come back in a week and to be sure to take each and follow the treatment closely during the week. If the condition is better controlled at the next visit, the relationship between adherence and response to medication should be reinforced and the length of time between visits increased. If the condition is still uncontrolled and the patient indicates full adherence, then an adjustment in treatment may be appropriate.

Often in practice it will not be clear if the patient has taken the treatment or not. A reasonable substitute is to base rewards on control of the condition. The patient should be given feedback about their response, with praise if they have done well or encouragement to do better if the condition is not controlled. Having patients monitor their own condition at home provides a useful basis for such discussions. Home monitoring has been shown to help improve adherence and lower blood pressure among patients with hypertension when combined with reinforcement from the physician[13] but does not improve adherence or blood pressure if the patient does this without subsequent discussion and reinforcement from the health care provider.[50] Finally, the patient can be rewarded for high adherence and good control by a negotiated decrease in visit frequency.

Social Support

Fostering social support for the patient constitutes the third route through which adherence can be enhanced.[53] The patient's family and friends can help or hinder adherence. Having a chronic disorder is a worrisome nuisance that most people would prefer to ignore. Worse, it can also drain family resources and reduce a person's self-esteem. Frequently patients' families are far from useful allies in helping them to cope with their treatments. The family may treat the patient as if he or she is ill, or fragile, or may convey the notion that the disorder is the patient's "fault" because they are not coping properly with stress.

A word from the physician to one or more members of the family may help them become "part of the solution." Unfortunately, our understanding of family dynamics in general, and the dynamics of a specific patient's family in particular, is very limited and involving the patient's family may have unpredictable effects. At least, the patient should be consulted before there is any attempt to involve his or her family in managing the patient's medical problems. With the patient's permission, then, the family can be asked to help by reminding the patient to take their medication at times when they are prone to forget, by providing positive reinforcement to the patient for following the treatment, by assisting the patient with monitoring (for example, taking blood pressure) at home, and by helping the patient to remember to attend appointments.

Improving Adherence with Nondrug Regimens

For "lifestyle" regimens, including prescriptions for dieting, exercise, smoking cessation, alcohol and other addictions, achieving and maintaining high adherence is generally much more difficult than for medications and the interventions that have some success are usually more complex and intensive than those for medications. Further, very few of these interventions have been validated in long-term studies that document improvements in clinical outcomes. It is beyond the scope of this paper to discuss these studies and interventions in detail, and readers are referred elsewhere for general reviews,[3–5,69] and specialized reviews on diet,[70–72] exercise for rehabilitation,[73] and smoking cessation.[74–76] It is worth noting that the benefits of diet and exercise for major health outcomes for patients with cardiovascular disease have not been as rigorously documented as for many medications.

Nonadherence and the Design and Execution of Clinical Research

In conducting *any* research involving treatments that are self-administered, adherence should be measured so that it can be taken into account as a co-variate.[77] If the research question is one of the efficacy of the treatment, nonadherent patients should be excluded from entry and methods of enhancing patient adherence should be included in the follow-up of patients in all groups being compared. Only if the objective of the research is to test the adherence effects of an intervention should strategies to enhance adherence be withheld from control group participants in clinical trials. In all studies, steps need to be taken to minimize the number of patients who are "lost to follow-up," whether or not patients continue on their assigned therapy. Analyses of data based on "compliers" are inherently flawed because nonadherers differ from adherers in important ways that go beyond merely forgoing the treatment.

Discussion

Because of the increasing number of efficacious self-administered treatments, nonadherence has become an increasingly important barrier to the preservation and restoration of health. Calls to "empower" patients and give them more responsibility for their own care serve to shift the focus from inadequate treatments and care delivery systems, and worse, blame patients for these problems.

Research into strategies to measure and enhance patient adherence with long-term regimens flourished in the 1970s and early 1980s, greatly stimulated by documentation of the benefits of antihypertensive therapy and the demonstration that nonadherence reduced the benefits for most patients to a modest fraction of that possible. Much useful information was generated by these studies, but they fell short of providing easily administered, highly effective monitoring and intervention strategies. Since the early 1980s, little important new information has been derived and the research effort has lagged.[78] With the recent advent of so many new, effective treatments for chronic medical disorders, there is substantial need and opportunity for innovation and new research into adherence. This may require interdisciplinary teams, including psychologists, sociologists, and medical scientists, to gain new understandings of the problems so that better ways of dealing with them can be derived. Alternatively, obviating the problems of adherence may have to await basic research leading to treatments that cure or treatment formulations that have ultra-prolonged actions, or that do not require self-administration, reducing the opportunities for nonadherence.

While we await better methods of helping patients to follow treatment prescriptions, practitioners can harness current best research knowledge on adherence through some relatively simple procedures.

When any therapy is prescribed, assisting the patient with adherence must be part of the treatment plan. Most adherence problems can be detected by watching for nonattendance or failure to respond to treatment or by asking those who do not respond about their adherence in a nonthreatening but direct way. In research, more accurate measurements are required and include home-visit pill counts, prescription refill monitoring, memory-cap medication containers, and drug or tracer levels in body fluids. Inadequate measurement and management of adherence in research can produce misleading results.

None of the strategies for improving adherence for long-term treatments is very effective on its own. A simple package that will work includes: keeping the regimen as simple as possible; giving clear instructions, with periodic checks to ensure understanding; calling the patient when an appointment is missed; discussing at each visit any problems the patient is having with the regimen; and congratulating patients for what they have been able to accomplish even if this is not perfect.

References

1. Haynes RB. Determinants of adherence: The disease and the mechanics of treatment. In Haynes RB, Taylor DW, Sackett DL (eds): *Adherence in Health Care*. Baltimore: Johns Hopkins University Press; 1979.
2. Haynes RB, Montague P, Oliver T. Interventions to assist patients to follow prescriptions for medications. The Cochrane Library. Oxford: *Update Software*. 1999;Issue 2 (in press).
3. Houston Miller N, Hill M, Kottke T, et al. The multilevel compliance challenge: Recommendations for a call to action. *Circulation* 1997;95:1085–1090.
4. Burke LE, Dunbar-Jacobs JM, Hill MN. Compliance with cardiovascular disease prevention strategies: A review of the research. *Ann Behav Med* 1997;19:239–263.
5. Roter DL, Hall JA, Merisca R, et al. Effectiveness of interventions to improve patient compliance. A meta-analysis. *Med Care* 1998;36:1138–1161.
6. Haynes RB, Taylor DW, Sackett DL, eds. *Adherence in Health Care*. Baltimore: Johns Hopkins University Press; 1979.
7. Mullen PD. Compliance becomes concordance. *BMJ* 1997;314:691–692.
8. Sackett DL, Snow JC. The magnitude of adherence and nonadherence. In Haynes RB, Taylor DW, Sackett DL (eds): *Adherence in Health Care*. Baltimore: Johns Hopkins University Press; 1979:11–22.
9. Carey R, Reid R, Ayers C, et al. The Charlottesville blood pressure survey: Value of repeated blood pressure measurements. *JAMA* 1976;236:847–851.
10. Wilber JA, Barrow JG. Hypertension—a community problem. *Am J Med* 1972;52:653–663.
11. Hedstrand H, Aberg H. Treatment of hypertension in middle-aged men. *Acta Med Scand* 1976;199:281–288.
12. Langfeld SB. Hypertension: Deficient care of the medically served. *Ann Intern Med* 1973;78:19–23.

13. Haynes RB, Sackett DL, Gibson ES, et al. Improvement of medication adherence in uncontrolled hypertension. *Lancet* 1976;1:1265–1268.
14. Sackett DL, Haynes RB, Gibson ES, et al. Randomized clinical trial of strategies for improving medication adherence in primary hypertension. *Lancet* 1975;1:1205–1207.
15. Garb JR, Stunkard AJ. Effectiveness of a self-help group in obesity control: A further assessment. *Arch Intern Med* 1974;134:716–720.
16. Wilson DM, Taylor DW, Gilbert JR, et al. A randomized trial of a family physician intervention for smoking cessation. *JAMA* 1988;260:1570–1574.
17. Birkett NJ, Evans CE, Haynes RB, et al. Hypertension control in two Canadian communities: Evidence for better treatment and overlabelling. *J Hypertension* 1986;4:369–374.
18. Baekeland F, Lundwall L, Shanahan TJ. Correlates of patient attrition in the outpatient treatment of alcoholism. *J Nerv Ment Dis* 1973;157:99–107.
19. Nelson A, Gold B, Hutchinson R, et al. Drug default among schizophrenic patients. *Am J Hosp Pharm* 1975;32:1237–1242.
20. Finnerty FA, Mattie EC. Hypertension in the inner city: Analysis of clinic dropouts. *Circulation* 1973;47:73–75.
21. Gates SJ, Colborn DK. Lowering appointment failures in a neighbourhood health centre. *Med Care* 1976;14:263–267.
22. Hoenig F, Ragg N. The non-attending psychiatric outpatient: An administrative problem. *Med Care* 1966;4:96–100.
23. Alpert JJ. Broken appointments. *Pediatrics* 1964;34:127–132.
24. Geersten HR, Gray RM, Ward JR. Patient nonadherence within the context of seeking medical care for arthritis. *J Chron Dis* 1973;26:689–698.
25. Brand F, Smith R, Brand P. Effect of economic barriers to medical care on patients' nonadherence. *Public Health Rep* 1977;92:72–78.
26. Clinite JC, Kabat HF. Prescribed drugs, errors during self-administration. *J Am Pharm Assoc* 1969;NS9:450–452.
27. Glick BS. Dropout in an outpatient, double-blind drug study. *Psychosomatics* 1965;6:44–48.
28. Gordis L, Markowitz M. Evaluation of the effectiveness of comprehensive and continuous pediatric care. *Pediatrics* 1971;48:766–776.
29. Hemminki E, Heikkila J. Elderly people's adherence with prescriptions, and quality of medication. *Scand J Soc Med* 1975;3:87–92.
30. Stuart RB. Behavioral control of overeating. *Behav Res Ther* 1967;5:357–365.
31. Gilbert JR, Evans CE, Haynes RB, et al. Predicting adherence with a regimen of digoxin therapy in family practice. *Can Med Assoc J* 1980;123:119–122.
32. Bowen RG, Rich R, Schlotfeldt RM. Effects of organized instruction for patients with the diagnosis of diabetes mellitus. *Nurs Res* 1961;10:151–159.
33. Gordis L, Markowitz M, Lilienfeld AM. Studies in the epidemiology and preventability of rheumatic fever iv) A quantitative determination of adherence in children on oral penicillin prophylaxis. *Pediatrics* 1969;43:173–182.
34. Ritson B. Involvement in treatment and its relation to outcome amongst alcoholics. *Br J Addict* 1969;64:23–29.
35. Haynes RB, Taylor DW, Sackett DL, et al. Can simple clinical measurements detect patient nonadherence? *Hypertension* 1980;2:757–764.
36. Stephenson BJ, Rowe BH, Macharia WM, et al. Is this patient taking their medication? *JAMA* 1993;269:2779–2781.
37. Urquhart J, De Klerk E. Contending paradigms for the interpretation of data on patient compliance with therapeutic drug regimens. *Stat Med* 1998; 17:251–267.

38. Frisk PA, Cooper JW, Campbell NA. Community-hospital pharmacist detection of drug-related problems upon patient admission to small hospitals. *Am J Hosp Pharm* 1977;34:738–742.
39. Hammel RW, Williams PO. Do Patients receive prescribed medication? *Am Pharm Assoc J* 1964;4:331–334.
40. McKenney JM, Slining JM, Henderson HR, et al. The effect of clinical pharmacy services on patients with essential hypertension. *Circulation* 1973;48:1104–1111.
41. Gupta RN, Haynes RB, Logan AG, et al. Liquid-chromatographic determination of nadolol in plasma. *Clin Chem* 1983;29:1085–1087.
42. Briggs WA, Lowenthal DT, Cirksena WJ, et al. Propranolol in hypertensive dialysis patients: Efficacy and adherence. *Clin Pharmacol Ther* 1975;18:606–612.
43. Porter AM. Drug defaulting in a general practice. *Br Med J* 1969;1:218–222.
44. Maenpaa H, Manninen V, Heinonen OP. Adherence with medication in the Helsinki Heart Study. *Eur J Clin Pharmacol* 1992;42:15–19
45. Feely M, Cooke J, Price D, et al. Low-dose phenobarbitone as an indicator of compliance with drug therapy. *Br J Clin Pharmacol* 1987;24:77–83.
46. Rudd P, Ahmed S, Zachary V, et al. Improved adherence measures: Applications in an ambulatory hypertensive drug trial. *Clin Pharmacol Ther* 1990;48:676–685.
47. Milgrom H, Bender B, Ackerson L, et al. Noncompliance and treatment failure in children with asthma. *J Allergy Clin Immunol* 1996;98:1051–1057.
48. Logan AG, Haynes RB. Determinants of physicians' competence in the management of hypertension. *J Hypertension* 1986;4(suppl 5):S367-S369.
49. Haynes RB, Wang E, Da Mota Gomes M: A critical review of interventions for improved adherence with prescribed medications. *Patient Educ Counsel* 1987;10:155–166.
50. Johnson AL, Taylor DW, Sackett DL, et al. Self-recording of blood pressure in the management of hypertension. *Can Med Assoc J* 1978;119:1034–1039.
51. Shepard DS, Foster SB, Stason WB, et al. Cost-effectiveness of interventions to improve adherence with antihypertensive therapy. *Prev Med* 1979;8:229.
52. Logan AG, Milne BJ, Achber C, et al. A comparison of community and occupationally oriented antihypertensive care. *J Occup Med* 1982;24:901–906.
53. Levine DM, Green LW, Deeds SG, et al. Health education for hypertensive patients. *JAMA* 1979;241:1700–1703.
54. Becker LA, Glanz K, Sobel E, et al. A randomized trial of special packaging for antihypertensive medications. *J Fam Pract* 1986;22:357–361.
55. Logan AS, Milne BJ, Achber C, et al. Treatment of hypertensive patients at the worksite by specially-trained nurses: A controlled trial. *Lancet* 1979;2:1175–1178.
56. Logan AS, Milne BJ, Achber C, et al. Cost-effectiveness of a worksite hypertension treatment program. *Hypertension* 1981;3:211–218.
57. Bass MJ, McWhinney IR, Donner A. Do family physicians need medical assistants to detect and manage hypertension? *Can Med Assoc J* 1986;134:1247–1255.
58. Brown BG, Bardsley J, Puolin D, et al. Moderate dose, three drug therapy with niacin, lovsastatin, and colestipol to reduce low-density lipoprotein cholesterol < 100 mg/dl in patients with hyperlipidemia and coronary heart disease. *Am J Cardiol* 1997;80:111–115.
59. Baird MG, Bentley-Taylor MM, Carruthers SG, et al. A study of the efficacy

tolerance and adherence of once-daily versus twice-daily metoprolol (Beta-locR) in hypertension. *Clin Invest Med* 1984;7:95–102.
60. Nessman DG, Carnahan JE, Nugent CA. Increasing adherence. Patient operated hypertension groups. *Arch Intern Med* 1980;140:1427–1431.
61. Swain MA, Steckel SB. Influencing adherence among hypertensives. *Res Nurs Health* 1981;4:213–218.
62. Morisky D. Five-year blood pressure control and mortality following health education for hypertensive patients. *Am J Publ Health* 1983;73:153–162.
63. Friedman RH, Kazis LE, Jette A, et al. A telecommunications system for monitoring and counseling patients with hypertension. Impact on medication adherence and blood pressure control. *Am J Hypertens* 1996;9:285–292.
64. Takala J, Niemela N, Rosti J, et al. Improving adherence with therapeutic regimens in hypertensive patients in a community health center. *Circulation* 1979;59:540–543.
65. Leventhal H, Cameron L. Behavioral theories and the problem of adherence. *Patient Educ Couns* 1987;10:117–138.
66. Tinkelman DG, Vanderpool GE, Carroell MS. Adherence differences following administration of theophylline at six and twelve hour intervals. *Ann Allergy* 1980;44:283–286.
67. Taggart AJ, Johnston GD, McDevitt DG. Does the frequency of daily dosage influence adherence with digoxin therapy? *Br J Clin Pharmacol* 1981;1:31–34.
68. Macharia WM, Leon G, Rowe BH, et al. An overview of interventions to improve appointment keeping for medical services. *JAMA* 1992;267:1813–1817.
69. Burke LE, Dunbar-Jacob J. Adherence to medication, diet, and activity recommendations: From assessment to maintenance. *J Cardiovasc Nurs* 1995;9:62–79.
70. Brownell KD, Cohen LR. Adherence to dietary regimens. 1: An overview of research. *Behav Med* 1995;20:149–154.
71. Brownell KD, Cohen LR. Adherence to dietary regimens. 2: Components of effective interventions. *Behav Med* 1995;20:155–164.
72. Harvey EL, Glenny A, Kirk SFL, et al. Improving health professionals' management and the organisation of care for overweight and obese people (Cochrane Review). In: The Cochrane Library, Issue 1, 1999. Oxford: *Update Software.*
73. Oldridge NB. Cardiac rehabilitation exercise programme. Compliance and compliance-enhancing strategies. *Sports Med* 1988;6:42–55.
74. Lancaster T, Silagy C, Fowler G, et al. Training health professionals in smoking cessation (Cochrane Review). In: The Cochrane Library, Issue 1, 1999. Oxford: *Update Software.*
75. Silagy C, Mant D, Fowler G, et al. Nicotine replacement therapy for smoking cessation (Cochrane Review). In: The Cochrane Library, Issue 1, 1999. Oxford: *Update Software.*
76. Silagy C, Ketteridge S. Physician advice for smoking cessation (Cochrane Review). In: The Cochrane Library, Issue 1, 1999. Oxford: *Update Software.*
77. Haynes RB, Dantes R. Patient adherence and the design and interpretation of clinical trials. *Controlled Clinical Trials* 1987;8:12–19.
78. Haynes RB. Patient adherence then and now [editorial]. *Patient Educ Counsel* 1987;10:103–105.
79. Haynes RB. Improving patient compliance in the management of hypertension. In Kaplan NM, Ram CVS (eds): *Individualized Therapy of Hypertension.* New York: Marcel Dekker, Inc, 1995:257–273.

Section II

Factors and Interventions Affecting Compliance

Chapter 1

Predicting Compliance:
How Are We Doing?

Deborah J. Bowen, PhD, Almut Helmes, MS, and Erika Lease, BA

Introduction to the Problem

The study of compliance and the predictors of compliance are of critical importance to current recommendations about health. Much research has been published about the study of compliance, and some of this research has helped to improve current practices in medicine and public health. More must be done, however, to learn the reasons for both compliance and noncompliance, and future research can make improvements by basing hypotheses in thoughtful, critical areas. This chapter will discuss issues in compliance, examine the published literature on predictors of compliance, and make recommendations for future research on compliance.

One of the difficulties in the field is the variance in estimates of compliance with professional directives to improve health and to reduce disease. Estimates of compliance range from 30% to 90% in the published literature (reviewed later). These estimates include compliance to disease or condition treatment activities, screening recommendations, and lifestyle or health behavior changes. This huge range is undoubtedly the result of numerous factors, many of them currently unknown to us. However, we propose that one factor is the use of differing definitions of compliance, and that these differing definitions are associated with differing levels of compliance.

This work was supported by several grants from the National Institutes of Health (N01-WH-2–2110, CA34847, CA79654).

From: Burke LE, Ockene IS (eds). *Compliance in Healthcare and Research.* Armonk, NY: Futura Publishing Company, Inc.; © 2001.

Differing Definitions of Compliance

A standard definition for compliance, and one that we will use in this chapter, is the degree to which an individual follows a specific recommendation. Specific definitions vary from study to study and from setting to setting. This variance is important because different predictors will be related to different outcomes. Some examples of the differing ways that compliance is predicted follow.

Available Technology

Differing technologies help to define the behaviors in which we are interested, and often provide differing patterns of behavioral outcomes. For example, O'Connell, et al.[1] have documented differences in measurement of relapse-related smoking cessation withdrawal symptoms. They compared the measurement as a recall of symptom patterns days later, versus real-time recording of symptoms using new electronic personal data recording systems. Using the recall method, the majority of relapse-related withdrawal symptoms were related to stress and negative affect. However, when the real-time monitoring devices for participants in smoking cessation studies were used to record their reasons for relapse, this pattern disappeared. It is unclear as to the reason for the difference in reporting, but this difference could make a dramatic change in the ways in which smoking cessation experts deal with relapse episodes.

Specific Spheres of Behavior

We know that complex behavior changes often require changes in several areas or spheres of daily life. For example, Whitaker, et al.[2] have documented the effects of changes in school lunch offerings on children's dietary habits overall. He found that, even with changes in lunch offerings and changes in consumption during lunch times, children's overall dietary intake did not change. Therefore, compliance with the intervention can show effects, but the effects may not carry over into other spheres of activity.

Usual Versus Specific Behavior

Research has documented the ways that human memory records information about health behaviors. For example, there are at least two and probably more methods of recording information regarding dietary habits: remembering the usual patterns of behavior and remembering the specific patterns that are tagged in place and time to situations, days, or other patterns.[3] These methods of remembering are reflected in the differing measurement tools used to measure dietary compliance. The food frequency questionnaire (FFQ) asks individuals to recall over the past three months the frequency of over one hundred foods consumed. These frequencies are then combined using several algorithms into nutrient estimates. The process by which individuals determine the frequency judgements on an FFQ is thought to be an estimate of the usual patterns of behavior in the rough time period, not the specific summation of several specific food consumption periods. In contrast, a 24-hour recall asks individuals to remember every food and drink item consumed over the past 24 hours, very specifically and precisely. Different memory processes are used to make these types of recall judgements and these dietary reporting methodologies often yield differing estimates of an individual's food intake. When dietary intake is defined using these two methods (usual intake versus specific intake), predictors of intake will likely differ also.

Correlates

Many studies in compliance use multiple measures of the participants' compliance to the regimen under study. For example, it is relatively common to use self-reported adherence and to add to the reports a biochemical marker of compliance. A common marker would be blood or urine levels of a metabolite of the drug or dietary element under study, such as the measurement of urinary micronutrients in a study of fruit and vegetable intake, or perhaps a marker of compliance that is known to correlate with the disease process, such as blood glucose for diabetic control. The patterns of compliance, however, can differ between the self-reported pattern and the biological measure, leading to differing conclusions about the level of compliance and the predictors of the compliance levels. For example, biochemical measures of drug metabolism can reflect compliance over a longer period of time and can be confounded by other exposures. Thus, the participant's self-report of compliance in the last week could be different from the blood measure of metabolism, and both could be "true" measures of compliance.

By Participants

Several investigators have documented the perspective of the patient in defining and understanding compliance. [4,5] This perspective often differs from the provider's or the researcher's, and can be a powerful influence in the achievement of ultimate compliance. For example, Leventhal[4] has documented the role of symptom experiences in patients' understanding of their illness label, and in their compliance with medical recommendations. Recently the authors of this chapter published on increases in symptom reporting during a placebo run-in period as a predictor of retention in a long-term clinical trial.[5] The more that people experienced symptoms and attributed them as side effects, the less likely they were to perform the requirements of the ongoing study. These studies indicate a lay person's understanding of health and illness can be important in predicting compliance.

Taken together, these differences make for a complicated definition and measurement task for understanding compliance. We feel that research on compliance is needed: not just *more* research but *more thoughtful* research on compliance must be funded and conducted. We have identified three gaps in the compliance literature that we see as important to address. We propose that careful consideration of these gaps will help move the field forward and will help to make sense of a large number of observations, both clinical and research oriented. These areas are: a lack of a population-based understanding of compliance, a lack of consistently asking why people comply with recommendations, and a lack of a unifying conceptual framework for predicting compliance. We will examine each in turn.

Lack of a Population-Based Analysis

The varying rates of compliance and the varying predictors of compliance should be considered in terms of the population measured and studied. We know that there are large differences between compliance in research settings and practice settings; these differences are due in part to the sample within the population being observed. A listing of the possible differences between research and practice settings is included in Table 1. The differences could include a broad inclusion of

Table 1

Compliance Setting Makes a Difference

Research	Practice
Screened participants	Non-screened participants
Motivated to be evaluated	No evaluation
Better compliance	Worse compliance

patients into a clinical setting, versus the careful screening and selection of participants into a randomized trial. Most trials have intensive screening procedures for each participant prior to trial entry. During these procedures, study staff explain the requirements of the research process and often mimic the necessary research procedures to fulfill trial requirements.[6] These screening procedures are meant to discourage any participant in a research project that cannot fulfill the minimal research requirements of record-keeping, etc. Most clinical settings, by contrast, do not directly discourage individuals from joining based on ability to follow procedures.

An example of the dramatic difference between compliance in a research and clinical setting is in compliance with vitamin recommendations. In population-based surveys, prevalent rates of vitamin consumption are approximately 45%, varying considerably by demographic group.[7] However, in a recently completed clinical trial of vitamin intake to prevent lung cancer, compliance rates were 88% across 7 years of intervention.[8] One of the major differences between these two settings is that the participants in the randomized trial were carefully selected for their ability to complete forms and perform the research requirements.

Even if compliance within research studies is considered, the specific research setting makes a difference in compliance rates. Some of the possible differences among research settings are presented in Table 2. These include the purpose of the study and the related demands on participants, and the intensity of the intervention or recommendation that is part of the study. An efficacy study is typically more intensive, requiring highly motivated participants and larger requirements of those participants. An effectiveness study is commonly less intensive and more targeted to individuals in a defined population who are not selected as stringently for their ability to perform the research requirements. An example of the differences between research settings is found in the literature on lowering dietary fat to reduce risk of cancer. In a recent randomized trial with intensive screening procedures and inter-

Table 2

Research Setting Makes a Difference

Efficacy Study	Effectiveness Study
Intensive screening	Less screening
Selected for ability	Not selected for ability
Better compliance	Worse compliance

vention activities, participants achieved a fat reduction of 11% of daily energy and maintained this decrease across the study period.[9] Contrast this finding with the 1.7% reduction in low-fat related behaviors achieved in an intervention using primary care physician practices as the delivery mechanism for a healthy-eating intervention.[10] The usefulness of these small changes across a population are supported by others.[11] Nevertheless, direct comparisons of the magnitude of these changes are likely to be confusing and misleading unless one uses a population-based analysis.

Asking WHY Individuals Comply with Recommendations

In addition to various definitions of compliance, there are also a variety of predictors of compliance. In order to better understand compliance we need these predictors to find out why individuals comply with recommendations. Examples for reasons (or predictors) for better compliance are treatment factors such as the size of pills, or demographic factors such as age or ethnic background. We need to first come up with ideas about possible predictors, formulate appropriate items to ask in questionnaires, and then calculate the influence of these predictors on compliance. Knowing which predictors play a role in compliance and which do not will help us in designing interventions to improve compliance rates and target specific interventions for specific populations. To get an idea of possible predictors, we examined what the field has done so far. We conducted a review of the published reviews in the compliance literature within the last 20 years. Our goal was to identify how research efforts were distributed across different categories of predictors of compliance.

Review Methodology

In our analysis, we included only review articles because we felt they gave the best overview of the literature for certain time points. We performed a computer search on the Medline database for the years 1978, 1983, 1988, 1993, and 1998, using "compliance" and "adherence" as our search terms. Choosing time points that were 5 years apart gave us the opportunity to look at the distribution of different topics within one year, but also to investigate the possible shift in topics from one year to another. We chose Medline over PsychINFO or other search engines because we were mostly interested in patients' compliance with health recommendations and we found Medline provided more relevant articles in this regard. We limited the search to review articles in English and were able to obtain reprints of all but four of the articles. In the actual analysis, we excluded articles that were either not review articles (eg, one article compared only three studies against each other) or did not have compliance or adherence as their main focus (eg, an article on exercise and weight control only once mentioned compli- ance). We selected the paragraphs in each identified article that re- viewed other articles on predictors of compliance. We only took the paragraphs into consideration that dealt with factors that influence compliance and did not include paragraphs that addressed ways to assess compliance or ways to change compliance. We divided the text about predictors into sections, each section only dealing with one spe- cific predictor. Within each section we then counted the number of lines. The line counts formed the basis for our analysis.

The next step in the analysis was to code each of the predictors into one of the following categories: demographics, treatment properties, psychological or behavioral models, and everything else that we found. We chose these categories because they seem to best capture the differ- ent approaches of the research effort to predictors on compliance so far. Demographics included sociodemographic information such as age, gender, education, income, etc. Examples for treatment properties were the duration of treatment, side effects, size of pills, physician-patient relationship, etc. The category of models contained sections that exam- ined the relationship of compliance with factors that were derived from models such as the Health Belief Model, the Social Learning Theory or the Self-Regulation Model. Finally, the "all else" category included all factors that did not fit into any of the other categories but also repre- sented factors that explain compliance or noncompliance with medical regimen. Examples for this last category are support from family, sever- ity of the disease, fear, or health knowledge.

For each article, we first added the number of lines for each cate- gory. We also added the number of lines of all four categories to get the total number of lines of the relevant paragraphs. We then calculated the percentage of line space by dividing the number of lines in each category by the total number of relevant lines per article. We then took a mean of all percentages in each category for each year.

Results of the Review

We found a total of 108 articles, 4 for 1978, 7 for 1983, 29 for 1988, 26 for 1993, and 42 for 1998 using the Medline search. Of these we excluded a total of 39 articles, because they did not meet our inclusion criteria or we could not obtain them. Therefore, we used data from the

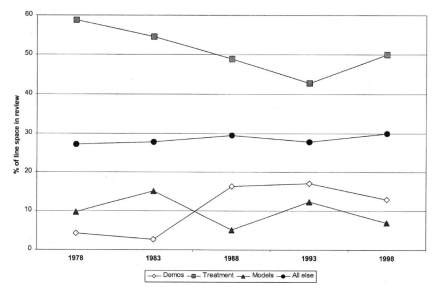

Figure 1. Graph of line space in compliance reviews over a 20-year period.

following number of review articles in the analysis: 4 for 1978[12–15], 6 for 1983[16–21], 13 for 1988[22–34], 13 for 1993[35–47], and 33 for 1998.[48–80]

Figure 1 shows the percentages of line space in each category for each year. In 1978, the treatment properties category was by far the most common category with 59% of line space, followed by "all else" with 27%, models with 10% and demographics with 4%. This pattern stayed almost the same into 1998. The only change in focus occurred between 1983 and 1988, when more emphasis was placed on demographics and less on models. The last year of our analysis, 1998, showed that 50% of review space focused on treatment properties, 30% on "all else", 13% on demographics and 7% on models.

These data indicate that the field focused mainly on treatment properties as predictors for compliance and that there has not been a lot of change in this focus over the last 20 years. The use of behavioral models as a strategy for guiding the selection of compliance predictors has not been a main area of attention. In fact, research in the field seems to be moving away from them.

How Shall We Ask WHY Individuals Comply?

In order to research questions of the reasons for compliance and noncompliance, one must have a predefined conceptual framework, used to design both intervention and evaluation. For example, if re-search suggests that the main reason for noncompliance with hormone replacement therapy is the fear of major and minor side effects associ-ated with taking hormones, then the investigators or clinicians must base both the assessment of issues at baseline and at subsequent follow-up points on the measurement of side effects and of the fear or worry of these effects. Often it is useful and even necessary to rely on a published model or picture of the issues to guide the assessment. The use of a model helps in several ways. First, most models have been researched and there are data to guide the selection of important variables included in the model. Other studies have developed measurement tools that can be imported or adapted for other settings. Finally, the use of a published and researched model will allow science to move forward so that we can identify the variables that do not predict compliance as well as those that do, and eliminate the useless ones from our under-standing of compliance. These functions indicate that using a model as a guide for measurement is important.

One difficulty with desiring and attempting to use a model is in the selection of the right model. There are many models in the literature and many of these claim to predict compliance and further the field. For example, a well-known and used reference book on compliance recently published its second edition.[81] In that edition over 17 models were cited and described in the first three chapters, each with its strengths and weaknesses. In our course on Health Promotion and Dis-ease Prevention taught in the Department of Health Services at the School of Public Health, University of Washington, over 20 models are referenced and discussed as part of the class requirements. The number of models grows every year and although there is considerable overlap among some of them, each claims to be better in its ability to predict compliance to medical recommendations.

It remains to the investigator or clinician to choose a framework from among those available or to identify, research, and create a better one. This process is often difficult and overwhelming. There are only a few clear rules for selection of the right framework. One is that there be data supporting the usefulness of a framework in predicting relevant health behavior or compliance; however, application of that rule to the specific setting is often difficult. For example, a researcher will often find that there are data supporting the usefulness of the model, but no data on the specific behavior in question. Therefore, the relevance of the model to the particular behavior is not known. Or, there will be some data found, but all in cross-sectional and longitudinal studies, not randomized intervention studies. Therefore, the usefulness of the model in a changing setting is unclear. Some models have more data to support them than do others. There are few direct empirical comparisons of the predictive value of two or more models, making direct comparisons difficult to achieve. Finally, there is much overlap between the variables in some of the models, and this overlap makes for very long questionnaires that seem redundant to participants.

One Solution to the Difficulty of Choosing a Model

Our research group at the FHCRC has struggled with these issues in our own research work. Because of these and other issues, we have attempted to synthesize the literature on models predicting compliance and health behavior change. We have identified a working model that pulls together many existing ideas and variables to produce a simplified framework that can be tested and researched in several settings.

This framework is summarized in Figure 2, a diagram of the framework that includes concepts from all the models we identified and reviewed, combined together to form an overview. For simplicity there are two categories of critical variables identified within the framework: Environmental and Personal. Personal variables focus on individuals' ideas and thoughts, while environmental variables are focused outside individuals. Each of these two categories of variables is presumed to influence individuals' health behaviors, through delivery and receipt of intervention and changes in framework variables. Also, we assume that these variables influence each other, but identification of these influences must wait for a full test of the framework.

Beliefs important to health behavior change range widely from beliefs about the importance of the health issue, to the causes and conse-

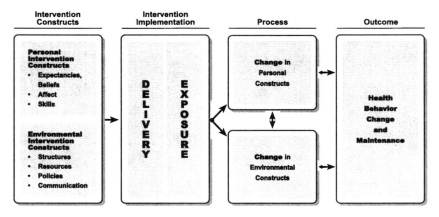

Figure 2. Evidence-based framework for health behavior change.

quences of the health issue, to beliefs about the role of other people and resources in the environment in supporting behavior change. Our model subsumes the concepts of motivation under beliefs. Affect addresses the positive and negative feelings participants have about the health promotion intervention. Skills needed for behavior change include skills specific to the behavior, as well as general skills to elicit social support, ask for help, etc. Structures that can play a role in changing or maintaining health behavior include physical structures, like clinics, kiosks, organizations, but also councils, communities, events, and activities. Resources come in many forms, including financial, social, and educational. Policies range from national laws regarding pricing, access, and regulation, to stated rules or preferences of local organizations such as schools, clubs, worksites, and food chains. Communications are equally far-ranging, from international news stories that include health promotion information and messages to exchanges between two people about the symptoms of an illness and the opportunities for care.

Any intervention must be implemented in order to have an effect. Implementation research divides this step into two parts, each measurable in the context of an intervention. The intervention strategies 1) must be delivered to the target population, and, 2) the target population must be exposed to the strategies. Delivery can often be measured simply by counts of material sent, by number of hours of contact time, by interventionists' logbooks or other record keeping, by direct observations of content delivered. Delivery, however, is only half of implementation. People must receive the delivered intervention elements in order to produce an effect. Envelopes can lay unopened, calls can go unanswered, and community activities can be avoided, creating a gap between delivery and exposure. Exposure can also be measured in multiple ways, by counting the number of people at events, by counting actions resulting from the delivery of an intervention material, or by simply asking target individuals if they have seen or been part of intervention strategies.

Finally, after intervention strategies have been delivered and exposure has occurred, we assume that key framework variables will change. Those changes will result in changes in the desired health behavior. The order in which these variables change, the importance of each variable in predicting outcome, the relationships among intervention delivery and exposure, and changes in key framework variables, are probably the least researched topics in this field and are currently not known for our model proposed here. This type of research, conducted using appropriate statistical techniques, should be a key part of every research project on health behavior and compliance interventions.

Application of Variables in the Framework to Compliance

There are data to support all of the variables in the model as predictors of compliance in diverse settings. For example, we found beliefs to be important in predicting compliance with trial requirements in a large randomized chemoprevention study. We tested the effects of two different types of incentives in a randomized factorial design to increase compliance with follow-up visit activities.[82] We found that when staff provided the incentives but did not attempt to increase participants' beliefs about the value of the participant's activities within the study, the incentives had no effect. However, when we provided incentives and also discussed with participants the importance of the participant role in the trial, then incentives had a positive effect on completion of trial requirements.

Affect has been shown to be important in several studies of compliance to recommendations. An example from our research is the role of affect in intentions to obtain breast cancer screening. Women who reported more concern about breast cancer risk and higher perceptions of risk reported higher intentions to obtain mammography screening, compared with women who reported low levels of concern and perceived risk.[83] This finding was true independent of actual breast cancer risk or family history of breast cancer. In other words, women's emotion about breast cancer risk was more motivating than the actual risk of breast cancer in encouraging screening compliance. This finding may be very important in situations where the fear of disease risk may be a critical factor in deciding whether or not to comply with the recommendation, such as the case of hormone replacement therapy for cardiovascular disease prevention, considering breast cancer risk as a factor as well.

On the group or community level the factors in this model may be very important to compliance. Several research projects have documented the role of the physician and the supporting office staff in encouraging smokers to quit smoking.[84] This model of structural advice and support can possibly be generalized to other compliance issues as well, especially those for which the office staff and chart-cueing mechanisms could be useful. Communications and policy changes can be useful motivators for compliance to recommendations. Changing communications in grocery stores to include the message of recommended consumption of at least five fruits and vegetables per day, and insuring that stores comply with the changed messages through national and local policies, has the potential to help consumers focus on this area as a positive change.

Conclusions and Future Directions

We conclude from this discussion that much is known, but there is much work to be done as well. Perhaps we are entering a new phase of research regarding compliance issues. Applying some of the ideas here might help research projects on compliance augment the literature in the area of study concerning why individuals comply with recommendations, in addition to documenting the existence or extent of compliance. Thinking carefully about the topics to be researched will help us to accept some novel ideas about compliance and eliminate others because they were not supported when examined empirically. It may be particularly important to pay attention to and to publish the ideas or strategies that do not bear up under empirical examination, in addition to the announcement of strategies that do improve compliance, so that we can discontinue efforts in those areas which are not helpful.

There are many things that can now be used clinically to improve compliance. We know many things about the treatment setting that can improve compliance, based on our review of the literature. These elements, documented in the reviews cited here, should be used to guide choices in practice. Altering advice about compliance, packaging and preparation of products, involvement of the provider, and discussions of symptoms, etc., are all a critical part of the activities in which we can engage now to improve compliance in research and clinical settings.

Policy makers can look to the future to fund innovative, cutting-edge compliance and health behavior change research and practice components. This should be carried through at the federal, state, and private levels. Policies to institute programs to improve compliance have the potential to improve cost outcomes as well as health outcomes in health care settings, and therefore are well worth the investment. Granting agencies should make sure that all relevant research projects include a compliance intervention and a compliance research track, insuring that we will gain in knowledge as we do basic biomedical and treatment research. Opening dialogues among these interest groups will insure that research on compliance is both practical and theoretical.

References

1. O'Connell KA, Gerkovich MM, Cook MR, et al. Coping in real time: Using Ecological Momentary Assessment techniques to assess coping with the urge to smoke. *Res Nurs Health* 1998;21:487–497.
2. Whitaker RC, Wright JA, Koepsell TD, et al. Randomized intervention to increase children's selection of low-fat foods in school lunches. *J Pediatr* 1994;125:535–540.

3. Smith A. Cognitive processes in long-term dietary recall. National Center for Health Statistics. *Vital Health Stat* 1991;6:1–34.
4. Leventhal H, Cameron L. Behavioral theories and the problem of compliance. *Patient Educ Couns* 1987;10:117–138.
5. Bowen DJ, Cartmel B, Barnett M, et al. Predictors of retention in two chemoprevention trials. *Ann Behavior Med* 1999
6. Meinert CL. *Clinical Trials: Design, Conduct, and Analysis.* New York: Oxford University Press, 1986.
7. Use of dietary supplements in the United States. Vital and Health Statistics from the Centers for Disease Control and Prevention / National Center for Health Statistics. Series 11, No. 244. June 1999.
8. Omenn GS, Goodman GE, Thornquist MD, et al. Effects of a combination of beta carotene and vitamin A on lung cancer and cardiovascular disease. *N Engl J Med* 1996;334:1150–1155.
9. Coates RJ, Bowen DJ, Kristal AR, et al. The Women's Health Trial Feasibility Study in Minority Populations: Changes in dietary intakes. *Am J Epidemiol* 1999;149:1104–1112.
10. Beresford SA, Curry SJ, Kristal AR, et al. A dietary intervention in primary care practice: The Eating Patterns Study. *Am J Public Health* 1997;87:610–616.
11. Rose G. Sick individuals and sick populations. *Intl J Epidemiol* 1985;14:32–38.
12. Gylding-Sabroe JP. Possible causes of treatment failure with the NSAID. *Rheumatol Rehabil.* 1978;90–93.
13. Haynes RB, Sackett DL, Taylor DW. Practical management of low compliance with antihypertensive therapy: A guide for the busy practitioner. *Clin Invest Med* 1978;1:175–180.
14. Mayo NE. Patient compliance: Practical implications for physical therapists. A review of the literature. *Phys Ther* 1978;58:1083–1090.
15. Taylor DW, Sackett DL, Haynes RB, et al. Compliance with antihypertensive drug therapy. *Ann N Y Acad Sci* 1978;304:390–403.
16. Bruhn JG. The application of theory in childhood asthma self-help programs. *J Allergy Clin Immunol* 1983;72:561–577.
17. Evans L, Spelman M. The problem of non-compliance with drug therapy. *Drugs* 1983;25:63–76.
18. Jones JG. Compliance with pediatric therapy. A selective review and recommendations. *Clin Pediatr (Phila)* 1983;22:262–265.
19. Levy RL. Social support and compliance: A selective review and critique of treatment integrity and outcome measurement. *Soc Sci Med* 1983;17:1329–1338.
20. Mitchell MF. Popular medical concepts in Jamaica and their impact on drug use. *West J Med* 1983;139:841–847.
21. Voyles JB, Menendez R. Role of patient compliance in the management of asthma. *J Asthma* 1983;20:411–418.
22. Comoss PM. Nursing strategies to improve compliance with life-style changes in a cardiac rehabilitation population. *J Cardiovasc Nurs* 1988;2:23–36.
23. Cramer JA, Russell ML. Compliance in epilepsy. Strategies to enhance adherence to a medical regimen. *Epilepsy Res Suppl* 1988;1:163–175.
24. Crapo PA. Use of alternative sweeteners in diabetic diet. *Diabetes Care* 1988;11:174–182.
25. Friedman M. Compliance with chronic disease regimens: Diabetes. *J Diabet Complications* 1988;2:140–144.

26. German PS. Compliance and chronic disease. *Hypertension* 1988;11:II56–60.
27. Green LW, Simons-Morton DG. Denial, delay and disappointment: Discovering and overcoming the causes of drug errors and missed appointments. *Epilepsy Res Suppl* 1988;1:7–21.
28. Klein LE. Compliance and blood pressure control. *Hypertension* 1988;11: II61–64.
29. Morrow D, Leirer V, Sheikh J. Adherence and medication instructions. Review and recommendations. *J Am Geriatr Soc* 1988;36:1147–1160.
30. Perel JM. Compliance during tricyclic antidepressant therapy: Pharmacokinetic and analytical issues. *Clin Chem* 1988;34:881–887.
31. Thompson PJ. Psychological aspects of non-compliance. *Epilepsy Res Suppl* 1988;1:71–75.
32. Vandereycken W, Meermann R. Chronic illness behavior and noncompliance with treatment: Pathways to an interactional approach. *Psychother Psychosom* 1988;50:182–191.
33. Weingarten MA, Cannon BS. Age as a major factor affecting adherence to medication for hypertension in a general practice population. *Fam Pract* 1988;5:294–296.
34. Witkowski JA. Compliance: The dermatologic patient. *Int J Dermatol* 1988; 27:608–611.
35. Berg JS, Dischler J, Wagner DJ, et al. Medication compliance: A healthcare problem. *Ann Pharmacother* 1993;27:S1–24.
36. Grange JM, Festenstein F. The human dimension of tuberculosis control. *Tuber Lung Dis* 1993;74:219–222.
37. Gritz ER, Bastani R. Cancer prevention—behavior changes: The short and the long of it. *Prev Med* 1993;22:676–688.
38. Horwitz RI, Horwitz SM. Adherence to treatment and health outcomes. *Arch Intern Med* 1993;153:1863–1868.
39. Kushner RF. Long-term compliance with a lipid-lowering diet. *Nutr Rev* 1993;51:16–18.
40. Lerman C, Schwartz M. Adherence and psychological adjustment among women at high risk for breast cancer. *Breast Cancer Res Treat* 1993;28: 145–155.
41. Luepker RV. Patient adherence: a 'risk factor' for cardiovascular disease. *Heart Dis Stroke* 1993;2:418–421.
42. Morris LS, Schulz RM. Medication compliance: The patient's perspective. *Clin Ther* 1993;15:593–606.
43. Rand CS. Measuring adherence with therapy for chronic diseases: Implications for the treatment of heterozygous familial hypercholesterolemia. *Am J Cardiol* 1993;72:68D-74D.
44. Schaub AF, Steiner A, Vetter W. Compliance to treatment. *Clin Exp Hypertens* 1993;15:1121–1130.
45. Sumartojo E. When tuberculosis treatment fails. A social behavioral account of patient adherence. *Am Rev Respir Dis* 1993;147:1311–1320.
46. ter Horst G, de Wit CA. Review of behavioural research in dentistry 1987–1992: Dental anxiety, dentist-patient relationship, compliance and dental attendance. *Int Dent J* 1993;43:265–278.
47. Trick LR. Patient compliance—don't count on it! *J Am Optom Assoc* 1993; 64:264–270.
48. Achieving long-term continuance of menopausal ERT/HRT: Consensus opinion of the North American Menopause Society. *Menopause* 1998;5: 69–76.

49. Abbott J, Gee L. Contemporary psychosocial issues in cystic fibrosis: Treatment adherence and quality of life. *Disabil Rehabil* 1998;20:262–271.
50. Allen H. Promoting compliance with antihypertensive medication. *Br J Nurs* 1998;7:1252–1258.
51. Baker F. Behavioral science applied to cancer screening. *Curr Opin Oncol* 1998;10:455–460.
52. Balkrishnan R. Predictors of medication adherence in the elderly. *Clin Ther* 1998;20:764–771.
53. Biddle SJ, Fox KR. Motivation for physical activity and weight management. *Int J Obes Relat Metab Disord* 1998;22(Suppl 2):S39–47.
54. Black B, Bruce ME. Treating tuberculosis: The essential role of social work. *Soc Work Health Care* 1998;26:51–68.
55. Boudes P. Drug compliance in therapeutic trials: A review. *Control Clin Trials* 1998;19:257–268.
56. Branden PS. Contraceptive choice and patient compliance. The health care provider's challenge. *J Nurse Midwifery* 1998;43:471–482.
57. Brandt P. Childhood diabetes: Behavioral research. *Annu Rev Nurs Res* 1998; 16:63–82.
58. Brasic JR, Will MV, Ahn SC, et al. A review of the literature and a preliminary study of family compliance in a developmental disabilities clinic. *Psychol Rep* 1998;82:275–286.
59. Chaulk CP, Kazandjian VA. Directly observed therapy for treatment completion of pulmonary tuberculosis: Consensus Statement of the Public Health Tuberculosis Guidelines Panel [published erratum appears in JAMA 1998 Jul 8;280(2):134]. *JAMA* 1998;279:943–948.
60. Cramer JA. Enhancing patient compliance in the elderly. Role of packaging aids and monitoring. *Drugs Aging* 1998;12:7–15.
61. Cramer JA, Rosenheck R. Compliance with medication regimens for mental and physical disorders. *Psychiatr Serv* 1998;49:196–201.
62. De Geest S, von Renteln-Kruse W, Steeman E, et al. Compliance issues with the geriatric population: Complexity with aging. *Nurs Clin North Am* 1998; 33:467–480.
63. Demyttenaere K. Noncompliance with antidepressants: Who's to blame? *Int Clin Psychopharmacol* 1998;13(Suppl 2):S19–25.
64. Griffin SJ. Lost to follow-up: The problem of defaulters from diabetes clinics. *Diabet Med* 1998;15(Suppl 3):S14–24.
65. Kehoe WA, Katz RC. Health behaviors and pharmacotherapy. *Ann Pharmacother* 1998;32:1076–1086.
66. King KM, Teo KK. Cardiac rehabilitation referral and attendance: Not one and the same. *Rehabil Nurs* 1998;23:246–251.
67. La Greca AM. It's "all in the family": Responsibility for diabetes care. *J Pediatr Endocrinol Metab* 1998;11(Suppl 2):379–385.
68. Lerner BH, Gulick RM, Dubler NN. Rethinking nonadherence: Historical perspectives on triple-drug therapy for HIV disease. *Ann Intern Med* 1998; 129:573–578.
69. Mallion JM, Baguet JP, Siche JP, et al. Compliance, electronic monitoring and antihypertensive drugs. *J Hypertens Suppl* 1998;16:S75-S79.
70. Marland G. Atypical neuroleptics: Use for schizophrenia. *Nurs Times* 1998; 94:61–62.
71. Pushpangadan M, Feely M. Once a day is best: Evidence or assumption? The relationship between compliance and dosage frequency in older people. *Drugs Aging* 1998;13:223–227.

72. Schmier JK, Leidy NK. The complexity of treatment adherence in adults with asthma: Challenges and opportunities. *J Asthma* 1998;35:455–472.
73. Shepherd M. The risks of polypharmacy. *Nurs Times* 1998;94:60–62.
74. Souery D, Mendlewicz J. Compliance and therapeutic issues in resistant depression. *Int Clin Psychopharmacol* 1998;13(Suppl 2):S13–S18.
75. Tseng AL. Compliance issues in the treatment of HIV infection. *Am J Health Syst Pharm* 1998;55:1817–1824.
76. Vidler V. Compliance with iron chelation therapy in beta thalassaemia. *Paediatr Nurs* 1998;10:17–18,20.
77. Wiecek A. Compliance of patients with arterial hypertension to therapeutic recommendations. *Przegl Lek* 1998;55:65–66.
78. Williams GH. Assessing patient wellness: New perspectives on quality of life and compliance. *Am J Hypertens* 1998;11:186S–191S.
79. Wilson TG, Jr. How patient compliance to suggested oral hygiene and maintenance affect periodontal therapy. *Dent Clin North Am* 1998;42:389–403.
80. Yasin S. Detecting and improving compliance. Is concordance the solution? *Aust Fam Physician* 1998;27:255–260.
81. Shumaker SA. *The handbook of health behavior change*, 2nd ed. New York: Springer Pub. Co.; 1998:xii, 607.
82. Bowen DJ, Thornquist M, Goodman G, et al. Effects of incentives on participation in a randomized chemoprevention trial. *J Health Psych* 1999;4:589–595.
83. Bowen DJ, Hickman KM, Powers D. Importance of psychological variables in understanding risk perceptions and breast cancer screening for African-American women. *Women's Health: Research on Gender, Behavior, and Policy* 1997;3&4:227–242.
84. Ockene JK, Lindsay EA, Hymowitz N, et al. Tobacco control activities of primary-care physicians in the Community Intervention Trial for Smoking Cessation. COMMIT Research Group. *Tob Control* 1997;6:S49–S56.

Chapter 2

Strategies to Increase Adherence to Treatment

Judith K. Ockene, PhD, MEd

Introduction

This chapter addresses the educational and behavioral strategies which can be used to increase adherence to cardiovascular risk reduction treatment. I will take a clinical approach, and report some data to help demonstrate major points. The topics that I will cover are: a review of the factors that affect adherence; theories and models of behavior change; constructs in social cognitive theory and strategies using those constructs to enhance adherence; a counseling model which we developed and have conducted research on at UMass Medical School, patient-centered counseling;[1] and evidence that the model produces behavior change and increases adherence to treatment when used as a brief intervention by physicians, nurses, and other health professionals.[2-4] I will conclude with a summary of my recommendations for increasing adherence to cardiovascular risk reduction treatment.

The strategies discussed here can be used for smoking cessation, dietary change, increasing physical activity, stress reduction, and alcohol use reduction. (Medication adherence will be addressed in Chapter 3.) Alcohol reduction is included because abuse of alcohol can have an effect on hypertension for hypertensive patients.

Factors Affecting Adherence

As noted previously, there are three groups or levels of factors that affect adherence: the individual—what he or she brings to treat-

From: Burke LE, Ockene IS (eds). *Compliance in Healthcare and Research.* Armonk, NY: Futura Publishing Company, Inc.; © 2001.

ment; the interpersonal—the people involved with that individual have a tremendous effect on whether he/she will adhere to treatment; and the environment or the context in which the individual lives, works, and participates. On the individual level, factors affecting adherence include: demographic, cognitive (knowledge), attitudinal (self-efficacy, outcome expectations), affective (eg, depression, anxiety), and behavioral (skills). The factors on the interpersonal level include relationships, communication (especially at the provider to patient level), and social support. On the environment level we cannot ignore that what surrounds the individual will greatly affect what happens to him or her, including whether or not he or she has access to various treatment options, and what the costs of those options are for the individual.

Theories of Change

I have two theories of change with which I like to work. You can choose whatever theory you want, as long as it works for you and helps you to explain to yourself what is happening in your interaction and work with patients. The first is social cognitive theory, developed by Dr. Albert Bandura and his colleagues.[5,6] I like it because to me it is an optimistic theory and acknowledges the resilience and flexibility which people have. It says that behavior is learned and can be unlearned. That's important for us to let our patients know. "You're not stuck because you have a particular behavior. It took you a lot of time to develop this behavior. Therefore, it will take you some time to change it or develop new behaviors." A second principle that I like about this theory is that it tells us that people learn best by active participation. Educational theory also tells us this (see discussion of patient-centered counseling model, below). However, physicians and other healthcare practitioners often are used to telling patients what to do. They do a lot of "advice" giving. "You need to do this, you need to do that." When it comes to behavior change, providers are often overwhelmed by the thought of needing to be able to tell patients exactly how to change behaviors. The truth is, they don't need to tell them how to change. Active participation means that there needs to be a dialogue between the patient and the provider. If I would like to help my patient change a particular behavior, then I need to engage him or her in a dialogue where he/she comes up with ways of making a change that fit for him or her. I will come back to that concept later, because that dialogue is one of the most important things we can do to enhance adherence to treatment regimens. We need to actively engage our patients in the planning process.

Social cognitive theory notes certain constructs that affect behavior and behavior change. These constructs are similar to the ones already noted as affecting whether an individual will change a behavior. For simplicity's sake we can fit these constructs into one of the three levels of factors we have noted: personal, interpersonal, and environmental. If we agree that these factors or constructs have an effect on behavior then we can ask ourselves, "What kinds of treatments can we use that take them into account?" As the two previous chapters have noted, there is not much research which demonstrates that, if you actually change the constructs or factors, you will see an effect on behavior. That is where some of the challenge to research lies today. However, we certainly do know, from a clinical perspective, that it helps to take those constructs or factors into account for our treatment strategies.

Another theory that is very useful in our work with patients, is stages of change theory, which has been described by Drs. James Prochaska and Carlo DiClemente.[7] That people who make changes go through stages of behavioral change is not a new concept. Other researchers also have noted that people go through various levels and stages of making behavioral changes.[8,9] I teach medical students in their first two years of medical school. When I present the concept of stages of change they say, "That really makes a lot of sense, it's intuitive". The overall concept is that change is a process, not a one-time event, and we can't expect people to make changes at a level for which they're not ready. Our interventions need to be directed to where the individual is. If I have a patient sitting in front of me, for example, and I say "It is important for you to stop smoking", and this individual has never thought about it, or has thought about it and has decided, "That's really not for me", this is a person who I must treat very differently than the person who has already thought about it, is taking some steps towards making changes, and feels confident about his ability to make that change. It is intuitive at some level, but we often forget about this process when we intervene with patients.

Constructs of Social Cognitive Theory, Interventions, Objectives and Treatment to Enhance Adherence

Factors or constructs in social cognitive theory can be grouped on the individual level, on the interpersonal level, and on the environmental level. (See Table 1.) On the individual level one factor is health knowledge. Knowledge is not the only thing that we need, but we sometimes assume patients know more than they do about a particular problem. Therefore, we at least need to assess, "How much does my

Table 1

SCT Constructs, Intervention Objectives, & Methods to Increase Adherence to Treatment on the Individual, Interpersonal, and Environmental Levels

Construct	Intervention Objectives	Methods
I. Individual		
Health Knowledge	Increase knowledge of CVD health risks and mechanisms	• Provide information • Assess relevance • Assess understanding
Self-Efficacy	Increase belief in ability to implement specific behavior in specific settings/ conditions	• Mastery experiences • Review past experiences • Focus on + experiences • Negotiate steps
Outcome Expectations	Increase belief in + effect of change (health, psychology, & social)	• Assess and identify expectations • Increase/reinforce + expectations • Reframe—expectations and problem solve
Self-Regulation • Self-Observation	Increase awareness of behavior and influences on it	• Self-monitoring log • Review patterns and provide feedback • Reinforce
• Goal Setting • Self-Reinforcement	Set proximal and distal goals Foster use of rewards contingent on change and maintenance	• Negotiate goals • Set realistic steps • Assess and negotiate rewards
II. Interpersonal		
Social Support • Provider • Home • Work • School • Organizations	Increase available social support for change of risk behavior	• Develop collaborative relationship with patient • Identify family/community sources of support • Provide information on community resources • Assist patient to develop assertiveness skills
III. Environmental		
Access and Costs	• Increase options (e.g., food) and awareness of them and availability of resources (e.g., for physical activity) • Develop governmental policies to increase options	• Provide info on appropriate options (e.g., food items) and sources of help

SCT = social cognitive theory; CVD = cardiovascular disease

patient know about this particular problem?" For example, we often think, "Smoking – It's in the media, it's all over, doesn't everybody know that it's harmful to you?" But some people may not know it, or may not relate it to themselves. It's important to at least assess with the person, "Do you understand the risks of smoking? Have you thought about this?" Do not assume that everybody knows the health and disease risks of smoking. A good example is pregnant women. We could assume that all pregnant women know that the effect of smoking on the fetus is very hazardous. Unfortunately, many, especially less educated women, don't know that fact. Another important piece of information is that if a woman stops smoking in the first trimester, the risk to the fetus is the same as for the woman who has never smoked. This fact is not well known. While information is not sufficient, it is necessary, and we need to assess knowledge and provide the necessary information. We should not assume that our patients understand the effect of what they're doing on their health or on the health of others.

Another construct on the individual level is self-efficacy. This is a term that psychologists and social scientists use a lot. It means that an individual believes in his/her ability to make a particular change in a particular setting. That's very important. Self-efficacy is not generalized. If I think that I'm capable, it doesn't mean I think that I'm capable in every setting for every particular behavior. Self-efficacy is a psychological and cognitive construct that has been demonstrated to be predictive of behavior change. If we believe that it's an important factor, then in our interventions we need to help our patients to increase their belief that they can make a particular change. Now, I don't mean that we want to say, "Oh yes, you can do it. Of course you can do it." That's not going to increase their belief. That's just telling them something. How can we help people increase their belief in their ability to do something? There are several ways. One, which we do a lot in patient-centered counseling, and is one of the basic principles of patient-centered counseling, is that we can help the individual explore past experiences that demonstrate his or her ability to make changes. For example, 80% of all smokers have stopped smoking at some point in the past.[10]

If I am working with a smoker, for example, I would ask him, "Do you think you can stop smoking?" And he might say, "Oh no. I've tried it before, and I was a failure." I might then say to him, "Tell me about that experience. How long were you off cigarettes?" He might answer, "I was off for only 3 weeks, and then I failed." Well, how do you think I'm going to respond to that particular statement, keeping self-efficacy in mind? "You stayed off for 3 weeks. That's a pretty long time. That's great! There are some people who can't stay off for 24 hours. You went back to smoking and that's okay. How did you manage to stay off for 3 weeks?" People can frame things in a very negative way, and I'm not suggesting that we want to be phony, or we want to say things that are not true. I'm suggesting that we can help the individual frame something in a way that can help to increase his sense of success.

Another construct is "outcome expectation." As Dr. Bowen noted in Chapter 1, it's a concept in other theories as well as Social Cognitive theory. The Health Belief Model talks a lot about expectations, that is, a belief that, "What I'm going to do is going to have a positive effect on me."[11] If I have a patient sitting in front of me who says, "If I stop smoking, it's not going to matter. I'm not going to get any healthier. I've already had my heart attack. It's not going to do anything about my heart attack. Why should I stop smoking?" If I thought the same thing, I would not want to stop smoking. Why do it if it's not going to have a positive effect on you or on your family? We need to know what the expectations are that the individual has regarding a particular behavior. The most important thing we can do is ask and listen. We want to know those expectations, and then we want to listen to the answers so that we can help that individual have positive and realistic expectations. Her expectations may be based on misinformation, so we need to identify them. We need to reinforce positive expectations. If they are not there, we can forget about that patient making any changes. Our job therefore will be to help that individual develop positive expectations. One way that I help patients to develop positive expectations is to ask them "What would be good for you if you did change this behavior? What benefit would you get from making this kind of a change?" Her expectations may not be what mine are, but I'd better know that they will be positive for her if I want to help her make a change. We need to help patients reframe expectations and problem-solve if they don't see anything positive about a change. Patients often say, "I don't really care about my own health, it doesn't really matter. I don't believe stopping smoking will have that much of an effect on me." Okay, "What do you see as a benefit in making this change?" "Well, I've been really concerned about my kids. They're concerned about my smoking. If I stop they will feel better." So that's an important expectation to help reinforce. If that's important to him, that's great. Let's work with that. The bottom line is that people need to believe that there's something positive that they're going to get out of the change. If they don't believe that there's anything positive to be gained, why should they adhere to a treatment?

People also need to know how to self-observe, self-monitor, and look at their own patterns of behavior. I have found, and I have worked in many randomized clinical trials (RCTs), as well as in my own clinical practice, it is often helpful for certain patients to record what they're doing for a brief period of time. I'm not saying your patient should keep a record for the next two months, because that is one way to increase nonadherence with that patient. It is very unlikely he will do that. What I do is find out, "How long do you think you can record for? One day? Two days?" People learn how to self-observe. It is very important to develop that as a skill because then they know how to self-correct; how to make changes if they are going down the wrong path. It is also important to negotiate goals. My goal may be very different from yours, and mine doesn't really matter if yours is not consistent with it. I may have a patient sitting in front of me whom I may want to stop smoking, but that may not be a goal that is consistent with how he sees himself. We need to develop goals that are realistic for the patient and that we can also be comfortable with. That means negotiating.

On the interpersonal level social support is an important factor. The collaborative relationship, based on communication and negotiation, is extremely important. We cannot say, "This is all your responsibility." Nor can we say, "This is all my responsibility." This is a partnership. We can work together to make sure that we come up with something that will work for you, and I can help you if you would like my help. Identification of sources of support is important. I find that physicians make very little use of community resources. In fact, they usually don't even know where they are. It is important and helpful to develop a list of community resources where patients can go for additional help.

I also find that physicians and other providers don't make use of available educational or treatment materials. For example, every pharmaceutical company that manufactures nicotine replacement therapy (NRT) has a telephone counseling line. I can't tell you how many times I ask providers, "Do you know that if your patient is using such and such NRT he can call a telephone counselor for help for no cost?" The answer is invariably, "No, I didn't know that." At least know the resources available so that you can provide them for your patient.

Patient-Centered Counseling

Let's put this all together into a patient-centered counseling mode. We have demonstrated evidence in three randomized clinical trials that the model is efficacious and effective: the diet RCT or WATCH[3], the alcohol RCT or Project Health[12], and the smoking RCT that we conducted.[13] First, I'll briefly review the patient-centered counseling model. As I've structured this chapter, I've given clues as to what is in the model. If we're going to ask providers such as physicians and nurses to use this model, there must be evidence that it works, and it is effective in helping patients make changes. If we want to have a far reach, our interventions need to be as brief as possible, especially if we expect physicians to use them. They need to be brief and fit within the context of a regular office visit. Patient-centered counseling takes up to about 10 minutes, but can take much less time. It can be tailored to fit within the time available.

Patient-centered counseling is very directive, "I would like to talk with you about your smoking today. Let's take a few minutes to talk about that. Is that okay with you?" It focuses on a particular problem. There is provision of information because, as providers, we have a responsibility to provide information to our patients. But there are also questions that physicians and other providers are taught to ask, which help move the patient along the continuum of change, and patients are provided feedback based on the answers. There are some important principles discussed earlier that I want to reinforce. (See Table 2.) We need to accept the patient where she is. We may wish she were further along, but we need to accept her where she is at. That is where we begin the dialogue. We need to accept what we do not know. It is often difficult for providers to accept that there may be things that we don't know. However, it can be overwhelming to think that you need to know everything about what's going to work with every one of your patients. I know I don't know what's going to work with all of my patients. I need to accept that and move on from there and acknowledge that my patient has many of the answers. To paraphrase Dr. William Osler, the father of modern medicine, "if you want to know about the patient, ask him." That's exactly what patient-centered counseling is. If you want to know about what's going to help your patient, ask him. Another principle is that we need to build self-efficacy by setting realistic expectations for ourselves and the patient. We also need to share responsibility.

There are five domains of questions that we use in patient-centered counseling. (See Table 3.) Think what you believe to be the most important things to consider if you were going to make changes in a behavior.

Table 2

Principles of Patient-Centered Counseling

Six General Principles:
- Accept patient where she is;
- Accept what you do not know;
- Acknowledge that the patient has the answers;
- Build self-efficacy;
- Set realistic expectations for self & patient; and
- Share responsibility

Table 3

Topic Areas for Patient-Centered Counseling

Uses questions related to five content areas:
- Desire and motivation to change behavior;
- Past experiences with the behavioral change;
- Factors that inhibit the change (barriers);
- Resources for change (strengths); and
- Plan for change and followup.

These are the ones that we've come up with as part of our patient-centered model: desire and motivation to change. "Would you like to change this behavior? Would you like to change any part of this behavior? Why? What's in it for you?" I can't tell you how many times I've asked physicians and other providers, "Have you asked your patients if they want to change this behavior and why?" Often the answer is, "No", which is quite amazing. Then it's important to ask, "What have been your past experiences with behavioral change?" (ie, smoking, weight change, diet, alcohol.) "Have you ever stopped smoking before?" It's very important to know what the past behavior of that patient has been. That's what's going to help you know what's going to help your patient now. "Yes, I quit smoking. I was off for 3 weeks." "What were some of the things that you did that helped you stop for those 3 weeks? What were some of the things that worked for you?" You would be surprised how well patients can come up with things that actually work for them if you ask them to think about it. Then, "What were some of the things that got in your way? Why did you go back to smoking?" If you know what gets in the way of success you can know how to plan for the problems in the future. We provide feedback to the patient; "it sounds like some of the things that were helpful to you were taking walks, and telling your wife that you were going to stop smoking. Those sound good and we can think about using them again. It sounds like one of the things that was a problem for you was when you got stressed and you needed that cigarette. Can you think of things that you could have done that would have helped you not take that cigarette?" The goal is to do some problem solving with the patient, and then make a plan for how to make the change.

Evidence that Patient-Centered Counseling Works

The evidence that patient-centered counseling works can be seen in several RCTs. One is the Physician-Delivered Smoking Intervention

Project, funded by the National Cancer Institute in 1986.[2] We tested a patient-centered counseling brief intervention to determine what kind of an effect it would have on the smoking behavior of patients being seen for a regular visit with their physicians in a primary care practice (internal medicine and family practice). These patients were randomized to three possible physician interventions. On possibility was that they received very direct personalized advice. The advice wasn't just "stop smoking," rather it was very relevant to what the patient presented with. The second possible condition was patient-centered counseling. The third was patient-centered counseling plus assessment of nicotine addiction and a prescription of NRT. At that time the only NRT that was available was nicotine-containing gum. All of the patients who were seen in a general medical practice were not there particularly for smoking intervention. This was not a special visit. The patients were screened and the physician was cued that a particular patient was a smoker. The patients received either very personalized advice, counseling, or counseling plus NRT. As a frame of reference for the results, in the general population of smokers about 3% of individuals stop smoking each year.[10] As can be seen in Figure 1, at 6 months we have a 9% cessation rate for advice. That intervention was about 5 minutes of

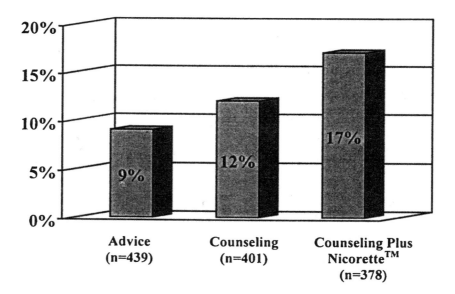

Physician-Intervention Condition

Figure 1. Physician-delivered smoking intervention project: 6-month self-reported smoking cessation rates.

very personalized advice. The second intervention, patient-centered counseling, took about 7 minutes producing a 12% rate, and the third intervention took about 9 minutes, producing a 17% rate. The rates at 12 months showed a significant difference in maintenance of change for three conditions of treatment.[13] This very brief intervention in the context of a regular medical visit produced significant differences. The training of physicians took about 2 hours; it should be noted that we didn't just teach physicians patient-centered counseling, we also provided them with reminders to intervene. We now teach patient-centered counseling to all of our medical students using about five modules during the first 2 years of medical school.

More works better than less. Would you be pleased if you spent an average of nine minutes with smokers and got a 17% cessation rate? I would be very pleased. And when we think about the fact that 80% of all adults see a physician each year,[14] it becomes very important to ask, what can we do in a very brief amount of time to help patients make changes? One of the things that we can do is learn how to ask the right questions and listen to the answers. For those providers who don't have enough time to do that, then we need to know what the resources are out there. Even intervening with a patient to refer him to someone else requires a patient-centered approach. I can't tell you how many times a patient will show up in my office and I'll ask, "What are you here for?" And he'll say, "Well, I don't really know. Dr. so-and-so told me to see you." That was not a good way to make a referral. So even referring a patient requires communication and understanding what will work well for that individual.

Summary and Recommendations

In summary, to enhance adherence we must start with the first encounter with the patient. It is not, "Well, I'll think about this five encounters down the road". It starts with that first meeting with the patient. We need to listen. We need to pick up on cues and be proactive with our patients. We need to be patient-centered and ask the right questions, even if we have just one or two minutes, a good question can at least get the patient thinking. "Have you thought about this? Is it a problem for you? Can we talk about it the next time you come in?" You don't need to take 9 or 10 minutes with each patient. You can take 1 minute and get him thinking about the possibilities and process of change. We need to provide information, be flexible, and be creative. Of course, we need to maintain our sense of humor because sometimes we get into some interesting and difficult situations and challenges.

Individuals need to have adequate information and believe in their ability to make changes. They need skills, support, and resources. Our interventions must be tailored to the individual, where he or she is at, and his or her social context. As we've heard before and as we know, one size does not fit all. Therefore, we need to know who the patient is sitting there in front of us. Patient-centered counseling, which emphasizes providing information, asking questions, and giving feedback, is an effective model which can increase adherence to cardiovascular risk reduction treatment.

References

1. Ockene J, Ockene I. Helping patients to reduce their risk for coronary heart disease: An overview. In Ockene I, Ockene J (eds): *Prevention of Coronary Heart Disease*. Boston: Little, Brown and Company; 1992:173–199.
2. Ockene J, Kristeller J, Goldberg R, et al. Increasing the efficacy of physician-delivered smoking intervention: A randomized clinical trial. *J Gen Intern Med* 1991;6:1–8.
3. Ockene I, Hebert J, Ockene J, et al. Effect of physician-delivered nutrition counseling training and a structured office-support program on saturated fat intake, weight, and serum lipid measurements in a hyperlipidemic population: Worcester Area Trial for Counseling in Hyperlipidemia (WATCH). *Arch Int Med* 1999;159:725–731.
4. Ockene J, Adams A, Hurley T, et al. Brief physician- and nurse practitioner-delivered counseling for high- risk drinkers: Does it work? *Arch Intern Med* (in press)
5. Bandura A. *Social Learning Theory*. Englewood Cliffs, NJ: Prentice-Hall; 1977.
6. Bandura A. *Self-efficacy: The Exercise of Control*. New York: WH Freeman and Company; 1997.
7. Prochaska J, DiClemente C. Stages and processes of self-change of smoking: Toward an integrative model of change. *J Consult Clin Psych* 1983;51: 390–395.
8. Horn D. A model for the study of personal choice health behavior. *J Health Educ* 1976;19:89–98.
9. Lichtenstein E, Brown R. Smoking cessation methods: Review and recommendations. In Miller W (ed): *The Addictive Behaviors: Treatment of Alcoholism, Drug Abuse, Smoking and Obesity*. New York: Pergamon Press; 1980.
10. U.S. Department of Health and Human Services. *Reducing the health consequences of smoking: 25 years of progress*. A report of the Surgeon General. U.S. Department of Health and Human Services, Public Health Service, Centers for Disease Control, Center for Chronic Disease Prevention and Health Promotion, Office on Smoking and Health. DHHS Publication No. (CDC) 89–8411, 1989.
11. Becker M. The health belief model and personal health behavior. *Hlth Educ Monographs* 1974;2:324–473.
12. Ockene J, Wheeler E, Adams A, et al. Provider training for patient-centered alcohol counseling in a primary care setting. *Arch Intern Med* 1997;157: 2334–2341.

13. Ockene J, Kristeller J, Pbert L, et al. The PDSIP: Can short-term interventions produce long-term effects for a general outpatient population. *Health Psychol* 1994;14(3):278–281.

14. U.S. Department of Health and Human Services. *Current estimates from the National Health Interview Survey, 1993 (Series 10: Data from the National Health Survey No. 190)*. Hyattsville, MD: Public Health Service, Centers for Disease Control, National Center for Health Statistics; 1994.

Chapter 3

Behavioral Strategies to Improve Medication-Taking Compliance

Elizabeth A. Schlenk, PhD, RN,
Lora E. Burke, PhD, MPH, RN, and
Cynthia Rand, PhD

Introduction

An underlying theme that pervades the work of clinicians and researchers in health care in general, and heart disease in particular, is a sense of frustration tempered with hope as we investigate new therapies. This is an exciting time in health care, as new breakthrough therapies are discovered that have the potential to markedly change the management of chronic diseases, such as heart disease, asthma, AIDS, and rheumatoid arthritis. However, the reality is that effective therapies often do not yield effective disease management, owing to the mediating variable of patient compliance (Figure 1). Even the best treatments will fail if patients are unwilling or unable to adhere with therapy. This chapter provides a brief overview of issues in noncompliance, including different types of compliance difficulties and strategies to modify patient compliance behavior.

Magnitude of Noncompliance

Overall, compliance research suggests that the magnitude of noncompliance and the forms of compliance problems are similar across

We wish to acknowledge Ms. Tracy Woloshyn, BSN, RN and Ms. Rachel Harvey, BSN, RN for their assistance in preparing this manuscript.
This study was supported in part by a grant from the National Institute of Nursing Research of the National Institutes of Health (5 P30 NR03924).

From: Burke LE, Ockene IS (eds). *Compliance in Healthcare and Research.* Armonk, NY: Futura Publishing Company, Inc.; © 2001.

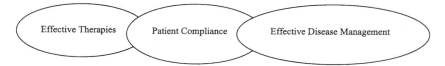

Figure 1. Model of disease management.

all chronic diseases. Using electronic monitoring of medication compliance, noncompliance rates averaging 50% have been reported for asthma,[1-5] hypertension,[6,7] and other chronic diseases.[8]

Asthma provides a well-studied model for examining patient compliance and compliance interventions because it is a chronic disease with an inflammatory component that requires prophylactic daily medication. Similar to patients with hypertension, patients with moderate to severe asthma must take daily medication even when they have no symptoms. Studies of compliance with asthma therapy have consistently found that the complexity of the prescribed regimen can influence rates of compliance. For example, Coutts et al.[9] investigated pediatric compliance with inhaled anti-inflammatory therapy with regimens of different prescribed daily frequency. Medication compliance was measured by an electronic metered dose inhaler (MDI) monitor called a Chronolog , which recorded the date and time of each use of the inhaler, and a self-report diary, which was completed by the parents of their children's compliance with the regimen. The investigators found that as prescribed regimen frequency increased compliance with the regimen decreased. The electronically recorded compliance was 71% for twice a day therapy but only 18% with the four times a day therapy. Two other common characteristics of patient compliance behavior were also observed in this study. First, self-reported compliance was generally high, especially for the twice a day and three times a day therapy. And second, there was a marked discrepancy between self-reported compliance and electronically or objectively measured compliance, with self-reported compliance significantly overestimated. Dunbar-Jacob and colleagues found the same discrepancy between self-reported compliance and electronically monitored compliance among patients taking lipid-lowering therapy.[10]

Form of therapy can also influence patient compliance. Kelloway et al.[11] conducted a pharmacy database review that examined compliance among adults and adolescents with three different forms of asthma therapy: (a) oral theophylline, (b) inhaled steroids, an anti-inflammatory medication, and (c) inhaled chromolyn, another anti-inflammatory medication. The results showed a significant difference between compliance with an oral regimen (79%) versus an inhaled regimen (inhaled steroid compliance 44% and inhaled cromolyn compliance 54%). This study illustrated another theme seen across many different therapies. The investigators found a marked discrepancy between adult compliance and adolescent compliance across all forms of medication, with refill rates for adolescents indicating significantly lower compliance with the prescribed asthma medication.

Impact of Noncompliance

Lewis[12] estimated that the costs of poor compliance to medication regimens are as high as $100 billion annually. Noncompliance can lead to disease exacerbation, additional diagnostic tests, hospitalizations, and even death.[13] The direct negative consequences of noncompliance with therapy was demonstrated by Milgrom et al.[14] in a study that measured compliance with an inhaled steroid regimen in a pediatric population using electronic monitors. Those subjects who had the lowest rate of electronically monitored compliance were the most likely to require a burst of prednisone, which is a reflection of an asthma exacerbation. The median compliance with inhaled steroids was 13.7% for those who experienced exacerbations requiring a burst of prednisone and 68.2% for those who did not.

Despite the potentially negative impact of noncompliance, many patients learn from some personal experiences that noncompliance may not lead to an immediate negative outcome in a direct and obvious way. Further, patients learn that sometimes compliance behavior does not result in improvement in their disease. As a result, patient's personal experiences may serve to reinforce noncompliance with therapy.

Types of Compliance Difficulties

Understanding the source of the compliance problem can assist health care providers to select the best strategies for improving that compliance. There are several different types of compliance difficulties.

Erratic Noncompliance

The first and most common type is erratic noncompliance, in which patients know what they are supposed to do, they basically agree with the regimen, but they fail to follow the therapy because it is difficult, complicated, or disruptions interfere with following the regimen. Some reasons for erratic noncompliance include a busy lifestyle, forgetfulness, a change in one's schedule, psychological distress, and running out of medication.[15-20]

The behavioral strategies used to remediate erratic noncompliance are ones that are geared towards simplifying the regimen,[9] prompting and cueing to increase attention to remembering the therapy,[21,22] and adherence aids that directly enhance one's ability to remember or to maintain the therapy.[23] Managed care policies, which allow patients to refill only one month of a prescription at a time and limit refills to one week prior to running out of medication, can contribute to erratic noncompliance. If patients' timing is not perfect, they will run out of medication. In this instance, patient compliance may be improved by systemic organizational changes that simplify and facilitate refilling prescriptions.

Unwitting Noncompliance

A second type of compliance difficulty is unwitting noncompliance, which is inevitably missed by its very nature. This is the type of compliance problem that neither the clinician nor the patient recognizes. Patients believe that they are complying appropriately, as does their health care provider. However, as a result of misunderstanding the regimen, incorrect administration technique, language barriers, and/or cognitive impairment, patients are incorrectly following the prescribed regimen.

Comprehension of the prescribed regimen is the first step in successfully complying with the regimen. One study reported that patients who were interviewed upon leaving a doctor's office had lost two-thirds of the information that they had received.[24] Several studies have reported that one-fifth to one-half of elderly patients have difficulty understanding or lack knowledge about their medication regimen.[16,25,26] A written medication schedule and instructions can enhance compliance.[27]

Particularly with more complicated regimens, patients may confuse the role and use of their medications. For example, patients with moderate to severe asthma are prescribed two forms of medication, a daily anti-inflammatory medication and a prn or "use as needed" bronchodilator to administer when they have symptoms. When patients are interviewed about their understanding of these two medications, there are gaps in their knowledge about which of these medications is prescribed to treat the symptoms of an asthma attack. In addition, the patient's understanding of "use as needed" is often poor. Some patients report that they take the daily medication "every day when needed." Indeed, Bender et al.[2] found that patients failed to take any inhaled corticosteroid doses on a median of 41.8% of days or inhaled beta-agonists on 28.1% of days despite prescribed daily use. Further, medication noncompliance was correlated with lower levels of asthma knowledge in this study. Thus, health care providers need to regularly review their patients' understanding of the regimen.

Patients must use the correct technique to effectively deliver the medication. For example, in asthma, MDI technique is fundamental to effective asthma management. Studies that examined patients' MDI technique have demonstrated that many patients have poor technique.[3,28] Further, when health care providers' MDI technique is assessed, they also show a lack of knowledge of the correct technique,[29,30] potentially contributing to patient's unwitting noncompliance.

Language barriers[1] and cognitive impairment[16,31] can contribute to patients not remembering the regimen. This problem can be identified if health care providers directly ask their patients to report their understanding of the regimen and to demonstrate their administration technique. This assessment should be done at every consultation because these behaviors can atrophy over time.

Intentional Noncompliance

The third type of compliance difficulty is "intelligent" or intentional noncompliance. Although it may not be wise to be noncompliant with the regimen, the patient makes a clear decision to alter or discontinue the therapy. Some reasons for intentional noncompliance include feeling better or believing that the medication is no longer needed, side effects, perceived ineffectiveness of therapy, complexity of the regimen, fear of addiction, and inability to afford the medication.[16, 32–39] Often these changes in therapy will not be reported to the health care provider because the patients feel that they will be judged negatively, or they want to please the health care provider. Patients may decide that they know what is best for them and they do not want to disappoint the health care provider who they perceive has made a wrong recommendation for therapy.

Patients frequently alter therapy because they feel better, they do not think they need the medication, or they think the medication is too much for them. There is a prevalent feeling in society, and particularly in pediatric management of diseases, that less medication is better. Patients sometimes believe that taking less medication is better because they are putting fewer chemicals into their body.

Fear of side effects, real or imagined, and perceived ineffectiveness of the therapy are other reasons given for not following the regimen. Patients may be more likely to use symptom-relieving drugs than preventive medications because they perceive greater efficacy for the therapy that provides symptom relief. For example, asthma research suggest that patients have better compliance with symptom-relieving bronchodilator medications than with preventive anti-inflammatory medications.[2,37]

Complexity of the regimen is associated with noncompliance. Asthma patients are recommended to follow a multi-component regimen consisting of monitoring peak flows, keeping an asthma diary, and using prophylactic medication up to four times a day. These are guideline-based practice recommendations from the National Heart, Lung, and Blood Institute that help patients manage their disease. However, this is a complicated regimen that can interfere with one's lifestyle. Patients may find a complex regimen burdensome, leading them to deliberately simplify the regimen.

A study examining pediatric asthma in the inner city revealed a common concern of mothers of children with asthma that their children would become addicted to the medication if they used the medication too much.[37] Patients' lay beliefs about medication and its effects can profoundly influence the way they use therapies. Studies of hypertension[40] and diabetes[41] have discovered similar lay beliefs that influence medication compliance. Knowing the community and the individual patient will assist health care providers to identify health beliefs that impact compliance.

Cost factors can also prevent full compliance. Patients find it difficult to admit to their health care provider that they cannot afford the medication. Thus, effective interviewing skills are needed to uncover financial reasons for noncompliance.

Summary

In summary, noncompliance with the medication regimen may result from several types of compliance problems. Effective strategies to improve patient compliance must necessarily be tailored to the form of compliance difficulty. Although behavioral strategies are important in promoting medication compliance, a review by the health care provider of pragmatic issues, such as comprehension of the regimen, mental status, and ability to pay for the medication is a necessary first step for all patients.

Compliance Across Populations

Compliance difficulties may differ across populations, specifically children and adolescents, the elderly, the mentally ill, and lower socio-

economic populations. These populations may need special consideration when selecting behavioral strategies. Compliance issues in pediatric populations involve compliance of both the parents and the
children. These two compliance curves overlap with parents managing
younger children's medications and providing less supervision as older
children become more autonomous and begin to assume greater self-
management of their own medications. Parents vary in the age at which
they allow children to take full responsibility for medication-taking. A
study of pediatric asthma in the inner city found that autonomy for
medication taking can occur in children as young as five and six years
of age.[42] Developmental issues and peer group influences can impact
adolescents' compliance behavior.[43] Understanding the transition process and developmental stage are critical to understanding compliance
in pediatric and adolescent patients.

Many elderly patients are not only managing their own chronic
illnesses, but the chronic illnesses of their partners as well. In addition,
they may be managing multiple therapeutic regimens. For example, an
elderly patient may be seeing a pulmonologist for asthma, a cardiologist for heart disease, and a rheumatologist for osteoarthritis. All of
these specialists may be prescribing medications. Compliance problems
may arise from multiple health care providers instructing and prescribing for the patient.[16] Thus, health care providers need to be aware of
all prescriptions before planning care.

Dementia[16,31] and substance abuse[44,45] have been shown to contribute to poor medication compliance. Several studies have found that
depression was associated with poor medication compliance.[46,47] These
latter findings suggest that compliance can be improved with the
proper diagnosis and treatment of depression.

Noncompliance cuts across ethnic and socioeconomic groups.
However, lower socioeconomic status does create additional financial
and social barriers to filling medication prescriptions and following
medication regimens.[38,39]

In summary, some patient populations are potentially at greater
risk for noncompliance to medication regimen than other groups. Compliance enhancing strategies should be tailored to meet the special
needs of children and adolescents, the elderly, the mentally ill, and
lower socioeconomic populations.

Clinical Approaches to Improve Medication Compliance

There are several educational, behavioral, and regimen-related
strategies that can be used to address these compliance problems (Table

Table 1

Clinical Approaches to Improve Medication Compliance

Educational Interventions
    Effective patient-provider communication
    Written instructions for medication use
    Instruction in and review of administration techniques
    Disease self-management programs
Behavioral Interventions
    Self-monitoring
    Cueing (reminders and prompts)
    Chaining
    Positive reinforcement
    Patient contracting
Therapy Tailoring
    Explore patient's schedule, beliefs, and preferences
    Simplify the dosing regimen
    Alter the administration route
    Use adherence aids

1). Although some of these strategies are framed within an asthma management model, they have application to other chronic diseases, including heart disease.

Educational Interventions

Knowledge of the regimen is crucial to compliance, although it does not guarantee compliance. Patients need information about the regimen as well as strategies to optimize compliance. Several studies have underscored the central role of effective patient-provider communication.[48,49] Increased attention by health care providers to their own and their patients' behavior may prevent misunderstandings about medications.

Written instructions about the regimen should be a core part of every interaction with the patient. A series of studies by Morrow and colleagues has focused on effective instruction formats for older patients. Comprehension and recall of medication information was facilitated significantly when medication-taking instructions were clear,[50] were structured in lists rather than paragraphs,[51] used pictorial icons in combination with written medication instructions,[52] and were consistent with patients' mental representations of taking medication.[53]

Patients need instruction in the use of any sort of equipment required as part of the regimen along with regular review of their administration technique, for example metered dose inhalers[54] and peak flow monitors[55] in asthma. This type of equipment allows patients to administer medications and to assess and record their health status.

Disease self-management programs are structured, community-based programs that integrate education with modeling and peer support. Disease self-management programs have been developed and found to be effective in enhancing the management of a range of chronic diseases, including asthma, hypertension and diabetes, arthritis, HIV infection, as well as chronic pain and chronic diseases more generally.[56-61]

Behavioral Interventions

Behavioral strategies, including self-monitoring, cueing, chaining, (that is, associating new behaviors with established ones), positive reinforcement, and patient contracting have been used to enhance medication compliance. [21,22,62-64] Frequently, these strategies are combined and included in multi-modal disease self-management interventions.

Therapy Tailoring

Tailoring the therapy to the patient is a strategy that is sometimes overlooked by health care providers. It is usually easier to change therapy than it is to change patient behavior. Health care providers may neglect negotiating with a patient a regimen that may be optimal from a behavioral perspective, although suboptimal from a pharmacological perspective. Whenever possible, negotiating a therapy that the patient is able to follow should be a first priority. Some examples of ways to tailor the therapy include exploring the patient's schedule, beliefs, and preferences, simplifying the dosing regimen, altering the administration route, and using adherence aids.[23, 65-67]

Clinical Trials of Compliance-Promotion Interventions

Few randomized controlled trials (RCT) have been conducted of interventions to improve medication compliance.[68] Haynes et al.[68] reported that only 13 studies met the criteria of randomization, use of a control group, assessment of compliance, and assessment of treatment effects. Of these studies, only seven showed improvements in compliance and only six showed improvements in treatment effects. In addition, these RCT were limited to hypertension, schizophrenia, asthma, epilepsy, and acute infections. The interventions that were successful in improving either compliance or clinical outcomes were complex, using some combination of more convenient care, information, counseling, reminders, self-monitoring, reinforcement, family therapy, and other forms of supervision. The effects on compliance were modest. Research should focus on the development and testing of innovative approaches to help patients follow prescribed medication regimens.

Summary

In summary, a variety of educational, behavioral, and regimen-related interventions are available to health care providers to promote medication compliance. A few of these intervention strategies have been systematically tested; however, they did not have robust effects on compliance. Additional clinical trials of compliance enhancing strategies are needed.

Conclusion

Compliance to medication regimen among persons with heart disease[69] and other chronic diseases is a significant problem. About half of patients have problems following their regimen, resulting in adverse consequences clinically and economically. Although several strategies have been evaluated for their ability to improve compliance, including educational, behavioral, and regimen-related interventions, very few randomized, controlled studies have been conducted. Therefore, the evidence supporting interventions is weak. Research endeavors are needed to better understand and improve compliance.

References

1. Apter AJ, Reisine ST, Affleck G, et al. Adherence with twice-daily dosing of inhaled steroids: Socioeconomic and health-belief differences. *Am J Respir Crit Care Med* 1998;157(6 Pt. 1):1810–1817.
2. Bender B, Milgrom H, Rand C, et al. Psychological factors associated with medication nonadherence in asthmatic children. *J Asthma* 1998;35(4): 347–353.
3. Berg J, Dunbar-Jacob J, Rohay JM. Compliance with inhaled medications: The relationship between diary and electronic monitor. *Ann Behav Med* 1998;20(1):36–38.
4. Bosley CM, Fosbury JA, Cochrane GM. The psychological factors associated with poor compliance with treatment in asthma. *Eur Respir J* 1995;8(6): 899–904.
5. Gibson NA, Ferguson AE, Aitchison TC, et al. Compliance with inhaled asthma medication in preschool children. *Thorax* 1995;50(12):1274–1279.

6. Lee JY, Kusek JW, Greene PG, et al. Assessing medication adherence by pill count and electronic monitoring in the African American Study of Kidney Disease and Hypertension (AASK) Pilot Study. *Am J Hypertens* 1996;9(8):719–725.

7. Mounier-Vehier C, Bernaud C, Carre A, et al. Compliance and hypertensive efficacy of amlodipine compared with nifedipine slow-release. *Am J Hypertens* 1998;11(4 Pt. 1):478–486.

8. Dunbar-Jacob J, Erlen JA, Schlenk EA, et al. Adherence in chronic disease. *Annu Rev Nurs Res* 2000;18:48–90.

9. Coutts JA, Gibson NA, Paton JY. Measuring compliance with inhaled medication in asthma. *Arch Dis Child* 1992;67(3):332–333.

10. Dunbar-Jacob J, Burke LE, Rohay JM, et al. Comparability of self-report, pill count, and electronically monitored adherence data. *Control Clin Trials* 1996;17(2S):80S.

11. Kelloway JS, Wyatt RA, Adlis SA. Comparison of patients' compliance with prescribed oral and inhaled asthma medications. *Arch Intern Med* 1994; 154(12):1349–1352.

12. Lewis A. Non-compliance: A $100 billion problem. *Remington Rep* 1997; 5(4):14–15.

13. Dunbar-Jacob J, Schlenk EA. Treatment adherence and clinical outcome: Can we make a difference? In: Resnick RJ, Rozensky RH, eds: *Health Psychology Through the Life Span: Practice and Research Opportunities* Washington DC: American Psychological Association; 1996:323–343.

14. Milgrom H, Bender B, Ackerson L, et al. Noncompliance and treatment failure in children with asthma. *J Allergy Clin Immunol* 1996;98(6 Pt. 1): 1051–1057.

15. Park DC, Herzog C, Leventhal H, et al. Medication adherence in rheumatoid arthritis patients: Older is wiser. *J Am Geriatr Soc* 1999;47(2):172–183.

16. Nikolaus T, Kruse W, Bach M, et al. Elderly patients' problems with medication: An in-hospital and follow-up study. *Eur J Clin Pharmacol* 1996;49(4): 255–259.

17. Dunbar-Jacob J. Understanding the reasons for patients' noncompliance and how these reasons impact therapeutic regimens and outcomes of care. Paper presented at a workshop, Pharmaceutical Care Programs: Their Role in Medication Compliance by EMMG, Kansas City; 1997.

18. DiMatteo MR, Sherbourne CD, Hays RD, et al. Physicians' characteristics influence patients' adherence to medical treatment: Results from the Medical Outcomes Study. *Health Psychol* 1993;12(2):93–102.

19. Avorn J, Monette J, Lacour A, et al. Persistence of use of lipid-lowering medications: A cross-national study. *JAMA* 1998;279(18):1458–1462.

20. Bailey JE, Lee MD, Somes GW, et al. Risk factors for antihypertensive medication refill failure by patients under Medicaid managed care. *Clin Ther* 1996;18(6):1252–1262.

21. Haynes RB, Sackett DL, Gibson ES, et al. Improvement of medication compliance in uncontrolled hypertension. *Lancet* 1976;1(7972):1265–1268.

22. Logan AG, Milne BJ, Achber C, et al. Work-site treatment of hypertension by specially trained nurses: A controlled trial. *Lancet* 1979;2(8153): 1175–1178.

23. Cramer JA. Enhancing patient compliance in the elderly: Role of packaging aids and monitoring. *Drugs Aging* 1998;12(1):7–15.

24. Joyce CR, Caple G, Mason M, et al. Quantitative study of doctor-patient communication. *Q J Med* 1969;38(150):183–194.

25. Blenkiron P. The elderly and their medication: Understanding and compliance in a family practice. *Postgrad Med J* 1996;72(853):671–676.
26. Lowe CJ, Raynor DK, Courtney EA, et al. Effects of self medication programme on knowledge of drugs and compliance with treatment in elderly patients. *Br Med J* 1995;310(6989):1229–1231.
27. Esposito L. The effects of medication education on adherence to medication regimens in an elderly population. *J Adv Nurs* 1995;21(5):935–943.
28. van Beerendonk I, Mesters I, Mudde AN, et al. Assessment of the inhalation technique in outpatients with asthma or chronic obstructive pulmonary disease using a metered-dose inhaler or dry powder device. *J Asthma* 1998; 35(3):273–279.
29. Plaza V, Sanchis J. Medical personnel and patient skill in the use of metered dose inhalers: A multicentric study. *Respiration* 1998;65(3):195–198.
30. Tsang KW, Lam WK, Ip M, et al. Inability of physicians to use metered-dose inhalers. *J Asthma* 1997;34(6):493–498.
31. Ruscin JM, Semla TP. Assessment of medication management skills in older outpatients. *Ann Pharmacother* 1996;30(10):1083–1088.
32. Branthwaite A, Pechere JC. Pan-European survey of patients' attitudes to antibiotics and antibiotic use. *J Int Med Res* 1996;24(3):229–238.
33. Chambers CV, Markson L, Diamon JJ, et al. Health beliefs and compliance with inhaled corticosteroids by asthmatic patients in primary care practices. *Respir Med* 1999;93(2):88–94.
34. Ferguson RP, Ziedins E, West Z, et al. Elderly drug choice survey. *J Geriatr Drug Ther* 1996;11(1):61–70.
35. Toyoshima H, Takahashi K, Akera T. The impact of side effects on hypertension management: A Japanese survey. *Clin Ther* 1997;19(6):1458–1469.
36. Montgomery SA, Kasper S. Comparison of compliance between serotonin reuptake inhibitors and tricyclic antidepressants: A meta-analysis. *Int Clin Psychopharmacol* 1995;9(Suppl. 4):33–40.
37. Butz AM, Malveaux FJ, Eggleston P, et al. Use of community health workers with inner-city children who have asthma. *Clin Pediatr* 1994;33(3):135–141.
38. Col N, Fanale JE, Kronholm P. The role of medication noncompliance and adverse drug reactions in hospitalizations of the elderly. *Arch Intern Med* 1990;150(4):841–845.
39. Watts RW, McLennan G, Bassham I, et al. Do patients with asthma fill their prescriptions? A primary compliance study. *Aust Fam Physician* 1997; 26(Suppl. 1):S4–S6.
40. Morrell RW, Park DC, Kidder DP, et al. Adherence to antihypertensive medications across the life span. *Gerontologist* 1997;37(5):609–619.
41. Charron-Prochownik D, Becker MH, Brown MB, et al. Understanding young children's health beliefs and diabetes regimen adherence. *Diabetes Educ* 1993;19(5):409–418.
42. Winkelstein M, Huss K, Butz A, et al. Factors associated with medication self-administration in children with asthma. *Clin Pediatr* In press.
43. Randolph C, Fraser B. Stressors and concerns in teen asthma. *Curr Probl Pediatr* 1999;29(3):82–93.
44. Ferrando SJ, Wall TL, Batki SL, et al. Psychiatric morbidity, illicit drug use and adherence to zidovudine (AZT) among injection drug users with HIV disease. *Am J Drug Alcohol Abuse* 1996;22(4):475–487.
45. Pablos-Mendez A, Knirsch CA, Barr RG, et al. Nonadherence in tuberculosis treatment: Predictors and consequences in New York City. *Am J Med* 1997;102(2):164–170.

46. Carney RM, Freedland KE, Eisen SA, et al. Major depression and medication adherence in elderly patients with coronary artery disease. *Health Psychol* 1995;14(1):88–90.
47. Spiers MV, Kutzik DM. Self-reported memory of medication use by the elderly. *Am J Health-Syst Pharm* 1995;52(9):985–990.
48. Hall JA, Roter DL, Milburn MA, et al. Patients' health as a predictor of physician and patient behavior in medical visits: A synthesis of four studies. *Med Care* 1996;34(12):1205–1218.
49. Roter DL, Stewart M, Putnam SM, et al. Communication patterns of primary care physicians. *JAMA* 1997;277(4):350–356.
50. Morrow D, Leirer V, Altieri P. List formats improve medication instructions for older adults. *Educ Gerontol* 1995;21(2):151–166.
51. Morrow DG, Leirer VO, Andrassy JM, et al. The influence of list format and category headers on age differences in understanding medication instructions. *Exp Aging Res* 1998;24(3):231–256.
52. Morrow DG, Hier CM, Menard WE, et al. Icons improve older and younger adults' comprehension of medication information. *J Gerontol B Psychol Sci Soc Sci* 1998;53B(4):P240–P254.
53. Morrow D, Leirer V, Altieri P, et al. Elders' schema for taking medication: Implications for instruction design. *J Gerontol* 1991;46(6):P378–P385.
54. van der Palen J, Klein JJ, Kerkhoff AH, et al. Inhalation technique of 166 adult asthmatics prior to and following a self-management program. *J Asthma* 1999;36(5):441–447.
55. Persaud DI, Barnett SE, Weller SC, et al. An asthma self-management program for children, including instruction in peak flow monitoring by school nurses. *J Asthma* 1996;33(1):37–43.
56. Allen RM, Jones MP. The validity and reliability of an asthma knowledge questionnaire used in the evaluation of a group asthma education self-management program for adults with asthma. *J Asthma* 1998;35(7):537–545.
57. Wang CY, Abbott LJ. Development of a community-based diabetes and hypertension preventive program. *Public Health Nurs* 1998;15(6):406–414.
58. Lorig K, Gonzalez VM, Ritter P. Community-based Spanish language arthritis education program: A randomized trial. *Med Care* 1999;37(9): 957–963.
59. Gifford AL, Sengupta S. Self-management health education for chronic HIV infection. *AIDS Care* 1999;11(1):115–130.
60. LeFort SM, Gray-Donald K, Rowat KM, et al. Randomized controlled trial of a community-based psychoeducation program for the self-management of chronic pain. *Pain* 1998;74(2–3):297–306.
61. Lorig KR, Sobel DS, Stewart AL, et al. Evidence suggesting that a chronic disease self-management program can improve health status while reducing hospitalization: A randomized trial. *Med Care* 1999;37(1):5–14.
62. Peterson GM, McLean S, Millingen KS. A randomized trial of strategies to improve patient compliance with anticonvulsant therapy. *Epilepsia* 1984; 25(4):412–417.
63. Bailey WC, Richards JM Jr., Brooks CM, et al. A randomized trial to improve self-management practices of adults with asthma. *Arch Intern Med* 1990; 150(8):1664–1668.
64. Schlenk EA. Patient contracting. In Fitzpatrick JJ (ed): *Encyclopedia of Nursing Research* New York: Springer; 1998:424–426.
65. Dunbar-Jacob J, Schlenk EA, Burke LE, et al. Predictors of patient adherence: Patient characteristics. In Shumaker SA, Schron EB, Ockene JK, McBee

WL (eds): *Handbook of Health Behavior Change* 2nd ed. New York: Springer; 1998:491–511.

66. Feldman R, Bacher M, Campbell N, et al. Adherence to pharmacologic management of hypertension. *Can J Public Health* 1998;89(5):I16-I18.

67. Heyscue BE, Levin GM, Merrick JP. Compliance with depot antipsychotic medication by patients attending outpatient clinics. *Psychiatr Serv* 1998; 49(9):1232–1234.

68. Haynes RB, McKibbon KA, Kanani R. Systematic review of randomised trials of interventions to assist patients to follow prescriptions for medications. *Lancet* 1996;348(9024):383–386.

69. Burke LE, Dunbar-Jacob JM, Hill MN. Compliance with cardiovascular disease prevention strategies: A review of the research. *Ann Behav Med* 1997;19(3):239–263

Section III

Multilevel Organizational Approaches to Compliance

Chapter 4

Provider Approaches to Improve Compliance

Ira S. Ockene, MD

Introduction

Previous chapters have addressed behavioral issues, but I really think that when we talk about patient centered counseling we are talking about a way of communicating with patients that applies equally well to medication-taking. This includes counseling with regard to the importance of taking medication, discussion of past problems, what helped, and so on. Although much of our work has been with physicians, I also want to point out that there is every reason to think that our findings are applicable to any provider.

A study was conducted where physicians were wired and it was noted how long they would allow a patient to talk before interrupting.[1] After asking a question such as "Why are you here", how many seconds do you think they allowed the patient to talk before interrupting? The answer is 18 seconds! I remember my relatives being horrified by this revelation, although being a physician I thought it was not surprising.

That's the background in which one works with physicians and it hasn't gotten any better since 1984.

This chapter presents work which is primarily derived from our nutrition studies, but which began with studies of smoking intervention. As Dr. Judy Ockene mentioned (see Chapter 2), we've now done successive studies on the use of patient-centered counseling for intervention in smoking, nutrition, and high-risk alcohol users in the Worcester area. I'll use as a model the Worcester-Area Trial For Counseling in Hyperlipidemia (WATCH).[2]

This controlled trial of physician-delivered dietary intervention

From: Burke LE, Ockene IS (eds). *Compliance in Healthcare and Research*. Armonk, NY: Futura Publishing Company, Inc.; © 2001.

included some 1278 patients who were in the top quarter of the LDL distribution. They were all patients of 45 internists at the Fallon Clinic, an HMO in Worcester, Massachusetts. These internists were randomized into three different groups: a control group of 15 physicians who were not trained in patient-centered counseling, and two other groups all of whose physicians were trained in patient centered counseling. The training took place in a single three-hour session, followed by a single individual visit by a simulated patient to the doctor in his or her office, to assess the physician's skill level, to answer any remaining questions, and to go over the study protocol.

One of the two groups of trained physicians was also given a very modest office support system, which included the provision of prompts and counseling algorithms whenever they saw a study patient, and also a simple dietary analysis tool which was filled out by the patient in the waiting room and brought in to the visit.[3]

Most physicians are unaware of the natural pattern of cholesterol and the way in which it varies by age and sex. Starting at around age 20, cholesterol and LDL raise very rapidly in both sexes. Generally, men have higher cholesterol at younger ages, and women at older ages. For reasons that are not well understood, middle aged men go through some climactic change such that their cholesterol levels stop rising. Thus, older women have much higher cholesterol values than older men, the average woman's cholesterol level being around 230 at age 70. As a consequence, if you treat a single number, for example 240 mg/dL, you'll find yourself treating an inordinate number of older women. This may or may not be the right thing to do.

Our patients averaged 49 years of age with mean cholesterols of 248 mg/dL and a mean LDL of 168 mg/dL, triglycerides a little elevated and HDL averaged 55 mg/dL in the women and 45 mg/dL in the men. The percentage of calories as fat was only 31%. (In the first National Health and Nutritional Examination Survey (NHANES 1), the percent of calories as fat was 40%, in NHANES 2 it was 38%, and in NHANES 3 fat consumption was down to 34% of calories, so only 31% of calories from fat and saturated fat at 11% is reasonable.) Body mass index averaged 27, indicating a culturally robust population with 28% of subjects classified as obese.

We were interested in two things. First, are doctors trainable? Second, assuming that doctors would in fact benefit from training, would they do what we asked them to do? And would their patients' diet show reductions in fat and saturated fat intake, with subsequent lower cholesterol levels?

We in fact found that physicians are trainable.[4] We found that counseling skills measured pre- and post-nutrition intervention training showed considerable improvement. Thus the likelihood of a physician discussing with a patient possible methods to deal with expected problems during a behavioral change increased from 3% preintervention to 44% postintervention, with similar increases demonstrated for other aspects of behavioral counseling. There are equivalent data from our group's alcohol intervention study. So physicians can definitely be trained to improve their counseling skills. The more important question, however, is whether or not these skills will be used in the busy environment in which physicians practice. In order to answer this question we carried out patient exit interviews (PEIs) in a random quarter of the patients in the WATCH study. As the patients left the physician's office, they were met by a trained interviewer who went through the 10 steps of the counseling sequence. As taught to the physicians, this sequence was to take no more then 7–9 minutes. The interviewer asked if the doctor had discussed the patient's cholesterol level, had discussed diet as it relates to cholesterol, had discussed resources and barriers to change, evaluated past attempts at change, negotiated future behavioral strategies, gave written educational material, recommended referral to a nutritionist (optional), and scheduled a follow-up appointment. What we saw here was really quite fascinating and it has implications for continuing medical education and the way it should be done.[5] (See Table 1.)

What we see here is that Condition 2 physicians, the group that were trained but not supported, did no better than the control physicians. On the other hand, the condition 3 physicians, receiving office support in addition to being trained, did significantly better, and in a very busy HMO environment carried out a surprising proportion of the counseling steps.

Table 1

| Condition | n | PEI Score (mean ± std. error) (max = 10) | |
		Unadjusted	Adjusted*
I	92	3.65 (0.28)	4.09 (0.38)
III	115	3.44 (0.25)	4.05 (0.73)
III	118	6.50 (0.25)	6.28 (0.27)**

*R^2 = .45, indicating that this proportion of total variability is accounted for by study factors. Adjusted results control for site, MD, and whether or not the PEI was conducted in person or by telephone. The least-square mean for this column is the condition-specific mean adjusted for these other factors.

**F-value for the test that the condition effects are equal = 14.39 (P < .0001)

(with permission, from Ockene et al (5))

Even though the condition 3 physicians did well, there is still lots of room for improvement. For example, patients were asked if the doctor had discussed problems making dietary change. That occurred 13% of the time in the control group, an identical 13% of the time in condition 2, and 37% of the time in condition 3. Now that's 3 times as often; which is a substantial improvement, but even so this important query is still being posed to the patient only one-third of the time, which is not very good. The other point I want to make is that these condition 2 doctors had all the tools available to them that the condition 3 doctors had. They had all of the materials in their office. They had the algorithms and the diet assessment forms, but to use them the physicians had to work out the logistics themselves, setting up a system that works. (I can tell you as a practicing physician that if I have to walk across the hall to get something it is not going to happen unless something serious will happen to the patient if I don't do it.)

The training session was held only once, at the beginning of the study. But patients were recruited for over 2 years—did the training effect hold up? Figure 1 shows the persistence of the training effect.

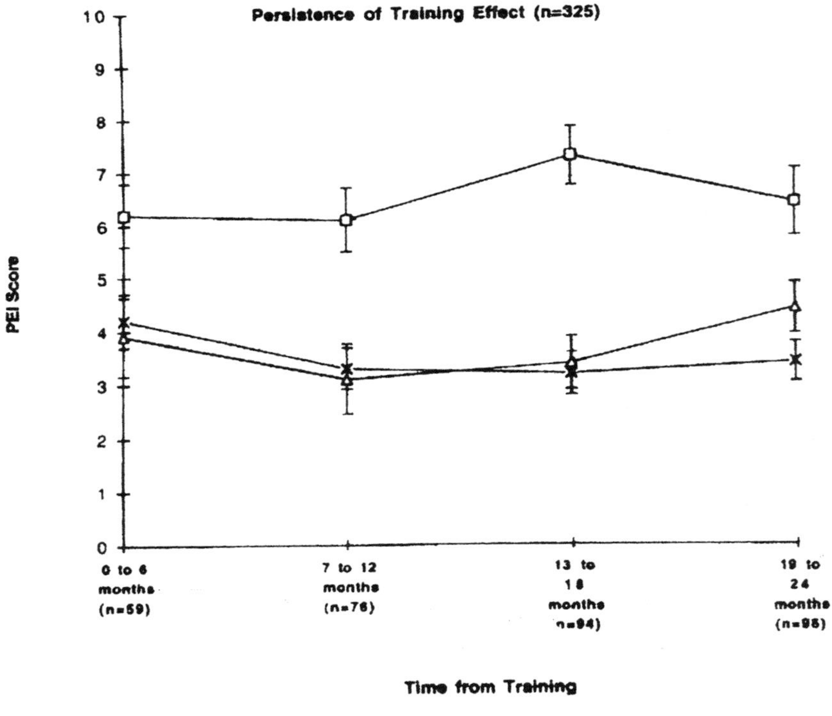

Figure 1. —△—, condition 1; —✖—, condition 2; —□—, condition 3.

During the entire 2-year period we continued to carry out the patient exit interviews, and as the figure shows, as long as we kept prompting the doctors, providing them with tools which reminded them what to do and made their job easier, they kept doing it. Dr. Judith Ockene saw the same effect in her Project Health Alcohol Intervention Study, and we conclude that this is a generalizable phenomenon.[6]

So we have come to several optimistic conclusions. First, these primary care internists want to do the right thing, and are interested in prevention, but they are very busy. Therefore we need to provide them not only with training but we must also make it exquisitely simple for the physicians to carry out the desired task. And second, we learned that as long as we keep providing them with the necessary tools, they will continue to deliver the intervention. On the less optimistic side, at best the desired intervention is well carried out only one-third of the time – a lot better than 10%–15% of the time, but hardly optimal.

It is important to remember that we are talking about 5 extra minutes of time. The control group physicians spent an average of 4 minutes discussing diet and suggesting changes, the condition 2 physicians spent 7 minutes and the condition 3 physicians spent 9 minutes. This is exactly in line with the training recommendations.

The physicians, even those in condition 3, did a poor job of follow-up. The number of repeat cholesterol measures and office visits was only minimally different from the control numbers, and far from optimal.

With regard to the risk factor outcomes, it is important to remember that this was a very modest intervention in a primary care population. What we see is that all of the significant changes were restricted to the condition 3 patients, which parallels the findings with regard to physician counseling behavior. The condition 2 patients, whose doctors were trained but not supported, demonstrated no significant changes as compared to the control group. In condition 3, however, a number of interesting changes were seen. The percent of calories from saturated fat fell by 1.1% as an absolute change. As these patients started at slightly under 11% of calories from saturated fat, there was a 10% reduction in saturated fat intake, a remarkable outcome for a 1 year follow-up given the trivial amount of time that was spent on the intervention. Even more interestingly, the patients in condition 3 lost on an average of 2.3 kilos—more or less 5 lbs.—in the course of a year, a striking outcome given that weight loss was not a specific goal of the intervention.

Most physicians are not aware of the manner in which small imbalances in caloric intake and expenditure result in weight change. How many calories do you have to eliminate each day to be five lbs. lighter at the end of a year? The average American gains 1 lb. a year between the ages of 20–45. How many calories do you have to add to gain a lb. a year? In fact there are approximately 3500 calories in a pound of fat. Thus taking in 10 calories a day more than is needed will result in a one pound weight gain over the course of a year. This is one-fifth of a small cookie per day. So, a loss of 5 pounds means a consistent negative balance of 50 calories per day, achieved by any combination of less caloric intake and higher caloric expenditure. The paradox of weight control is that the changes that people need to make are so trivial that everyone can surely do it, but of course in reality few people can sustain even these trivial changes over the long course. One of the mistakes we made in this study is that we weren't smart enough to have physical activity recommendations as part of the exit interview. Thus I don't know what the doctors said about physical activity but it is my belief that no doctor is capable of talking about diet without adding on "By the way you should try walking around the block."

The lipid changes were modest although they came very close to achieving statistical significance. There was a 3.8 mg/dL decrease in LDL-cholesterol ($P = 0.10$), a small decrease but important on a population basis, and especially when one considers the minimal effort involved. In fact, because more patients in the control group were placed on lipid-lowering medication than were patients in group 3, the overall cost of the intervention was only $1.86 per patient/yr, or 49 cents per 1 mg/dL LDL lowering per patient.

So providers can develop patient counseling skills, and the counseling effect has been seen in interventions for smoking, alcohol and nutrition. Furthermore, the importance of office support has also been shown in our group's alcohol intervention study.[6] These results highlight the difference between acuity and importance. Prevention is always of high importance, but low acuity. Appendicitis is high acuity – if you don't do something the patient will be dead the next day. That's never true of prevention. You don't have to do anything, and as a consequence it always falls to the bottom of your priority list during the visit. We need to develop systems that move prevention higher on that list, and make it happen. I'd like to make a few other points about the WATCH study. There was a very interesting interaction between the nutrition classes to which patients could be referred and the physician intervention itself, with those patients doing best who were in physician condition 3 *and* were in the nutritionist-led classes. However, very few patients were sent to the classes. In fact only 14% were referred and only 7% ever actually attended the classes. The other effect that was very interesting was that patients with lesser levels of education responded better than those with greater levels of education. Dr. Haynes mentioned that education is not a major factor in adherence. This may be true on an individual level, but I think that education is an extraordinary factor on the societal level. There is an obvious inverse relationship between smoking and education level, and this is also true of obesity. Why in our study the less educated persons did better is a matter of conjecture, but I personally believe that if I see a well-educated person who eats a very high-fat diet and smokes despite all he sees in the newspaper and the peer pressure to which he is subjected by his equally-educated friends, he will be a difficult patient in whom to induce change.

As a consequence of these findings and the realization that our efforts led to better but still far from adequate results we initiated WATCH 2. We are now in the first year of this study, in which all providers are in condition 3. They all are being trained and all will be given office support. Half of the patients are randomized to a nutrition-based intervention that involves a computerized tracking system that we've set up that interacts with the hospitals registration system and the medical center laboratory system and essentially watches what the physicians are doing with the hyperlipidemic patients in the study. If by the end of 3 months in the study a patient has not received a repeat lipid profile the system drops the doctor an email saying "Dear doctor, your patient was supposed to have had a lipid profile done by this time but has not – therefore we are going to do it – is that okay?" The doctor retains veto power, but if the test is not vetoed it will happen. If that lipid returns showing an LDL level that is not yet at goal the system refers the patient to a nutrition lipid intervention group with the same note to the doctor. In essence we've changed the paradigm from one where the physician has to do something active to make an intervention happen to one where the indicated test or referral happens automatically, but the physician retains veto power. When we set up the study people told us that physicians are very possessive of their professional rights and would not agree to this. In fact, the reaction was quite the contrary. It was too good. The uniform reaction of the primary care doctors was "Thank God, one less thing I have to think about!" And that's truly not what we wanted. But it's the way it is in modern primary care medicine. I might also mention that in the first study I don't remember ever having a complaint from or a problem with any physician. In this study it has taken five training sessions to get all the doctors trained, and there is a continuous sense that they are bombarded, that they are abused, and that life is much more difficult now then it was 7–8 years ago. This is a reality that we have to deal with.

One final point. You have to provide evidence to physicians in order to achieve change. But the evidence that we see in a large study is not apparent in a one-to-one physician-patient relationship. If you succeed in getting your average hyperlipidemic patient to lose 5 lbs, in the midst of all of your patients you probably won't be aware it has happened. If you get 15% of your patients in any given year to quit smoking, that is really quite good, but your perception will be that you are a dismal failure – 85% of the time you fail. It is very important to realize that this is the case. All of us need to have and to teach a public health orientation, so that we provide the feedback that says "hey, you're doing a great job" so that the physician in his or her office understand the importance of their preventive efforts and perceives the public health value.

References

1. Beckman HB, Frankel RM. The effect of physician behavior on the collection of data. *Ann Intern Med* 1984;101:692–696.
2. Ockene IS, Hebert JR, Ockene JK, et al. Effect of Physician-delivered Nutrition Counseling Training and an Office Support Program On Saturated Fat Intake, Weight, and Serum Lipid Measurements In a Hyperlipidemic Population: The Worcester-Area Trial For Counseling in Hyperlipidemia (WATCH). *Arch Intern Med* 1999;159:725–731.
3. Ammerman A, Haines P, DeVellis R, et al. A brief dietary assessment to guide cholesterol reduction in low-income individuals: Design and validation. *J Am Diet Assoc* 1991;91:1385–1390.
4. Ockene JK, Ockene IS, Quirk ME, et al. Physician training for patient-centered nutrition counseling in a lipid intervention trial. *Prev Med* 1995;24:563–570.
5. Ockene IS, Hebert JR, Ockene JK, et al. Effectiveness of Physician Training and a Structured Office Practice Setting on Physician-Delivered Nutrition Counseling: The Worcester-Area Trial For Counseling in Hyperlipidemia (WATCH). *Am J Prev Med* 1996;12:252–258.
6. Ockene JK, Adams A, Hurley TG, et al. Brief physician and nurse practitioner-delivered counseling for high risk drinkers: Does it work? *Arch Intern Med* 1999;159(18):2198–2205.

Chapter 5

Organizational Approaches to Improve Compliance

Thomas E. Kottke, MD, MSPH,
Leif I. Solberg, MD, and Milo L. Brekke, PhD

"Occupational organization . . . constitutes a dimension quite as distinct and fully as important as its knowledge."

Eliot Freidson, 1970[1]

Introduction

Eliot Freidson's 30-year-old observation that organization of a medical practice will determine which services are delivered is as true today as it was at the time Freidson wrote it. Translation of medical knowledge to improved patient health requires at least the willingness and ability of a health care professional to prescribe preventive services and advise lifestyle changes. Ira and Judith Ockene[2] for example, and the team of Robert DeBusk and Nancy Houston-Miller[3–5] have designed and tested innovative demonstration projects that prove that a systematic approach to preventive cardiology interventions can lower patient risk. However, few investigators have taken on the task of testing how programs such as these can be disseminated across the entire spectrum of medical practices.

In this chapter we focus on reviewing our own efforts to define the organizational factors that influence the delivery of preventive services, and we review our efforts to modify these factors to disseminate the delivery of preventive cardiology and other preventive services. We present both observational and trial data to support our conclusions

Supported in part by AHCPR Grant HS08091

From: Burke LE, Ockene IS (eds). *Compliance in Healthcare and Research.* Armonk, NY: Futura Publishing Company, Inc.; © 2001.

about whether and how the important factors can be changed. Finally, we speculate about what will be required if we are to create a health care environment where professionals can and will deliver preventive cardiology services at optimal rates.

Generating a List of Critical Factors that Promote and Impede the Delivery of Preventive Cardiology Services

When we assumed responsibility for the University of Minnesota Heart Attack Prevention Workshops in 1981, the post-workshop evaluations were enthusiastic, but the attendees found it nearly impossible to implement the innovations that we demonstrated at the workshop. Upon returning home they found themselves unable to convince their colleagues that their enthusiasm for disease prevention justified action. They also told us that "even when we agree where we want to be, we can't figure out how to get there from here." Clearly, more than the knowledge and skills that we taught were needed if we were going to implement preventive cardiology in clinical practice.

At the request of Henry Blackburn, we began to work on a paper that came to be titled, "The Systematic Practice of Preventive Cardiology."[6] Using a technique called comparative analysis, we investigated four services: two preventive cardiology services that were not widely adopted (nutritional advice and advice to quit smoking), a preventive cardiology service that had been adopted because of a concerted international effort (hypertension treatment and control), and a cardiology intervention that had rapidly spread despite little convincing evidence of efficacy, percutaneous coronary angioplasty. We identified, in addition to *knowledge of benefit* and *skills*, seven other factors that influenced the ability of a physician to deliver preventive services (Table 1).

As the result of more than a decade of subsequent experience with trials to implement preventive services in clinical practice, we would suggest that there are at least two additional factors that predict whether a physician will provide preventive cardiology services: whether the physician's practice has a method of undertaking and achieving planned organizational change, and whether there is leadership at all levels in the health care delivery system to guide and nourish the delivery of preventive cardiology services. (While we prefer to work from this list, many other lists or models have been proposed. We believe that it is preferable for the preventive cardiology implementer to generate their own list or model so that it can contributes to their ability to organize their experience and build from it.)

Table 1

Barriers to Physicians' Implementation of Preventive Services

---

Knowledge of benefit: The physician does not understand or accept how the patient's health will benefit from the preventive intervention.

Skills: The physician lacks the skills to deliver the intervention effectively.

Organization: There is no system to cue the physician to intervene or to follow patients who have received an intervention. Physicians lack guidelines for intervention.

Adequate return: The intervention loses money for the physician or requires financial subsidy.

Perceived patient demand: The physician does not believe that patients want the intervention.

Perceived effectiveness: The physician does not believe that intervention actually changes patient behavior or risk.

Perceived legitimacy: The physician does not believe that preventive intervention is part of a professional role.

Confidence: The physician lacks confidence to deliver the preventive intervention.

Commitment: The physician lacks commitment to deliver the intervention and to practice preventively.

From: Kottke TE, Blackburn H, Brekke ML, Solberg LI. The systematic practice of preventive cardiology. Am J Cardiol 1987;59:690–694, with permission.

Addressing the Physician Recruitment Problem

Early in our dissemination trials we recognized that we were faced with a separate but related problem: attracting the physician's attention to preventive cardiology. Even if you knew what to teach, how could you teach it if the physician wouldn't sit down and listen to you?

When we mailed our Heart Attack Prevention Workshop brochure to physicians only about 5% on the list would register. To fill our workshop, we simply mailed to a very large number of physicians. When we first implemented the Doctors Helping Smokers trial[7] by recruiting and randomizing individual physicians, our experience with the Heart Attack Prevention Workshops was repeated; we were only able to recruit 5% of physicians in the target group.[8] We recognized that this was a significant problem because preventive cardiology services cannot be delivered to a population if only 5% of the doctors are active.

As a result of demonstration projects that we were conducting in our own practices at this time, we were becoming increasingly aware of the importance and benefit of involving all of the practice personnel in the innovation process.[9] We came to recognize that a large proportion of doctors would provide preventive cardiology services if it were convenient to do so even if they wouldn't attend a preventive cardiology workshop. Based on this observation, we reorganized Doctors Helping Smokers to recruit clinics rather than individual doctors and were able to gain involvement of over 55% of the physicians.[8] We were also able to significantly increase the proportion of patients who reported that they had received support with their smoking cessation efforts.[10]

Distinguishing Between the Efficacy Testing Paradigm and the Action Research Paradigm

At the time that we wrote the Doctors Helping Smokers trial it was generally expected that all projects would define a hypothesis and a methods to test it that would remain unchanged throughout the entire period of the trial. However, our experience was beginning to teach us that the clinical trial paradigm to test the efficacy of interventions is not directly applicable to solve problems of organizational development.[11] Both the process of conducting the Doctors Helping Smokers trial itself and the process of helping the participating clinics emphasized to us that we needed to develop a data-driven iterative process by which learning could be incorporated into the decision process and actions adjusted in response to new knowledge. In other words, we needed a research methodology that would allow us to do many small studies within the context of a larger trial. The participating clinics also needed a similar tool to assist them in their organizational changes to incorporate preventive services into clinical practice.

We had reviewed many models of organizational readiness for change, but most of these were checklists that defined whether or not an organization was likely to be able to accomplish change at a particular point in time. They did not address the issue of what one should do to help an organization become more capable at instituting planned change. We were looking for a dynamic strategy and concluded that we needed an iterative data-driven process. We discovered that we were looking for the research and intervention methodology that Lewin had developed and called "action research" more than 40 years earlier.[12] The philosophical underpinnings of this methodology have been explored more recently by Argyris, Putnam, and Smith.[13]

Fortuitously, the concepts of Continuous Quality Improvement (CQI) and Total Quality Management (TQM) were also rediscovered by American business at about this time. While the overly exuberant enthusiasm for these techniques has tempered as the users have learned the limitations of these techniques, the acceptance of CQI and TQM as valid organizational development tools meant that we no longer had to simultaneously promote the concept that preventive services delivery required a multicomponent intervention while promoting the concept that any trial of organizational development for preventive services delivery needed the ability to be modified in response to new information even while the trial was underway.

A Randomized Trial to Implement Preventive Services Systems: The IMPROVE Project

We began to conceptualize the IMPROVE project in 1990 and the Agency for Health Care Policy and Research funded it as an investigator-initiated trial (RO1HS08091) in 1993. The primary hypothesis of this randomized controlled trial was that managed-care organizations can improve the delivery rates of preventive services by teaching clinics to apply continuous quality improvement to the task of developing preventive services delivery systems.[14] To test this hypothesis, we randomized 22 matched pairs of clinics in the Twin Cities area of Minnesota to intervention and control arms of the study. We followed the delivery rates of eight services as indicators of trial success: screening for hypertension, hypercholesterolemia and tobacco use; screening for breast cancer with clinical breast examination; screening for breast cancer with mammography; screening for cervical cancer; immunization against influenza, and immunization against pneumococcus. The 22 clinics in the intervention group were offered training in the use of continuous quality improvement and were encouraged to develop preventive services systems that included the 10 components listed in Table 2.[14,15]

All 44 clinics that entered the trial completed it, and while the trial did not result in increased service rates (unpublished data), it did provide us with a great deal of information about medical practice organization as it applies to the delivery of preventive services. We learned that, with the exception of pneumococcus immunization, about two-thirds of patients were already up-to-date on preventive services at the time of their visit to their doctor.[16] Although lower SES patients were as likely to receive a preventive service recommendation as any other patient,[17] only about one-third of the patients who were not up-to-date on a service were offered the service during the visit.[16]

While the clinicians endorsed the value of preventive services and endorsed general statements about the need to improve the way in which preventive services were delivered, a majority did not see a need to improve specific services. There was little association between attitudes about the value of preventive services and the rates at which they were being delivered,[18] and there were no "star practices" that

Table 2

Suggested Components of a Preventive Services Delivery System

Essential

Guidelines. A clinic-wide written policy that has been specifically accepted by all clinicians as a common approach to preventive services.

Screening. A routine way to identify the preventive services needs of patients as they are seen in the clinic.

Status summary. A medical flow sheet summarizing the date of all preventive services or data on risk factor changes.

Follow-up. A routine timely way to inform patients of test results, to reinforce behavior changes, and to reinvolve patients who don't return.

Important

Reminders. A routine way to remind clinic staff or clinicians that a particular patient may be in need of something for a preventive service.

Resources. Educational or referral information for patient or health care personnel that is organized to be readily available when needed.

Counseling. A nonphysician who can provide patients with information and problem-solving assistance beyond brief advice.

Useful

Outreach. An organized way to offer preventive services to nonpatients or to involve a patient's family members in the patient's care

Prevention visit. An office visit designed primarily to identify and address prevention issues, either alone or as part of a "checkup."

Patient activation. An activity that informs patients of the clinic's prevention guidelines while encouraging them to actively stay up-to-date.

From: Solberg LI, Kottke TE, Brekke ML, Calomeni CA, Conn SA, Davidson G. Using continuous quality improvement to increase preventive services in clinical practice-going beyond guidelines. Prev Med 1996;25(3):259–267, with permission.

were outstanding for all eight services. None of the practices had service delivery systems that could be described as anywhere near complete[19], and a practice that was in the top quartile for the delivery of one service was no more likely than chance alone to be in the top quartile for the delivery of another service (unpublished data). While enthusiastic about participating in the trial, the participating clinicians tended to have limited experience in the use of continuous quality improvement.[20]

We found an association between the delivery of a preventive service and patient satisfaction with that particular service, but this association appeared to be too weak to trigger clinician action.[21] About one-third of the patients agreed with the statement, "I wish my clinic would do more about making sure I stay healthy" but one-third were indifferent, and one-third disagreed.

The participating clinicians liked working with the IMPROVE project staff, and the managed care organizations that sponsored the project were also viewed in a positive light. (unpublished data). Clinics in the intervention group took significant steps to organize preventive services delivery systems, but these systems were incomplete[22], and many of the intervention group clinics had not implemented their preventive services systems by the time of the postintervention assessment.

As a group, the participating clinics experienced a high level of turmoil during the project due to mergers, buy-outs, and clinic reorganizations.[23,24] Anecdotal reports suggest that this turmoil distracted the participating clinicians from the task of developing preventive services delivery systems.

Conclusions

Although our understanding of preventive services delivery has improved markedly since Freidson recorded his observation, our profession still does not understand occupational organization to the extent that preventive services delivery programs of documented efficacy can be disseminated at will. We would encourage the reader not to be discouraged by this fact, however. A group of 12 veteran guideline implementers from the Twin Cities that we are in the process of systematically debriefing are all optimistic about their understanding of the organizational systems that will be required to disseminate preventive services systems. They have developed a list of more than 87 variables in 5 categories that they believe influence their ability to implement a guideline, and have identified 25 strategies that they use to actually implement guidelines; while their understanding is incomplete, each one of them appears to believe that they can and will accomplish their mission. Although their task is complex, they appear to prefer being faced with a complex task that can eventually be solved through a process of careful trial, error, observation, and retrial than to be faced with a simple enigma that is destined to remain unsolved forever.

Distilling 20 years of program dissemination research into a few bullet points, we would emphasize the following:

About Clinicians And Preventive Services

- Although very few clinicians will travel to attend a preventive cardiology workshop, the majority of clinicians will participate if there is a clinic-wide system to deliver the services.

- Evidence-based guidelines are acceptable to clinicians and help them agree upon which services to deliver.
- Clinicians already believe that preventive cardiology services have value. Therefore, cajoling them about the importance of preventive services cannot be expected to significantly change behavior.
- Clinicians do not sense missed opportunities to provide preventive services. If a cueing system were in place to help them sense these occasions, they would probably deliver more services.
- Clinicians find that continuous quality improvement is a useful organizational problem-solving tool. In fact, after learning the technique to develop preventive cardiology service delivery systems, they also will use it to address a diverse array of other problems that they face in their practices.

About Disseminating Preventive Cardiology Services

- We are unaware of any model that perfectly explains organizational behavior. Therefore we believe that every individual who is working to disseminate preventive cardiology services needs to adopt a strategy that will help them learn from their experience. We suggest that the best strategy is one that allows the individual to continually embellish a personally meaningful model by both borrowing from the experience of others and incorporating one's own experience.
- While the paradigm for efficacy testing trials and the action science paradigm share many similarities, they also have critical differences. The task of disseminating preventive cardiology services will not be successful if a strict efficacy testing paradigm is used as the model for intervention.
- The *need* for preventive services delivery systems in medical practices is universal. The *form* that the system must take in any particular medical group will be defined by the physical and social environment of the group.
- Although there tends to be a positive association between preventive services and patient satisfaction, other factors, particularly timeliness of appointment availability, are far stronger determinants of patient satisfaction. Because acute care and preventive cardiology services compete for the same appointment slots, emphasizing patient satisfaction in

general cannot be expected to increase the rates at which preventive services are delivered.

- Cooperation among health plans is probably a critical requirement for preventive services delivery. If competing plans promulgate different service requirements, it is most likely that clinicians will respond to none of them.
- The agenda for preventive cardiology services needs to be promoted at every level. This includes the level of the patient, the clinician, the health plan, and the corporate or government purchaser of health services.
- Experienced guideline implementers in the Twin Cities of Minnesota are very optimistic about their ability to modify medical practice to improve patient care.
- The compliance burden falls on no one in particular and everyone in general. If every party does their part, the burden of delivering preventive cardiology services need not be onerous for anyone. If even one party fails to do their part, services are likely not to be delivered.

References

1. Freidson E. Profession of Medicine. A Study of the Sociology of Applied Knowledge. New York: Dodd, Mead & Company, 1970; xi.
2. Ockene IS, Hebert JR, Ockene JK, et al. Effect of physician-delivered nutrition counseling training and an office-support program on saturated fat intake, weight, and serum lipid measurements in a hyperlipidemic population: Worcester Area Trial for Counseling in Hyperlipidemia (WATCH). *Arch Intern Med* 1999;159:725–731.
3. DeBusk RF, Miller NH, Superko HR, et al. A case-management system for coronary risk factor modification after acute myocardial infarction. *Ann Intern Med* 1994;120:721–729.
4. DeBusk RF. MULTIFIT: A new approach to risk factor modification. *Cardiol Clin* 1996;14:143–157.
5. Houston-Miller N, Smith PM, DeBusk RF, et al. Smoking cessation in hospitalized patients. Results of a randomized trial. *Arch Intern Med* 1997;157: 409–415.
6. Kottke TE, Blackburn H, Brekke ML, et al. The systematic practice of preventive cardiology. *Am J Cardiol* 1987;59:690–694.
7. Kottke TE, Brekke ML, Solberg LI, et al. A randomized trial to increase smoking intervention by physicians: Doctors Helping Smokers, Round 1. *JAMA* 1989;261:2101–2106.
8. Kottke TE, Solberg LI, Conn S, et al. A comparison of two methods to recruit physicians to deliver smoking cessation interventions. *Arch Intern Med* 1990;150:1477–1481.
9. Solberg LI, Maxwell PL, Kottke TE, et al. A systematic primary care office-based smoking cessation program. *J Fam Pract* 1990;30:647–654.
10. Kottke TE, Solberg LI, Brekke ML, et al. A controlled trial to integrate

smoking cessation advice into primary care practice: Doctors helping smokers, Round III. *J Fam Pract* 1992;34:701–708.

11. Kottke TE, Solberg LI, Brekke ML. Beyond efficacy testing: Introducing preventive cardiology into primary care. In Stone EJ, Van Citters RL, Pearson TA (eds): Preventive Cardiology: Perspectives in Physician Education. *Am J Prev Med* 1990;6:77–83.

12. Lewin, K. Action research and minority problems. *J Soc Issues* 1946;2:34–46.

13. Argyris C, Putnam R, Smith DM. Action Science. San Francisco: Jossey-Bass, 1985.

14. Solberg LI, Kottke TE, Brekke ML, et al. Using continuous quality improvement to increase preventive services in clinical practice—going beyond guidelines. *Prev Med* 1996;25:259–267.

15. Solberg LI, Kottke TE, Conn SA, et al. Delivering clinical preventive services is a systems problem. *Ann Behav Med* 1997;19:271–278.

16. Kottke TE, Solberg LI, Brekke ML, et al. Delivery rates for preventive services in 44 Mid-Western clinics. *Mayo Clin Proc* 1997;72:515–523.

17. Solberg LI, Kottke TE, Brekke ML. Are physicians less likely to recommend preventive services to low-SES patients? *Prev Med* 1997;26:350–357.

18. Solberg LI, Brekke ML, Kottke TE. How important are clinician and nurse attitudes to the delivery of clinical preventive services? *J Fam Pract* 1997; 44:451–461.

19. Solberg LI, Kottke TE, Brekke ML, et al. The case of the missing clinical preventive services systems. *Eff Clin Pract* 1998;1:33–38.

20. Solberg LI, Brekke ML, Kottke TE, et al. Continuous quality improvement in primary care: What's happening. *Med Care* 1998;36:625–635.

21. Kottke TE, Solberg LI, Brekke ML, et al. Will patient satisfaction set the preventive services implementation agenda? *Am J Prev Med* 1997;13: 309–316.

22. Solberg LI, Kottke TE, Brekke ML. Will primary care clinics organize themselves to improve the delivery of preventive services? A randomized controlled trial. *Prev Med* 1998;27:623–631.

23. Magnan S, Solberg LI, Giles K, et al. Primary care, process improvement, and turmoil. *J Amb Care Manage* 1997;20:32–38.

24. Magnan S, Solberg LI, Kottke TE, et al. IMPROVE: Bridge over troubled waters. *Jt Comm J Qual Improv* 1998;24:566–578.

Section IV

Measurement of Compliance

Chapter 6

Conceptual and Methodological Problems

Jacqueline Dunbar-Jacob, PhD, RN, FAAN and Susan Sereika, PhD

Introduction

The progress of science is dependent upon good observation and precise measurement.[1] This generalization applies fully to an understanding of patient adherence/compliance. Indeed, an understanding of patient compliance can be no better than the method of assessing it. The assessment of compliance, however, raises several conceptual and methodological issues. These issues include the variety of measurement strategies used, the variety in definitions of adherence, the correspondence between measures, the accuracy of measures, the acceptability of measures, and the nature of the data yielded. These issues affect the interpretation of studies of compliance as well as the structure of research or clinical assessment of compliance. Each of these issues are discussed below.

Definitions of Compliance

The first issue addresses the definition of compliance. Philosophically, compliance has many meanings for individuals. While the term compliance is most commonly used and produces the greatest yield in literature searches, *compliance* has often been conceptualized as obedience. That is, the physician prescribes and the patient obeys. This interpretation is similar to that used in the early psychology studies on compliance where obedience and compliance were used interchangea-

From: Burke LE, Ockene IS (eds). *Compliance in Healthcare and Research.* Armonk, NY: Futura Publishing Company, Inc.; © 2001.

bly.[2] In these cases, compliance or obedience "refers to situations in which we execute certain behaviors because we are asked to or pressured into making them, even though we may not want to."[3] To avoid an emphasis on obedience, an alternative term, *adherence*, has been suggested. The interpretation of the term adherence denotes the idea of sticking to it, as does the term *therapeutic alliance*, which places an emphasis on following a jointly (patient-provider) prescribed regimen. Other approaches may be more behavioral, noting the proportion of the regimen carried out regardless of the circumstance. The philosophical conceptualization of compliance is likely to influence the definition of compliance selected for any study.

The theoretical perspective of a study or compliance program will also influence the definition of compliance selected. There are few studies that specifically address compliance. Of those studies which define compliance, we find two general definitions. One specifies the *intention* to engage in a recommended behavior, while the other specifies the *performance* of the recommended behavior. Examples of theories in each category include the Health Belief Model, the Theory of Reasoned Action versus Self-Efficacy Theory, and the Common Sense Model of Illness.

While influenced by the philosophical and theoretical perspectives on compliance, the operational definitions are typically behavioral in nature. This behavioral definition often follows the work of Haynes, who defined compliance as "the extent to which a person's behavior coincides with medical or health advice."[4] Thus, behavioral definitions have evolved which examine the proportion of the regimen using counts, which has been carried out over a specified period of time. This has particularly been the case in studies of medication and exercise compliance. In the area of dietary compliance, time sampling strategies have been used to estimate compliance using diaries or frequencies which estimate current compliance based on food histories. In each of these cases, summary data are provided yielding information on the percent of the regimen carried out or the proportion of persons who exceed some preestablished criterion for good compliance.

The criteria typically set are based upon the work of Haynes, et al.[5] in the first randomized controlled intervention study which addressed compliance in uncontrolled hypertension. Haynes and colleagues set a level of 80% of medication taken for good compliance. In the absence of data on the extent of compliance necessary to achieve a desirable therapeutic outcome for most medications, this level of compliance has been widely, although not universally, adopted as a common standard. Common standards to define compliance have not been set for dietary or exercise compliance. The use of a common standard is helpful in comparing the proportion of good compliers across studies.

What is missing from this method of summary data is the pattern of compliance which leads to the overall percent of the regimen carried out. Indeed, multiple patterns can contribute to a similar compliance rate. An example based upon diary recordings in one of our studies can be seen in Figure 1.

The definitions of compliance behavior patterns also yield differing ways of conceptualizing and reporting compliance. Termination of the regimen is one behavior of significance. This may also be referred to as 'drop out' or 'regimen withdrawal.' As a portion of individuals stop treatment but resume at a later point, two other terms define this pattern – 'temporary drop out' (withdrawal) or 'regimen holiday'. Typically the holiday defines a shorter period off-treatment than temporary drop out; however, no commonly used definitions exist for either. Thus, the terms may have different meanings in different studies or programs.

Also of interest is the missed 'dose' or event. There are no standards for defining the missed dose. It may be captured by self-report, with attendant recall problems, or by a pill count which reports the total number of doses omitted over a period of time. However, efforts to compensate for missed doses by taking extra doses subsequently masks the problem of missed doses. With the use of event monitoring, missed doses can also be defined as the omission of dosing within therapeutically sound temporal or interdose intervals. Unfortunately there is insufficient data available to establish the boundaries for these intervals. As Urquart[6] noted, both the onset of action as well as the

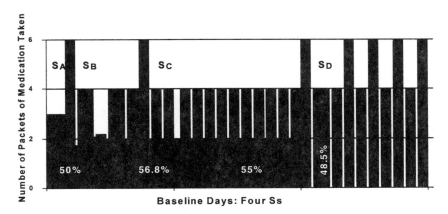

Figure 1. Variations in reported adherence patterns during daily recording: four Ss taking one-half prescribed dose of six packets per day.

duration of action is important in determining the relevant interval boundaries.

The converse to missed doses is the issue of extra doses or events. Do extra events constitute a compliance problem? For medication purposes, extra doses are more likely to produce a compliance problem. The question is open for exercise—how does one define and classify exercise beyond the prescription. The case is similar in the dietary arena. How then are extra events counted in the calculation of compliance? Extra events may erase missed events, may count as non-compliant events, or they may be ignored. How extra doses are addressed will impact the final summary of compliance. Unfortunately, the issue of extra events is rarely addressed in studies of compliance.

The patient or research subject generally does not present with only one pattern. More typically, multiple behaviors are found over time within the person. An example can be seen in the following individual from our research program who is on a once-a-day dose (see Figure 2). As can be seen, doses are missed, extra doses are taken, and holidays appear. Out of the 20 days covered in this graph, 14 doses have been taken, for a compliance rate of 70%. If one examines the number of days in which any number of doses were taken, the compliance rate is 55%. If one examines the number of days in which the correct dose was taken (one and only one), the compliance rate is 45%. Thus, how the pattern of compliance is addressed can significantly impact the estimation of compliance.

Indeed doses may be missed on a single occasion or for a period of time, extra doses may be taken, or doses may be spaced too close

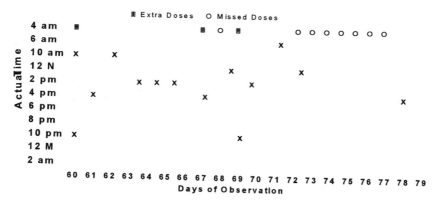

Figure 2. Once-a-day dosing prescription.

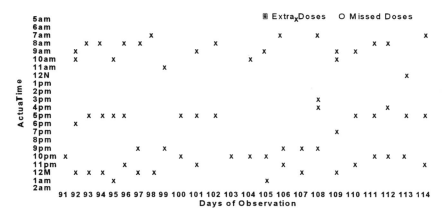

Figure 3. Three-times-a-day dosing prescription.

together or too far apart. This can be seen in Figure 3, where a subject within our research program is on a three-times-daily prescription. As can be seen, the patient may still take extra doses, eg, day 92, omit single doses (day 99), take two of three doses (day 104), take two doses too close together (day 105), or take an extra dose (day 109). As with the previous case, the treatment of these behaviors can yield differing compliance rates.

A further pattern of adherence, a temporal pattern, has also been identified.[7] This pattern has been called the 'white coat' pattern of compliance and assumes a scallop shape.[8] That is, individuals comply well just prior to and just following a clinical visit with a decline in compliance between visits. The time at which the individual is assessed will impact then their reported compliance, while summarizations over time will obscure this pattern. With each of these patterns of compliance, different rates of compliance can be obtained depending upon how these patterns are defined, if at all, and how they are treated in the summary data. The particular difficulty in group studies is that the differences in reported compliance rates may impact the interpretation of the outcome.

Measurement Strategies

The issue of assessment is further complicated by the variation in strategies of measurement. As we examine the literature on adherence over the past 25 years, we find that multiple methods of assessment have been used and the studies compared without regard for the method. Yet these measures address diverse aspects of managing a regimen. The five general categories of measurements incorporate a variety of strategies. These measurements include self-report strategies, behavioral counts, electronic monitors, biological indicators, and direct observation.

Perhaps the most common measurement strategy is the self-report of compliance. Within this category are interviews, both time structured and global, questionnaires, and diaries. More recent techniques include the use of the Internet or the telephone to record self-reported behavior. These methods assess the patient's recall of, and willingness to report, their regimen behaviors. Our own data suggested that in a 7-day recall of medication taking, subjects were able to recall backwards 1 to 3 days. Beyond 1 to 3 days, specific details could not be recalled. Typically, the self-report methods are thought to provide a systematic bias toward the over-reporting of good adherence. With the exception of the daily diary, self-reporting does not provide data on the patterns of compliance and to some extent relies on the patient's definition of compliance.

Behavioral counts form a second category of assessment methodology. Behavioral counts include such strategies as pill counts, calorie counts, and/or exercise frequency. These strategies are related to self-report measures and indeed may overlap with them. For example, the pill count is dependent upon the patient bringing pills back to the clinician and not removing pills to ensure a positive assessment. The use of calorie or other nutrient counts is dependent upon the willingness to record eating behaviors. The recall of eating behaviors must be recorded in a timely fashion, and must involve the ability to assess the composition of foods. Therefore, such behaviors may be subject to recall, a willingness to disclose information, and/or to accuracy in assessing one's own behavior. Again, with the exception of the use of the diary, behavioral counts do not provide information on the patterns of compliance.

Related to the behavioral counts is the use of electronic monitors. This third category of assessment is used to monitor medication adherence, exercise adherence, and blood sugar monitoring. Daily diaries with timed prompts and electronically recorded reports are also used. These strategies yield event data over time and are not dependent upon recall or willingness to report. Efforts to trick the system and over-report adherence are often detectable as entries are timed. Consequently, missed events will be noted, as will extra entries within a brief period of time.

Biological indicators of compliance are also used. This fourth category of assessment typically reports on the detection of the treatment, its metabolite, or the outcome of a treatment regimen. Little attention is typically given to the individual physiological variations in the metabolism of treatment or the clinical effect of the regimen. Further, there are essentially no data provided on the proportion of the regimen complied with, nor on any daily variations in compliance. Assessment generally is made of a brief and relatively recent time period related to the duration of action of the treatment.

The last category of compliance assessment methods is that of direct observation. This is a less frequently used strategy outside of the monitoring of appointment keeping. It has been used, though, in Directly Observed Therapy (DOT) in the management of tuberculosis and in the assessment of supervised exercise compliance. The advantage of this strategy is that is permits a direct assessment of whether the regimen was carried out on an event-by-event basis. It is however costly, unless the regimen is designed to be supervised, as in the case of some exercise programs.

Each of these measurement strategies assess different aspects of regimen behavior. How compliance is assessed has the potential to affect the reported compliance rates and may affect, therefore, the reported outcomes of interventions as well as predictor studies. The key issue is how comparable these measures are in their estimates of compliance.

Correspondence Between and Accuracy of Compliance Measures

The variations in measures and definitions are important only if they are poorly related to each other. Our own research suggests that the correlation between measures is poor. For example, we carried out an examination of compliance on a once a day medication for lipid lowering or placebo, using three measures of compliance, electronic event monitor, pill count, and 7-day recall.[9] The differences in reported compliance were significantly different ($x^2 = 29.27$, $P \leq 0.00005$) even with the measures made in the same population, on the same regimen, over the same period of time. Recall reported the highest compliance and electronic monitor the lowest. The question then is, which measure is more accurate. In this study the *only* measure that was associated with clinical outcome (cholesterol lowering) was the electronic event monitor. The association was $r_s = 0.26$, $P \leq 0.043$. An examination of the compliance the week before the determination of the cholesterol value showed an even higher association, ($r_s = 0.34$, $P \leq 0.009$). Thus, at least in this study, it appears that the electronic monitor provided a more accurate assessment of compliance than either self-report or pill count.

The poor correspondence between measures was further supported in our examination of compliance among patients being treated for rheumatoid arthritis.[10] In this case self-report and electronically monitored adherence approached zero associations (r_s = -0.07 to $+0.04$).[10] Daily diary data were also compared with the electronic monitor. In this case the kappa coefficient was 0.241, a relatively poor association. Furthermore, each measure had its own set of associated predictor variables.[11] Gender, employment status, income, support, and symptom severity were associated with monitored adherence. Age and cost of medications were associated with interview elicited compliance. Thus, there is at least some beginning data to indicate that the different measures may lead to different findings with regard to factors associated with compliance.

Overall, these data suggest that different measures of compliance may not be comparable and further may have different relationships to clinical outcomes and to predictor variables. This raises the question of whether we can compare findings across studies when different measures of compliance are used. The data also suggest that further examination of compliance measures and clinical outcomes may be useful in identifying meaningful measures.

Acceptability of Measures

The poor correspondence between measures may be due to real differences in what is being assessed by each measure. But differences may also be due to the different subsets of a population who respond to the various measures. For example, in a study of a group of patients with rheumatoid arthritis we assessed adherence, as noted previously, with a daily diary, a telephone interview and an electronic monitor. Of the sample, 89% completed the telephone interview addressing a one-month period of time, 75.6% completed daily diaries for an average of 263 days, and 75% used and returned an electronic event monitor for an average of 257 days. Differences in the composition of each sample may lead to differences in reported rates of compliance.

The extent of completion by participating subjects can potentially further impact the reported compliance. In the above mentioned study 24% refused and did not keep the diary at all, 59% kept it for at least 6 months, and 42% kept it for the full 12 months of the study. Interestingly, differences were not found between the sociodemographic characteristics of the users and refusers, nor were any differences found between these groups in compliance assessed by the electronic monitor. With the electronic event monitor 23% failed to return the monitor for a variety of reasons, so no data were available for them. Another 12.6%

used the monitor for just one month before abandoning it; the remaining 64.4% continued to use the monitor and to return it. Thus, while superficially it appears that the monitor and the daily diary had similar numbers use them (75%) for a similar period of time (257 vs. 263 days), more data were actually available from the monitor than from the diary over the 12 months of the study. In addition to any differences due to the measures themselves, the different contributions to the overall summary data on compliance could have led to the differences in the reported compliance.

Cost and Ease of Administration

Each of the issues previously raised regarding the measurement of compliance address the ability to accurately and reliably capture and interpret data. A further pragmatic issue remains, that of the cost and ease of administration. The acceptability data, which were presented here, suggests that the most complete data can be captured through self-report methods and that this is also a relatively inexpensive measure. The problem with this strategy is that it does not appear to have the accuracy that can be found with other methods. Methods of capturing accurate self-report data rely heavily on the ability of persons to recall routine events in their lives over a significant period of time or to be willing to provide ongoing and accurate data on paper and pencil event measures. These methods cannot be done unobtrusively. Less obtrusive are the biological methods and the pill count strategies. These strategies offer limited information and, at least with the biological methods, tend to be time restricted. Pill counts require access to the dispensing information over time and thus have limited application. The costs of biological methods need to be compared with the quality of the information offered. The electronic event monitors are likely the most accurate with the greatest detail in the information offered,[12] but costs per unit of assessment remain high. Thus, the choice of assessment method remains a decision between cost, ease of administering, and in terms of detail and accuracy, the information requirements.

The Nature Of Compliance Data

In addition to the variability in reported compliance that arises from the definitions chosen and the measurement method used, including the level of detail provided by each measure, differences can be attributable to the summary statistics used in analyzing the data. While this will be treated more thoroughly in the chapter on analysis in this monograph (see Chapter 9), it is useful here to point out the underlying nature of group compliance data. A review of studies which published the distribution of compliance data within their populations indicates that in general, compliance assumes a J-shaped distribution.[13] This distribution is resistant to efforts to normalize it. An example of this distribution can be found in Figure 4.

These data were drawn from our studies of persons with rheumatoid arthritis. The data were collected via electronic monitor and were defined as the proportion of prescribed pills that were taken, referred to here as comparable to a pill count method. As can be seen the majority of the patients adhered above the 90% level with the remaining distributed along the remaining percentage levels. This distribution is found for each of the measures of compliance, although the median may be higher or lower and the lowest compliance point may vary.[13]

Interestingly, this distribution appears to persist over time. In an examination of the packet count compliance data within the Lipid Research Clinics Coronary Primary Prevention Trial, the J-shaped distribution was consistent over the seven years of participant follow-up. These data can be seen in Figure 5, which presents the distribution for years 1, 4, and 7.[13]

Given the robustness of the distribution across measures and over time, and its resistance to transformation, the traditional parametric analyses and presentation of means and standardizations are not useful. More helpful is the presentation of medians and ranges and the use of nonparametric analyses. Therefore, one needs to examine, in studies of adherence, the nature of the summary and analytic statistics that are used. Different compliance rates for a group may be put forward when the mean versus the median is presented.

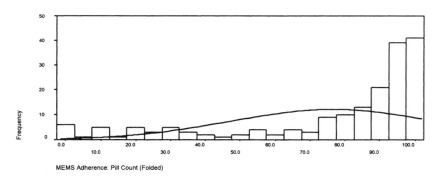

MEMS Adherence: Pill Count (Folded)

Figure 4. Electronically monitored adherence (pill count).

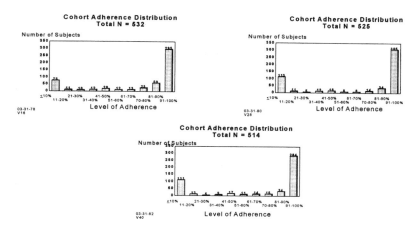

Figure 5. Distribution of levels of adherence over time: LRC-CPPT cohort.

Summary

Overall, a number of issues are pertinent to an examination of the measurement of compliance. Of particular note are the multiple factors that can lead to differences in reported rates of compliance. These include the definitions chosen, the attention to patterns of compliance over time, the choice of measurement method, and the analytic strategy for summarizing the data. Unfortunately, the measures do not appear to have a high degree of correspondence. Given this finding, it is not surprising that there are some data suggesting that the measures may yield different predictors and further may be differentially associated with clinical outcomes. The choice of measures will be influenced by costs and ease of administration, but there is an indication that the quality of the measures themselves ought to be considered. Given the variations in measures, definitions, and summary strategies in investigations of compliance, this chapter suggests that measurements need to be accounted for in the interpretation and comparison of compliance studies.

References

1. Derry G (ed): What Science Is and How It Works. Princeton, NJ: Princeton University Press. 1999;64.
2. Milgram S. Behavioral study of obedience. *J Abnorm Soc Psychol* 1963;67: 371–378.

3. Houston JP (ed): Motivation. New York: Macmillan Publishing Company; 1985:293.
4. Haynes RB. Introduction. In Haynes RB, Taylor DW, Sackett DL (eds): Compliance in Health Care. Baltimore: The Johns Hopkins University Press, 1979:1.
5. Haynes RB, Sackett DL, Gibson ES, et al. Improvement of medication compliance in uncontrolled hypertension. *Lancet* 1976;1:1265–1268.
6. Urquart J. Personal communication. 1999.
7. Cramer JA, Scheyer RD, Mattson RH. Compliance declines between clinic visits. *Arch Int Med* 1990;150:1509–1510.
8. Feinstein AR. On white-coat effects and electronic monitoring of compliance. *Arch Int Med* 1990; 150:1377–1378.
9. Dunbar-Jacob J, Burke LE, Rohay JM, et al. Comparability of self-report, pill count, and electronically monitored adherence data. *Controlled Clinical Trials*, 1996;7(2 Suppl):S80.
10. Dunbar-Jacob J, Sereika S, Burke LE, et al. Do patients do what they say they do: Adherence in patients with rheumatoid arthritis. Presented at Friends of the National Center for Nursing Research Day, Washington, DC. 1994.
11. Dunbar-Jacob J, Sereika S, Rohay JM, et al. Predictors of adherence: Differences by measurement method. *Ann Behav Med* 1995;17(Suppl), S. p. 196.
12. Dunbar-Jacob J, Sereika S, Rohay JM, et al. Electronic methods of assessing adherence to medical regimens. In Krantz D, Baum A (eds): Technology and Methods in Behavioral Medicine. Mahwah, NJ: Lawrence Erlbaum Associates; 1995:95–113.
13. Dunbar-Jacob J, Sereika S, Rohay JM, et al. J-shaped curve of the compliance distribution: Revisited. *Controlled Clinical Trials* 1994;15(Suppl. 3):120.

Chapter 7

Biological Measures

John Urquhart, MD, FRCP(Edin)

Introduction

As this chapter will show, the promise of making reliable estimates of past drug exposure in ambulatory patients, based on observations of the patient—physical examination or chemical analysis of blood, other biological fluids, or tissues—is beset by obstacles that preclude general utility, with the possibility of exceptions in the case of a few drugs that have unusual characteristics. It is instructive to understand why the role of biological markers is so limited.

Definitions

To begin, clarity demands a definition of "patient compliance with prescribed drug regimens." To that end, it is useful to consider the key steps in ambulatory pharmacotherapy, which, like most things, has a beginning, a middle, and an end. The beginning occurs with the patient's acceptance, or not, of the principle and the regimen of treatment. The middle involves the execution of the regimen. The end comes when prescriber, some other caregiver, or the patient, opts to discontinue the treatment. The beginning and end are inherently dichotomous, although they may involve some hesitation, manifest by irregular dosing during a relatively brief period. The middle is an ongoing process, with a wide spectrum of possible deviations from the prescribed regimen, which of course specifies both a quantity of drugs to be taken and a frequency of dosing or an interval between doses, depending on how the prescription is written. Some prescriptions may be even more specific, in designating a specific relation to meals, administration of other

From: Burke LE, Ockene IS (eds). *Compliance in Healthcare and Research*. Armonk, NY: Futura Publishing Company, Inc.; © 2001.

drugs, or clock times for dosing. Whatever the degree of specificity of timing instructions, however, a prescribed regimen of drug administration defines a time series of dosing events. The patient's actual dosing history constitutes another time series of events, and it is the comparison of those two time series that allows one to quantify "patient compliance with the prescribed drug regimen."[1]

Formally, one can say that patient compliance is the extent to which the patient's actual dosing history corresponds to the prescribed drug regimen.[1] In this sense, "patient compliance with the prescribed drug regimen" can be viewed as a quality parameter in ambulatory care, on the assumption that the pharmaceutical in question has been rationally prescribed, and that the recommended regimen is optimal, or nearly so, for the patient. Naturally, these assumptions are not always valid. Indeed, one scientific dividend of research on patient compliance is recognition of the importance of the question "how much compliance is enough?"[2] Implicit in the question is the recognition that pharmaceuticals differ considerably in the margin for errors in drug regimen execution that they permit without subsequent loss of therapeutic activity, or even triggering of a hazardous reaction to a drug holiday.[1-3] By the same token, the question challenges the presumption of optimality of recommended drug regimens.

There has been a great deal of controversy about terminology in research in the field we are considering. Given the ongoing controversy about "compliance" versus "adherence" versus "concordance", it is useful to take a step backwards and recognize that the primary data one needs to gather concerns dosing histories of ambulatory patients, and translation of those data into a record of the patient's exposure to drug. The difference between a 'dosing history' and 'exposure to drug' has to do with the occurrence of drug-drug and drug-food interactions that may modify drug absorption enough to change dose-effect relations. A useful terminologic compromise is to use the term 'adherence' as a blanket term for all three phases of ambulatory pharmacotherapy, recognizing that ambulatory pharmacotherapy can be undermined by nonacceptance, by poor execution, and/or by early termination. 'Compliance' refers, in this definitional scheme, specifically to the execution of the accepted, prescribed drug regimen, and the extent to which the patient's actual dosing history corresponds to the prescribed drug regimen. Naturally, this definition was not operational until it became technically possible to compile dosing histories of ambulatory patients in a reliable manner. That advance was made possible by electronic monitoring methods, which are discussed in Chapter 8.[4] My task in this chapter is to consider what may be gleaned from biological measurements linked to variable exposure to prescription drugs.

Asking the Patient

Some may think that self-reports are beyond the scope of 'biological markers,' but the repetitive act of self-administration of prescription drugs leaves a memory trace, which is a biological phenomenon. Certainly, asking the patient has a basic simplicity, although the patient can easily exaggerate, censor evidence for poor compliance, or otherwise obscure the actual dosing history. There is no better account of both the utility and limits of what can be learned by asking the patient than in the first-ever clinical study that sought to use variable patient compliance as an explanatory variable in trials analysis, by Wood, Simpson, Feinstein, and others in the late 1950s.[5] Unfortunately, this publication is too early for inclusion in computerized literature searches, so it has been overlooked by many. I reviewed this work a few years ago; the reader may turn to that review for many of the key details, or, better, to the original reports discussed therein.[6]

The problem that Wood, et al. studied was how best to use prophylactic antimicrobial agents to prevent streptococcal infections and their triggering of recurrent, acute rheumatic fever. They compared three regimens to which patients were randomly assigned: a monthly injection, professionally administered, of depot penicillin; a once-daily oral administration of penicillin; a once-daily oral administration of sulfadiazine. The study lasted 5 years and involved approximately 140 patients in each of the three groups. They recognized that compliance (which they termed 'fidelity', a term that did not last) with the self-administered oral regimens would be a key issue. They considered but rejected reliance on returned tablet counts, on the grounds that patients could easily create a false record of good compliance by simply discarding or hoarding untaken doses before returning the drug container to the investigative staff at each of the monthly follow-up visits. In this judgment, they were far ahead of their time, for many clinical researchers still persevere in the use of this method, which has since been thoroughly discredited.[7,8]

So, Wood, et al. opted to ask the patients at each visit, searching always for inconsistencies with earlier reports. Every half-year, a review was made of the past 6 months' dosing, also searching for inconsistencies. At the end of the study, the researchers were able to classify patients with three groups: "good," "poor," and "uncertain." Half the patients were classified as "good, with a quarter of the patients in each the other two categories. For analysis, they combined the 2nd and 3rd categories into one. The results showed strikingly higher incidences of recurrent streptococcal infections among the "poor" than among the "good" compliers with each of the two oral regimens.

In the injection group, only 6% of the patients had some missed doses, and the streptococcal infection rate was very low—an important result because the randomization of treatment assignment assured that the injection group included its share of patients who brought with them whatever social, behavioral, and other nonspecific factors one might suppose would be involved in poor compliance with the oral regimens and/or poor response to antimicrobial therapy. Thus, the low incidence of recurrent infection in the injection group demonstrated that consistent exposure to penicillin was highly effective in preventing recurrent streptococcal infections and rheumatic fever, irrespective of social, behavioral, or other factors. That observation, in turn, supports the conclusion that inconsistent exposure to penicillin or sulfadiazine was the responsible factor for the high rates of streptococcal infection in the poor compliers with the two oral regimens. A further finding was that the incidence of streptococcal infections among the 'good' compliers with the oral regimens was appreciably higher than among recipients of the monthly depot injections, which, considered together with results of follow-up studies done by the same researchers,[6] support the conclusion that even nominally good compliers with the oral regimen may still have an occasional lapse in dosing, undetected by interview methods, that affords an opportunity for reinfection.

A striking finding, not highlighted by the authors, was that the patients who were poorly compliant with the oral sulfadiazine regimen had a very low rate of recurrent acute rheumatic fever, despite their high rate of streptococcal infections. In contrast, patients poorly compliant with the oral penicillin regimen had high rates of both streptococcal infection and acute rheumatic fever. This finding is probably the first demonstration of a "forgiving drug regimen," because something associated with the sulfadiazine treatment, even when poorly complied with, seems to have disrupted the usual link between streptococcal infection and acute rheumatic fever.

Two noteworthy aspects of this pioneering study are still applicable today. One is that the assessment of compliance by interview methods is limited to a two- or three-point scale, which of course cannot deal with some of the more subtle aspects of how isolated dosing lapses may undermine treatment effectiveness. The other aspect is that interviewing is not cheap. If one assumes, eg, that the interviewer spent 5 minutes at each monthly visit with each of the 280 patients assigned to the oral regimens, the total expenditure of time to collect data over the course of the 5-year study was on the order of $280 \times 5 \times 12 \times 5$ = ca. 84000 minutes, or ca. 1400 hours. Currently, \$60.00/hr might be a reasonable estimate for the fully burdened salary of a skilled interviewer, so the cost to collect such data today would be ca. \$84000, or \$300 per patient.

Physical Signs of Drug Action

One of the most strikingly clear-cut physical signs of drug action is the pupillary constriction that occurs with the administration of the antiglaucoma drug, pilocarpine. Yet despite its clear-cut nature, it well illustrates the obstacles that complicate interpretation of a biological marker of drug regimen compliance. The field of glaucoma is of particular interest because concerns about patient noncompliance with sight-preserving drug regimens already in the 1970s triggered the development of the first electronic monitors.

For over a century, until the mid-1970s, pilocarpine was the first-line agent in the management of elevated intra-ocular pressure, in order to prevent optic nerve damage and blindness due to glaucoma. The advent of the beta-receptor blocker, timolol maleate, displaced pilocarpine from first-line use, although the agent still enjoys some clinical use. The actions of pilocarpine, applied as a 1%–2% eyedrop, mimic those of the parasympathetic nervous system, so the agent is sometimes referred to as a parasympathomimetic. Its three most prominent actions are: (a) reduction in intra-ocular pressure, lasting 6–8 hours; (b) maximal constriction of the pupil (also called miosis) lasting 1–2 hours; (c) induction of focal changes in the lens that induce myopia – an effect which lasts several hours, but is absent in older patients who become unresponsive as they develop presbyopia, which dictates their need for bifocal lenses. The miotic effect of pilocarpine is seen at all ages, and occurs irrespective of the duration of pilocarpine treatment. The pupil reduces to so-called 'pin-point' diameter during the peak of pilocarpine's miotic action.

A glaucoma patient who administers an eyedrop in the hour or so prior to a scheduled visit to the ophthalmologist will thus present to the examining physician with maximal miosis. What does that observation tell the astute clinician about the patient's compliance with the prescribed, four-times-a-day dosing regimen? One aspect of the answer has to do with timing, the other with the specificity of the effect. The typical patient with chronic, open-angle glaucoma (the most common form is seen quarterly or semi-annually, which represent ca. 2000–4000 hours between visits. The observation of miosis during a visit indicates that the patient took an eyedrop sometime within the two hours prior to the visit, which is of course a tiny fraction of the long interval between visits. Furthermore, as we now know from electronic monitoring studies, compliance in the day or two prior to a scheduled visit is often much better than usually-prevailing compliance—a phenomenon that Alvan Feinstein has termed "white-coat compliance," based on findings by Kass, et al. in glaucoma patients using eyedrops and by Cramer et al. in patients taking oral medications.[9–11] Thus, the observation of miosis during a scheduled visit is likely to be a misleading indicator of usually-prevailing compliance, and is a contributor to the prevailing overestimation of compliance by clinicians.[9]

A further limitation arises because morphine and related narcotics can also induce profound miosis, so miosis is not specific for pilocarpine. Yet another twist in this story is that the delivery system form of pilocarpine, which delivers the drug at a constant, low-rate from a membrane insert under the eyelid, is capable of lowering intra-ocular pressure without inducing miosis.[12] The total dose of pilocarpine provided by the delivery system is a small fraction of the dose provided by eyedrops, and so the delivery system form of pilocarpine is able to control intra-ocular pressure without miosis. That unprecedented dissocation between the miotic and ocular hypotensive actions of pilocarpine created considerable confusion in the marketplace when the delivery system form of the drug first appeared, because many ophthalmologists concluded that the delivery system form of the drug was not working because there was no miosis.

Another example of an ophthalmologic marker of drug exposure is provided by timolol maleate eyedrops, which supplanted pilocarpine as first-line therapy for management of ocular hypertension and glaucoma. The first few doses of timolol maleate have a much larger ocular hypotensive effect than doses given after many days of consistent treatment. This partial waning of drug effect, called 'partial tolerance', has a somewhat paradoxical effect, for the patient who takes little or no medication except in the "white-coat" run-up to a scheduled visit will manifest a lower intra-ocular pressure during the visit than patients who systematically follow the prescribed drug regimen. An unwary ophthalmologist may be tempted to lavish inappropriate praise on the white-coat complier for the gratifyingly low intra-ocular pressure.

Biochemical Evidence of Drug Action

The first cholesterol-lowering drug to be proven effective in reducing the risk of coronary artery disease was cholestyramine, an agent that acts by binding bile acids in the gastrointestinal tract and preventing their absorption. This epochal point was established in the Lipid Research Clinics—Coronary Primary Prevention Study (LRC-CPPT), which studied 3806 patients in a randomized, placebo-controlled trial for 10 years.[13] Cholestyramine is, in effect, a locally-acting agent, not subject to the pharmacokinetic variability of absorption into the blood stream and distribution throughout to the body. Indeed, as was shown in the analysis of LRC-CPPT results,[13] both the cholesterol-lowering and coronary risk-reducing effects of cholestyramine depend on the average amount of drug the patients took. Compliance with the cholest-yramine and placebo regimens was estimated by counting returned, unused packets of drug or placebo in this exceptionally highly disci-plined trial, in which no patients were lost to follow-up during the study. Unlike the perfunctory attention given to counting returned dos-age forms in most trials, in which dumping or hoarding of untaken drug is prevalent, the packet counts in LRC-CPPT indicated that half the patients had taken nearly all prescribed doses, and the remaining half divided almost equally between patients who took about half the doses and patients who took less than a third of the doses. Over 30 million packets were dispensed, about one-third of which were re-turned unused and counted—a formidable, not inexpensive task.

On average, there was a linear relation between the average amount of cholestyramine taken and the two principal effects of the drug: cholesterol reduction and coronary risk reduction.[14] The overall average coronary risk reduction was 19%; in the 50.8% of patients whose packet counts indicated full compliance with active drug, the average reduction in coronary risk was 39%, and the coronary risk-reducing effects of the drug were proportionally lower in those who complied partially or poorly.[14] A similarly linear relationship was found between drug intake and cholesterol reduction, but the percent-age reduction in cholesterol levels was almost exactly half the magni-tude of the reduction in coronary risk, dose for dose. In the placebo group, no effect of variable compliance on either coronary risk or cho-lesterol levels was found, which means that there was no evident ancil-lary mechanism, aside from the dose-dependent actions of the drug, mediated through its effects on cholesterol levels, that modified coro-nary risk.[14]

The linear relationship between average cholestyramine dose and the average reductions in coronary risk and cholesterol levels is strik-ing, and, in the absence of any linkage between compliance with pla-cebo and these endpoints, reinforces the statistically rather shaky con-clusion drawn from the intention-to-treat analysis,[15] which of course ignores the compliance data. The compliance-stratified efficacy data gave rise to the slogan that "a 1% reduction in cholesterol levels gives a 2% reduction in coronary risk", which has been useful in communicat-ing to the general public the importance of cholesterol reduction.

The striking, linear relation between average cholestyramine dose and the average reductions in cholesterol level and coronary risk is the most extensive body of dose-response data for any drug.[14] Usually, of course, dose-response studies are purposefully designed, carefully controlled, relatively small studies in which various doses are given to limited numbers of trial volunteers in specially designed sequences, as the corresponding effects are observed. In the LRC-CPPT, the dose-response relations of cholestyramine arose from a huge natural experiment, in which 3806 patients, each for their own reasons, opted to take all, some, or little of the drug or its placebo. Lacking the protection provided by randomized assignment of drug and dose, we must remain uncertain about concluding that the different levels of observed response were caused by the associated, different doses of drug. The finding that there was no evident association between compliance with the trial placebo and either cholesterol reduction or coronary risk reduction goes a long way to resolving those doubts, as have the results of subsequent trials of other types of cholesterol-lowering drugs, all of which appear to be consistent with the view that dose-dependent reductions in cholesterol levels act through a consistent relation between cholesterol levels and coronary risk. The details are complicated by the fact that coronary risk reduction is inversely related to the high-density fraction (HDL) of cholesterol, and that some drugs, eg, gemfibrozil, have a dual effect because they act both to increase HDL-cholesterol and decrease other fractions.[16]

There has been a great deal of controversy about the interpretation of the natural experiment in dose-ranging created by variable compliance with protocol-specified drug regimens. The matter is reviewed in the papers from the Limburg Compliance Symposium.[17] Suffice it to say that, as medical progress makes it increasingly more difficult, for both ethical and practical reasons, to carry out trials that include placebos, we will sooner or later be forced to have to glean as much information as possible from the natural experiment in dose-ranging, created by patients' own choices of drug intake. It is a recognized statistical challenge and research priority to find the best ways to "mine" the natural experiment for all that it can reliably teach about the dose-dependent actions of drugs.[18–20]

In the present context, one might reasonably conclude that the uniquely well-established dose-response relations between cholestyramine dose and cholesterol reduction would allow us to turn this relationship around and use an individual patient's changes in cholesterol level to indicate that patient's level of compliance with the cholestyramine regimen. Furthermore, if this maneuver could work in any situation, it ought to be optimal in the case of cholestyramine, because of its having the best-documented dose-response relation plus the fact that the relation is essentially linear. So here we should have the optimal circumstances for a biological marker. Figure 1 shows the individual data from one of the centers (Stanford) that constituted a 15% subset of the entire trial population. As the figure shows, the between-patient variability is far too great to use cholesterol levels as a marker of compliance with the cholestyramine regimen.

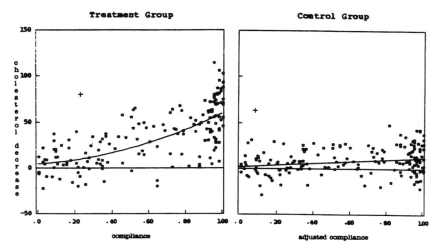

Figure 1. Relations between measured compliance with cholestyramine (left panel) or placebo (right panel) and cholesterol concentrations in plasma in individual trial volunteers (points) and on average (solid line). The points designated by a cross represent extreme outliers and were omitted from the curve-fitting procedure. (Reproduced, with permission, from Reference 18.)

Deliberate Use of a Chemical Marker

Feely and colleagues, working at Leeds in the UK, have succeeded in validating low-dose phenobarbital as a marker of drug regimen compliance.[21] Their approach is to add a very low dose (2 mg) of phenobarbital to dosage forms of drugs that a patient is taking for therapeutic purposes—not a trivial task, certainly, but not impossible—and then to sample the patient's plasma at intervals to measure phenobarbital concentration. Several exceptional characteristics of phenobarbital have made this approach possible. One is its very slow turnover in the body: its plasma half-life is sufficiently long that a single measurement of phenobarbital concentration in plasma reflects aggregate drug intake during the prior 2 weeks. Another feature of phenobarbital is its exceptionally low variability in absorption and distribution in the body, so that the dose-concentration relation is highly predictable. The validation studies that Pullar and Feely have done[21] serve as a model for what has to be done to validate any other substance that one might consider using as a chemical marker.

Even so, there is a zone of ambiguity in intermediate levels of measured concentrations of phenobarbital in plasma that could signify either that the patient is a partial complier or a full complier with an unusually high clearance of phenobarbital from plasma. By policy, Feely et al. opted to give patients with such values the benefit of the doubt, by classifying them as good compliers with high clearance values.[21] In any case, Feely et al. have adduced an impressive body of work of evidence to support use of phenobarbital as a chemical marker for compliance assessment, and then proceeded to use the method in an array of disease conditions. Among other things, they have provided the most definitive, damning evidence for the unreliability of returned tablet counts,[7] plus they have shown how clinically unrecognized noncompliance can confound the management of oral anticoagulant therapy, rheumatoid arthritis, thyroid conditions, and so forth.[22-24] More or less coincident with the work of Pullar and Feely was that of Maenpaa and others to develop low-dose digoxin as a chemical marker, in conjunction with the Helsinki Heart Study.[25] Digoxin has a considerably shorter plasma half-life than phenobarbital, so its use tends to be more confounded by white-coat compliance than is the case with phenobarbital.

The main limitation of the marker method is that it provides no information on the timing of doses. Thus, while the marker method proves ingestion but does not show dosing timing, the electronic monitoring methods show timing but do not prove ingestion. Recognition of the importance of dose-timing information is growing as work in the compliance field shifts from simple descriptions of the prevalence and clinical correlates of poor compliance in various fields of ambulatory care, toward interventions to improve compliance.[26]

Overview

Biological variability in drug response is the main obstacle to using biological markers of compliance. A basic introduction to the sources of variance in drug response is a paper written about a decade ago by Carl Peck and the late John Harter.[27] Unfortunately, their work was published in a setting and under a title that almost completely camouflaged their valuable contribution. Anyone considering work to try to qualify a biological marker should begin with the Harter-Peck model, with consideration of some extensions of the Harter-Peck work that take into account the types of nonlinearities commonly encountered in pharmacodynamics.[28] Harter and Peck were probably correct in ranking the variation created by variable patient compliance as a source of variance in drug response co-equal to that created by pharmacokinetics,[27] but therein of course lies the difficulty in trying to estimate compliance from measured drug response: there is simply too much variance from other sources to permit reliable assessment.

Conclusion

The idea of using biological markers to indicate compliance is superficially appealing, but encounters insuperable obstacles created by variability that arises from multiple sources. Specific exceptions, eg, low-dose phenobarbital used as a specific chemical marker, added to drug dosage forms, have provided valuable research information, but the lack of dose-timing information limits their value in interventions to improve compliance.

References

1. Urquhart J, de Klerk E. Contending paradigms for the interpretation of data on patient compliance with therapeutic drug regimens. *Stat Med* 1998; 17:251–267.
2. Norell SE. Methods in assessing drug compliance. *Acta Med Scand* 1984; Suppl 683:35–40.
3. Urquhart J. The electronic medication event monitor—lessons for pharmaco-therapy. *Clin Pharmacokinet* 1997;32:345–356.
4. Burke L. Electronic Measures. In Burke LE, Ockene IS (eds): Compliance in Healthcare and Research. Armonk, NY: 2001.
5. Wood HF, Simpson R, Feinstein AR, et al. Rheumatic fever in children and adolescents: A long-term epidemiologic study of subsequent prophylaxis, streptococcal infections, and clinical sequelae. I. Description of the investigative techniques and of the population studied. *Ann Int Med* 1964;60 (suppl 5):6–17.
6. Urquhart J. Ascertaining how much compliance is enough with outpatient antibiotic regimens. *Postgrad Med J* 1993;68 (Suppl 3),S49-S59.
7. Pullar T, Kumar S, Tindall H, et al. Time to stop counting the tablets? *Clin Pharmacol Ther* 1989;46:163–168.
8. Rudd P, Byyny RL, Zachary V, et al. The natural history of medication compliance in a drug trial: limitations of pill counts. *Clin Pharmacol Ther* 1989;46:169–176.
9. Feinstein AR. On white-coat effects and the electronic monitoring of compliance. *Arch Intern Med* 1990;150:1377–1378.
10. Kass MA, Gordon M, Meltzer DW. Can ophthalmologists correctly identify patients defaulting from pilocarpine therapy? *Am J Ophthalmol* 1986;101: 524–530.
11. Cramer JA, Scheyer RD, Mattson RH. Compliance declines between clinic visits. *Arch Int Med* 1990;150:1509–1510.
12. Urquhart J. Development of the OCUSERT® pilocarpine ocular therapeutic systems—a case history in ophthalmic product development. In Ophthalmic Drug Delivery Systems, Joseph Robinson (ed): Washington, DC: APHA Academy of Pharmaceutical Sciences; 1980:105–118.
13. The Lipid Research Clinics Coronary Primary Prevention Trial results: (I) Reduction in incidence of coronary heart disease; (II) The relationship of reduction in incidence of coronary heart disease to cholesterol lowering. *JAMA* 1984;251:351–374.
14. Urquhart J. Patient compliance as an explanatory variable in four selected

cardiovascular trials. In Patient Compliance in Medical Practice and Clinical Trials. Cramer JA, Spilker B (eds): New York: Raven Press; 1991:301–322.
15. Meier P. Discussion. *J Am Stat Assoc* 1991;86 (413):19–22.
16. Manninen V, Elo MO, Frick H, et al. Lipid alterations and decline in the incidence of coronary heart disease in the Helsinki Heart Study. *JAMA* 1988;260:641–651.
17. Papers from the Limburg Compliance Symposium. *Stat Med* 1998:17.
18. Efron B, Feldman D. Compliance as an explanatory variable in clinical trials. *J Am Stat Assoc* 1991;86 (413):7–17.
19. Rubin D. Comment: Dose-response estimands. *J Am Stat Assoc* 1991;86 (413): 22–24.
20. Cox D. Discussion of the Limburg Compliance Symposium. *Stat Med* 1998; 17:387.
21. Feely M, Cooke J, Price D, et al. Low-dose phenobarbitone as an indicator of compliance with drug therapy. *Br J Clin Pharmacol* 1987;24:77–83.
22. Kumar S, Haigh JRM, Rhodes LE, et al. Poor compliance is a major factor in unstable outpatient control of anticoagulant therapy. Thrombosis Haemostasis 1989;62:729–732.
23. Pullar T, Peaker S, Martin MFR, et al. The use of a pharmacological indicator to investigate compliance in patients with a poor response to antirheumatic therapy. *Brit J Rheumatol* 1988;27:381–384.
24. Penn ND, Speaker S, Griffiths AP, et al. Use of a pharmacological indicator to monitor compliance with thyroxine. *Eur J Clin Pharmacol* 1988;35: 327–329.
25. Maenpää, Javela K, Pikkarainen J, et al. Minimal doses of digoxin: A new marker for compliance to medication. *Europ Heart J* 1987;8 (suppl I):31–37.
26. Cramer JA, Rosenheck R. Enhancing medication compliance for people with serious mental disease. *J Nervous Mental Dis* 1999;187:53–54.
27. Harter JG, Peck CC. Chronobiology: Suggestions for integrating it into drug development. *Ann NY Acad Sci* 1991;618:563–571.
28. Urquhart J. Pharmacodynamics of variable patient compliance: Implications for pharmaceutical value. *Adv Drug Delivery Revs* 1998;33:207–219.

Chapter 8

Electronic Measurement

Lora E. Burke, PhD, MPH, RN

Introduction

Patient compliance with treatment is essential to achieve optimal cardiovascular risk reduction. However, until recently, assessment of patient compliance with treatment regimens has been less than precise due to measurement limitations. The commonly used methods have relied on patient self report through interviews, questionnaires, and diaries, or on pill counts, the method used more often in clinical trials. Less frequently, active compounds or a biological tracer have been measured in urine or blood. There are inherent weaknesses in each of these methods, eg, (1) dependence on patient recall of previous medication-taking events or other behaviors such as exercise; (2) patient censoring of a report; (3) the potential influence of diary recording on the behavior being monitored; (4) patient hoarding or dumping of pills prior to the follow-up clinic visit; and (5) the problem that "spot checks" of serum drug concentration or chemical markers may not reflect long-term compliance.[1-3] In summary, the major issue of measuring compliance is that problems with compliance diminish under scrutiny.[4] Once patients know they are being monitored, whether through direct questioning or indirect observation, their answers may not be representative of actual behavior, or their behavior may change.

Significance of the Problem

The limitations of traditional measures of compliance have been highlighted by the arrival of electronic methods of measurement. The

This paper was supported in part by the National Heart, Lung, and Blood Institute (HL07560).

From: Burke LE, Ockene IS (eds). *Compliance in Healthcare and Research*. Armonk, NY: Futura Publishing Company, Inc.; © 2001.

discrepancy between medication adherence measured by electronic event monitoring (EEM) and self-report (SR) was reported by Straka et al. in 1997.[5] In their study of isosorbide dinitrate prescribed three times daily, the researchers reported that compared to EEM, diaries overestimated compliance in 67% of the study participants.[5] Dunbar-Jacob and colleagues extended this work in their comparison of SR, pill counts (PC), and EEM of adherence to lovastatin, a once-daily medication.[6] They reported mean compliance by SR was 97%, PC 95%, and EEM 84%.[6] It is noteworthy that the setting for this study was a clinical trial, a setting in which optimum compliance is often assumed. Berg and colleagues examined another dimension of medication-taking behavior, the inter-dosing intervals of using inhaled medication.[7] When they examined the self-reported intervals recorded in a daily diary and the intervals measured by the Metered Dose Inhaler Chronolog, the correlation was .44, weaker than the moderate correlation of .55 found when the number of administrations was compared.[7,8] Both findings highlight the discrepancy between self-reported behavior and electronic monitoring. The aims of this chapter are to review the methods of electronic monitoring available to measure adherence to medication-taking and physical activity regimens, to discuss the indications for their use, and to present the advantages and disadvantages of these methods. The use of electronic diaries for self-reporting smoking cessation and eating behaviors will be discussed briefly.

Electronic Monitoring of Medication-Taking Behavior

Electronic monitoring is a somewhat novel approach to indirectly monitoring a person's medication-taking behavior in an objective manner. A 'medication event' is a set of actions taken with a medication container that is critical to the taking of the medication, or at least for removing the dose from the container.[3] The medication packaging contains a microprocessor that records the time and date the container was opened or a medication released, referred to as 'time-stamping.'[3] This technology has been applied to various medication packaging.[3,9,10]

Methods Available

The first application of this device in the 1970s was in eyedrop dispensers where the joint occurrence of cap removal and dispenser inversion were registered as a presumptive dose of the medication.[9] The microprocessor, which today is the size of a large coin, is able to record several thousand events over a period of approximately 2 years.

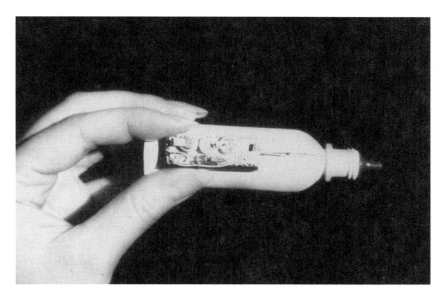

Figure 1. Eyedrop dispenser. The circuitry is tucked inside the cul-de-sac in the container away from the eyedrop solution. The simultaneous occurrence of the cap being removed and the bottle inverted triggers the recording of date/time. Copyright AARDEX Ltd, reproduced with their permission.

See Figures 1 (eye drop dispenser) and 2 (Aprex MEMS cap/bottle, [Aprex Corp., Fremont, CA]) for a pictorial display of this technology used in an eye drop dispenser and in a medication bottle cap. In medication bottle caps the microprocessor time-stamps the opening/closing of the bottle, in blister packs, the removal of the tablet; in pill ring dispensers, the removal of the birth control pill; and in the Chronolog nebulizer, the release of the aerosol medication. As there are multiple formats for the use of this technology, so are there numerous purposes for their use.

Purpose of EEM

The purpose of using an EEM is to document a reliable chronology of medication events, which can be interpreted as a history of drug dosing or exposure.[2,3] From this history, one can compare the actual dosing history with the prescribed regimen, eg., identify dosing errors by examining the interval between doses and relate this to the prescribed dosing frequency and inter-dosing interval. Additionally, the monitor can detect drug holidays, a lapse in dosing of 3 or more

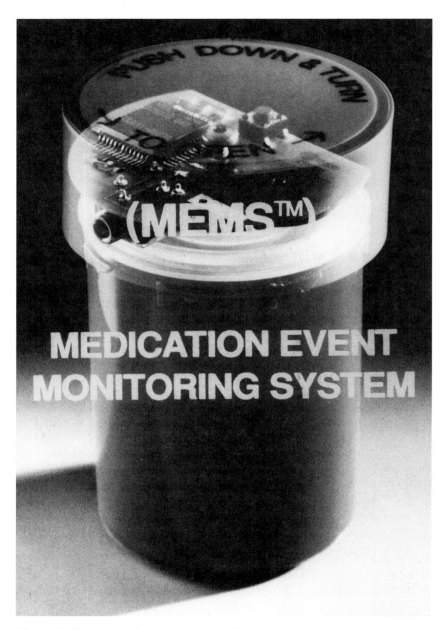

Figure 2. The micro-circuitry of the medication event monitoring device contained inside the medication bottle cap. Copyright AARDEX Ltd, reproduced with their permission.

days.[9,11] Furthermore, varying patterns in adherence can be detected, eg., increased compliance immediately preceding a clinic appointment or on different days of the week[12], and help distinguish between pharmacological nonresponse and noncompliance. Use of these monitors eliminates the sole use of inaccurate methodologies such as self-report (eg., diaries, interviews, and questionnaires) and pill counts. Additional uses include pre-randomization screening for compliers, determination of optimal dosing, the degree of compliance required for a desired effect, and occurrence of clinical events related to changes in dosing pattern.[2,3,9] In summary, this method goes beyond establishing the presence or absence of compliance, but rather aims to determine if adverse events occur following skipped doses or extra doses. Electronic monitoring allows a detailed examination of the pattern of medication-taking as it relates to the clinical course.

Use and Interpretation of Drug Chronology Data

Depending on the question being asked, there are various approaches to summarizing the drug administration history. Four commonly used approaches and the reason for each follows.

1. *percentage of prescribed doses*—to evaluate the impact of variable compliance on bulk pharmaceutical consumption.[3] This is based on the calculation of the number of prescribed doses taken out of the total number prescribed and converted to a percentage figure, eg., 72% compliance.
2. *administration chronologies* (the intervals between doses and subsequent clinical events)—to evaluate the adequacy of the therapeutic response, or distinguish between pharmacological nonresponse and noncompliance, or determine the minimum compliance needed for a good outcome.[3,9,11]
3. *periods of short-interval administration & absence of drug administration for three or more days (drug holidays)* —to predict the likelihood of adverse reactions following increased dosage or absence of dosage. Drug holidays may trigger adverse rebound or recurrent first-dose effects.[13,14]
4. *chronology of dose administration*—to assess patient behavior and determine how to improve compliance. Examination of within-day patterns of medication-taking (eg. morning-evening), between-day patterns (eg. weekday-weekend), patterns proximate-remote from scheduled visits and over the course of treatment duration.[2,3,15]

Procedures for Using EEM

Initialization

The first step in using the medication event monitor is to initialize the microprocessor by encoding the intended user's identifying information on the enclosed microprocessor memory. This information includes patient name or identification number, name of physician, name of drug, and dosing information (number of tablets per dose), frequency of dose, and therapeutic range or duration of drug. The monitor and medication are given to the individual and on subsequent visits the data are downloaded through a communicator, which electronically reads and transfers data (See Figure 3). Initializing the monitor's microprocessor is not absolutely necessary but following this procedure prior to its use ensures that the identifying information is on the monitor

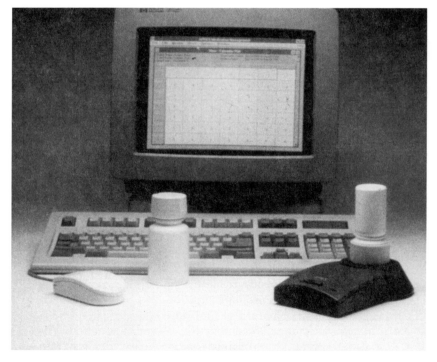

Figure 3. Standard setup for initializing or downloading data from the microprocessor. The bottle is inverted so the cap can sit on the communicator, which translates data from the micro-processor to the computer for instant display on the screen. Copyright AARDEX Ltd, reproduced with their permission.

and, more importantly, that the monitor is operating. If one is not able to encode the identifying information on the monitor, one can use the monitor's serial number and assign the patient or study participant to that number.

Downloading Data

The same procedure that is used in initializing the monitor is followed for downloading data. The monitor is placed on the communicator, which is connected to the personal computer or laptop. The communicator electronically reads and transfers the data that are stored in the monitor to the computer (See Figure 4). The (proprietary) software processes and quickly analyzes the data retrieved from the communicator. The data can be displayed instantly on the monitor screen, or printed on hard copy. This process can take place at remote sites, such as a clinic or a patient's home. Following this procedure, the data file can be converted to an ASCII format and exported to a statistical package for group analysis.

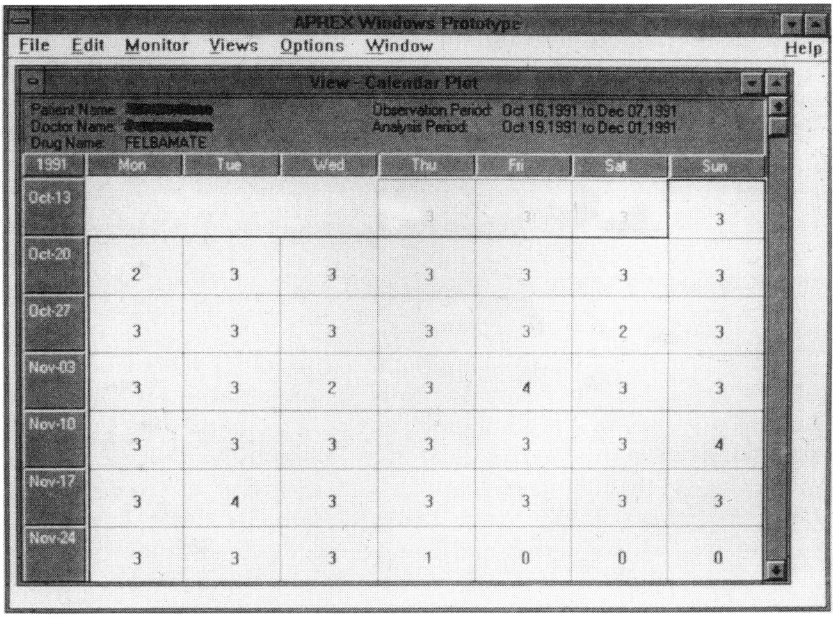

APREX Windows Prototype
File Edit Monitor Views Options Window   Help

View – Calendar Plot

Patient Name:
Doctor Name:
Drug Name: FELBAMATE

Observation Period: Oct 16,1991 to Dec 07,1991
Analysis Period: Oct 19,1991 to Dec 01,1991

1991	Mon	Tue	Wed	Thu	Fri	Sat	Sun
Oct-13				3	3	3	3
Oct-20	2	3	3	3	3	3	3
Oct-27	3	3	3	3	3	2	3
Nov-03	3	3	2	3	4	3	3
Nov-10	3	3	3	3	3	3	4
Nov-17	3	4	3	3	3	3	3
Nov-24	3	3	3	1	0	0	0

Figure 4. Calendar plot display. This display provides only the frequency of cap openings for each 24–hour period. Copyright AARDEX Ltd, reproduced with their permission.

EEM Data Formats

An array of formats for data presentation is available, which may vary slightly by manufacturer. The following terms describe these formats.

Dose Frequency

This format is limited in that it presents only frequency data, ie, the number of medication events for each 24-hour period are displayed on a calendar plot. Thus, no data on inter-dosing interval are provided. See Figure 4 for a display of these data.

Dose Time

The data are displayed on an 'event list,' which provides the date and time of each presumptive dose, the interval in day/hours/minutes since the previous dose (removal of bottle cap), and if there were any multiple open/close events that were filtered. Events are filtered if multiple repetitive openings occur with less than 30-second intervals between the cap removal and replacement; these are noted in the next column as a filtered event (See Figure 5). The event list is a continuous display for the entire monitored period, or specified periods may be selected by date.

Dose Interval

This format consists of a bar graph or chronology plot that displays the dosing intervals in hours and thus shows variations in doses and also the presence of drug holidays. In Figures 6 and 7, the European day/month format is on the horizontal axis and the 24-hour clock is on the vertical axis. Figure 6 graphically depicts the pattern of varying dosing, eg., the morning dose is taken later on weekends. In Figure 7 one can see that the individual was taking the medication regularly until the beginning of March. From that point on the compliance begins to deteriorate and later the participant withdrew from the study, suggesting that the previous decline in compliance may have served as a warning sign of the impending study withdrawal. (Personal communication, April 1999, John Urquhart)

APREX MEMS View™ v1.61
May 28, 1998 13:52

Patient	C7321		ID	7
Physician			Time zone U.S.A. Pacific	
Clinic			Site	
Drug	HIV Medication			
Duration of Action	8 hours			
Regimen	Take 1 tablet(s) of HIV Medication every 8 hour(s).			

Event List				
Date	Time hh:mm	Interval dd:hh:mm	Multiple Open/Close	Notes
02/04/97	19:50			
02/05/97	05:56	00:10:06		
	13:58	00:08:02		
	20:13	00:06:15		
02/06/97	05:52	00:09:39		
	14:03	00:08:11		
	20:24	00:06:21		
02/07/97	05:37	00:09:13		
	13:53	00:08:16		
	20:30	00:06:37		
02/08/97	06:35	00:10:05		
	14:08	00:07:33		
	20:24	00:06:16		
02/09/97	05:58	00:09:34		
	14:30	00:08:32		
	20:11	00:05:41		
02/10/97	07:29	00:11:18		
	14:52	00:07:23		
	20:16	00:05:24		
02/11/97	06:23	00:10:07		
	14:24	00:08:01		
	20:13	00:05:49		
02/12/97	06:03	00:09:50		
	14:12	00:08:09		
	19:42	00:05:30		
02/13/97	06:14	00:10:32		
	14:09	00:07:55		
	20:01	00:05:52		
02/14/97	05:43	00:09:42		
	13:48	00:08:05		
	19:48	00:06:00		
02/15/97	06:13	00:10:25		
	14:13	00:08:00		
	20:26	00:06:13		
02/16/97	06:07	00:09:41		
	14:52	00:08:45		
	19:59	00:05:07		
02/17/97	06:03	00:10:04		
	14:21	00:08:18		

Patient File: 74221FF4.AP4   Page 1 of 4

Figure 5. Event list displays the date and time of each presumptive dose, the interval in day/hours/minutes since the previous dose (opening), and if there were any multiple open/close events less than 30 seconds apart. The event list is continuous for the entire monitored period. Copyright AARDEX Ltd, reproduced with their permission.

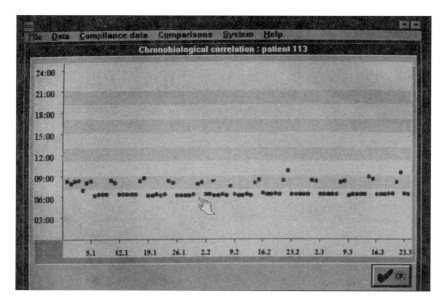

Figure 6. Chronology plot with the 24-hour clock time on the vertical axis and the European day/month format on the horizontal axis. The patient took all scheduled doses but sleeps a few hours later on the weekend. Copyright AARDEX Ltd, reproduced with their permission.

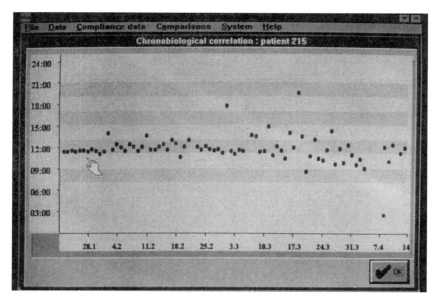

Figure 7. Chronology plot in same format as Figure 6. Participant in a clinical trial takes medication regularly in Jan/Feb; by early March individual's medication taking is erratic and person withdraws from trial at the end of the period represented on the plot. Copyright AARDEX Ltd, reproduced with their permission.

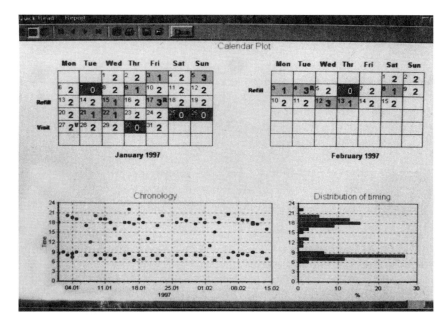

Figure 8. Composite of data displays: calendar plot, chronology plot, and a histogram showing the distribution of dosing times. Copyright AARDEX Ltd, reproduced with their permission.

Dose Timing

This format includes a scatter plot or histogram of the data's distribution of dosing times, which allows one to identify the number of days the medication is taken at a specific time, eg., 1000, 1200, and how this varies across days (See Figure 8).

EEM Data Storage

Current medication event monitors have a non-volatile memory that prevents the loss of stored data in case there is a loss of battery power. However, if a battery failure occurs, new data will not be recorded until the battery is replaced. The typical battery has an 18- to 24-month shelf-life and should record approximately 1800 events. The data file can be converted to an ASCII file.

Costs of EEM

As is the case with other technology based products, the size and the costs of these devices have been dramatically reduced in the past two decades. Purchasing or leasing arrangements of electronic monitors varies with the manufacturer or supplier and the type of monitor device. The same applies to costs, eg., the cost of a medication bottle cap is different from a monthly blister pack. Use of these devices is still relatively limited and thus costs remain higher than might be if the volume of use was higher. The approximate cost for use of an electronic monitor in a medication bottle cap is $60 and the cost of a monthly blister pack is $32. The software that analyzes the data and the hardware, i. e., the communicator which electronically reads and transfers the data, may be purchased or leased. The users of these devices may elect a plan to have the proprietor handle the data, eg., the user sends the downloaded data file to the company to have a report compiled, which is then sent to the user. This arrangement is more commonly used in clinical settings where personnel with the requisite expertise or time may not be available, especially when monitoring is not done in high volume. The greater volume of monitors used in a research setting requires that trained staff be present to manage the data through all stages of the process. In this setting, it is more economical to purchase the required software and hardware.

Manufacturers should be contacted regarding cost and purchasing or leasing arrangements of the specific monitors and associated equipment. It should be noted that the technology is not limited to the devices or formats described here, for example, monitoring of adherence with topical medication, such as creams or salves can be designed. The researcher or clinician can discuss the desired application and specific design with the manufacturers's representative. A wide array of bottles is currently available and this will increase as the demand for varied formats and their use increases.

Advantages

The strength of the electronic medication event monitors is that they are objective and unobtrusive. The date and time of each "medication event" is recorded into the memory of the device and protected from subsequent tampering or alteration.[9] If an individual opens and closes the bottle repetitively at less than 30 second intervals, the events are noted on the data list as a filtered event. This type of activity might suggest that a person was trying to open the bottle as many times as the frequency of the prescribed medication, not realizing that the counter was also recording date and time of openings. This might be suspect if there were few or no openings in the period preceding the filtered events and the multiple openings occurred immediately prior to a clinic visit, suggesting possible tampering with the device. This type of behavior is comparable to the patient dumping pills prior to a clinic visit when a pill count is expected. However, unlike pill dumping, the electronic monitor captures the multiple openings. Actual falsification of the data with these devices would have to occur in real time and would be difficult if not impossible for the patient to do.[9] The blister pack has an additional advantage in that it records the actual time each dose is removed from the package. The memory capacity allows data collection for approximately 24 months, thus not necessitating frequent clinic visits for data download. Finally, the advantage of the electronic monitor over self-report methods is that it can detect drug holidays and differentiate the non-complier from the non-responder.

Disadvantages

The weakness of the compliance monitors is that a medication event represents a presumptive dose, there is no evidence that the patient removed the medication from the bottle, or took the medication upon its removal. However, these episodes would represent additional omissions of drug administration. It is generally thought that few doses following a cap opening are not ingested and that the monitors capture an accurate picture of medication compliance, mainly capturing delayed or omitted doses.

Additional factors may represent disadvantages of this method of compliance measurement. Some patients may have well-established habits of medication-taking and refuse to use the special bottle and cap, eg., wishing to use a weekly or daily pill organizer instead. Because the bottle is larger than the standard pharmacy issue bottle, individuals who require multiple dosing throughout the day may refuse to carry the larger bottle. This should be less of a problem today as pharmaceuticals aim to reduce the dosing frequency. If the patient requires medication while at work and at home and this becomes an issue, two monitors can be provided and the data files later merged. The limited types of dispensers available today is temporary and will change with technological advances, increased use of these devices, and requests for more diversified formats.

In summary, electronic monitoring for medication-taking assessment provides the researcher or clinician a detailed picture of adherence patterns and an opportunity to evaluate the effectiveness of adherence enhancing interventions. For the clinician, it also allows an examination of the occurrence of clinical events in relation to changes in adherence patterns. Furthermore, it provides detailed information on the patient's adherence pattern, which can be taken into consideration when prescribing drug therapy.

Thus far this chapter has focused on electronic monitoring of medication-taking behavior. The focus will now shift to another behavior, exercise and physical activity, and the monitoring devices used to measure compliance in this behavioral domain. Following this discussion there will be a brief review of electronic diaries used to record self-reported behavior related to smoking cessation and dietary management.

Electronic Monitoring of Physical Activity

The literature suggests that exercise adherence rates are lower than that for pharmacological therapies because of the increased behavioral demands to maintain this regimen. Measurement of adherence to exercise in most settings has been limited to self-report and direct observation, with the latter requiring the participant to exercise in supervised groups, a condition which may contribute to nonadherence.[16,17] Furthermore, direct observation limits the range of physical activity in which one may engage. These methods have been improved upon by the addition of a microprocessor that measures and sequentially stores heart rate data, which allows an examination of the proportion of time the individual exercises within the prescribed heart rate, a proxy adherence indicator.[18,19] In the past decade electronic monitors have become available which provide additional detail on exercise and adherence patterns.

Methods Available

There are three types of monitors available that directly record dimensions of physical activity: (1) heart rate and motion sensors; (2) accelerometers that detect body motion in one or more planes; and (3) actigraph monitors that sense temperature, light, and acceleration. The Vitalog (Vitalog Corporation, Mountain View, CA) is a portable solid-state recorder-display system that measures, analyzes, and sequentially stores heart rate. The recorder uses an analog R-R interval detector to calculate heart rate and a motion sensor to record bodily movement.[17] Two studies reported on its use to record heart rate as an indirect measure of physical activity.[18,19] More precise estimates of energy expenditure are provided by a combination of heart rate and bodily motion data.

More recently, the Caltrac and Tri-Trac Accelerometers (Hemokinetics, Inc., Madison, WI) have provided a portable and an objective means of directly measuring the intensity and frequency of body move-

ments.[20,21] The Caltrac estimates energy expenditure through its measurement of the body's vertical acceleration and deceleration.[20] The
Tri-Trac has three separate accelerometers to register the body's acceler-
ations and decelerations in three planes, horizontal, vertical, and lat-
eral.[21] This device, which operates on a 9-volt battery with a lithium
back-up battery, determines total activity count per time sample based
on the relationship between energy expenditure, mass, and velocity.
A software program converts the units of integrated acceleration into
caloric expenditure (kilocalories), which is calculated from regression
equations (height, weight, age, and gender).

A validation study reported that the Caltrac's energy estimation,
expressed as caloric expenditure, was less accurate at higher speeds of
exercise and consistently overestimated energy expenditure in a sample
of normal and overweight individuals walking on a treadmill.[20] Bouten
and colleagues[21] reported a correlation of 0.95 between the triaxial accelerometer output of all three measurement directions and the metabolic cost of physical activity as measured by indirect calorimetry and
sleeping metabolic rate. Two studies reported on the comparability of
self-report and accelerometer measurements for activity.[22,23] Schlenk
et al. reported an agreement of 86.2% between self-report exercise logs
and the triaxial accelerometer.[23] Jakicic reported that participants in a
behavioral weight control program over-reported the weekly frequency
and total time spent in exercise compared to the accelerometer data.[23,24]
These data support the use of the accelerometer as a second measure
of exercise adherence.

Actigraph (Ambulatory Monitoring, Inc., Ardsley, NY) monitors
are devices worn on the wrist or ankle and sense and store motor
activity or body movement to reflect sleep/wake states and provide
information regarding circadian rhythm. The device also records
changes in ambient illumination and temperature from the skin surface
or a rectal probe. A Mini-Motionlogger Actigraph is a miniaturized
version that is similar to a wrist watch and records data that can be
analyzed for activity levels. The device is fully waterproof and can run
for 30 days with options for expanded battery power. An additional
accelerometer-based activity monitor is available for use and can measure a wide range of wrist, waist, or ankle activity in free-ranging persons (Computer-Science and Applications, Inc., Shalimar, FL).[25] Validation studies have reported that the Actigraph differentiated between
physical and sedentary activities and that Actigraph counts were significantly correlated with oxygen uptake and heart rate. However, the
wrist may not be the best placement for indexing daily activity intensity.[26]

Currently, the most affordable and widely used device to measure
exercise adherence seems to be the Tri-Trac accelerometer.[21–24] Other

features make it attractive for use in exercise adherence studies. The battery pack for the Tri-Trac ergometer is approximately five by three inches in size and easily fits into a pocket on a belt, thus allowing a free range of activity. An alternative is to place the battery pack in a fanny pack so that the battery pack rests on the hip, a manner preferred by some individuals (personal communication, E. Schlenk, April 1999). The investigator sets the device to sample data at prespecified intervals, eg., from every 1 to 15 minutes. Data can be sampled for prolonged periods, i.e., if sampled at 1-minute intervals the battery life will allow 30 days of recording and at least 60 days for 2-minute interval sampling. The device has a nonvolatile memory, which prevents loss of stored data should the battery fail.

Initialization of the ergometer is done in a manner similar to what has been previously described for the medication event monitors, utilizing an IBM-compatible personal computer and proprietor specific software. The data are downloaded in the same manner and are displayed on three different graphs, one showing motion recorded in each of the three dimensions, one a composite activity graph, and one displaying the total kilocalories per measurement interval. These procedures can be performed in a clinic or with a laptop computer off site.

Advantages

Like the medication event monitors, these devices provide a second source of data to validate self-reported exercise. Other benefits include the ability of the user to preset the interval for data sampling and also the ability to sample for prolonged periods. The lithium battery backup provides a safety margin for data storage and the ergometer's size and portability make it practical for regular use.

Disadvantages

The primary limitation of these devices is cost. The activity accelerometers cost approximately $250 to $300 and the software an additional $500. The actigraph monitors cost is significantly greater. This factor is the most prohibitive in terms of allowing more widespread use of these monitors. Investigators may purchase a limited number of the devices and take measurements periodically over a relatively brief period, eg., 7 days every 6 months in a longitudinal study, or may monitor a randomly selected subsample, depending on the size of the study. An additional issue is having the participant wear the device during their waking hours for a week. Some may feel uncomfortable doing so and may not use it. However, this does not seem to be a major concern among users.

Electronic Methods for Self-Report

Self-monitoring of overt behaviors, self-ratings of symptoms with exertion or pre- and post-medication, or of cognitions and affective responses have become frequently used methods of behavioral assessments.[27] Other studies require detailed records over prolonged periods of time, eg., recording of food intake and its fat grams and caloric value in behavioral weight control programs, or tobacco craving and number of cigarettes smoked each day. Compliance to these requested recordings can be measured to some extent by the returned records but the time the actual recording occurred is unknown. It is not unheard of to observe a study participant complete the last few days of a diary in the clinic waiting room. An alternative to the paper and pencil method of self-report is the use of hand-held computers. The use of such a device would provide an opportunity to objectively assess under naturalistic conditions the degree of compliance to the recording schedule. Two studies reported the comparative use of hand-held computer or electronic recording devices with paper and pencil recordings.[27,28] Herman, Peters, and Blanchard[27] reported that the actual level of adherence to the recording schedule during use of the hand-held computer was considerably less than during the paper and pencil use. When participants were informed there was a clock in the device, adherence improved but was still lower than with the traditional method.[27] In a pilot study testing the use of electronic patient diaries Donovan et al. reported no significant difference in the number of days completed between use of the electronic versus the paper and pencil diary format but found 89% of the self reports recorded in the electronic diaries were more accurate in the timing schedule compared to 78% of the paper and pencil format.[28] More participants (57%) preferred the use of the electronic diary than the paper and pencil diary (35%). These studies demonstrate the feasibility and acceptability by patients of using electronic formats for self-report data collection. Additional work in this area has been done in smoking cessation research where the value of real time data collection has been emphasized.[29]

Methods Available

Two devices are commercially available and will be described briefly. Similar to the medication event monitors, these devices can be programmed to use in an intervention but the discussion here is limited to their use for self-reported adherence. The LifeSign (PICS, Inc., Reston, VA) is a compact electronic recording device approximately the

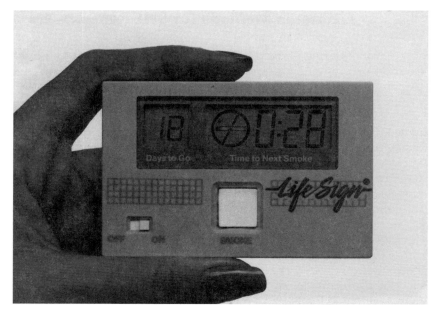

Figure 9. Lifeline device for self-monitoring of tobacco use and to provide cues to guide smoking cessation treatment; can download/upload data to PC through standard interface. Copyright PICS, Inc., reproduced with their permission.

size of a credit card and one-half inch think (See Figure 9). The individual records each time a tobacco product is used by pushing one button. The DietMate (PICS, Inc., Reston, VA) is a larger electronic recording device, approximately 4 by 7 inches, and is more sophisticated in its programming (See Figure 10). The device does not have a full keyboard but has four direction keys, yes/no, and alphanumeric display of approximately 10 lines. There are 1000 food items in the database and programming capability for a weight loss, cholesterol-lowering, and a combined cholesterol and sodium lowering diet plan. Assessment questions and personalized monitoring can be programmed to determine if the participant is following the treatment protocol. Both of these devices can upload and download data to a personal computer through a standard interface.

Advantages

The primary advantage of using the electronic recording devices is that data are collected in real time, at the time of the symptom or

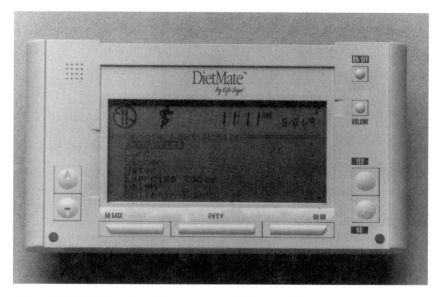

Figure 10. DietMate has 200 menus available, 1000 food items in database; diets programmed for weight loss, cholesterol-lowering, and sodium and cholesterol-lowering. Copyright PICS, Inc., reproduced with their permission.

behavior performance. This immediate recording eliminates one of the biggest threats to the validity of self-report data, recall bias. An individual can record only what he or she recalls and thus the amount of time that lapses between the actual behavior and the recording influences what is recorded. Other intervening factors may influence a person's retrospective view of a symptom or a specific behavior performed when an individual is looking back over several hours or days. If the person is recording the data in a delayed manner this is documented in an electronic diary and provides another indicator of adherence. Finally, the data recorded in an electronic device are stored in memory and thus cannot be altered or erased by the individual.

Disadvantages

Similar to the other devices discussed, the hand held computer may present a challenge to those uncomfortable with computers and its accompanying technology. Since the data being collected are self-report, the person may still censor the data. Cost remains an issue with these devices and like other products referred to in this chapter, this will change as the use of these monitors increases.

Summary

This chapter has reviewed an array of modalities available for the researcher and clinician to use in gaining a detailed picture of an individual or group's adherence to a treatment protocol. One of the primary purposes of this monitoring is not just to identify whether or not an individual is compliant, but rather to observe the varying patterns of adherence and relate this to antecedent or subsequent events in an individual's lifestyle and clinical picture. Identification of a problem requires an accurate, valid, and reliable assessment. The use of electronic devices is paramount to achieving this. However, one needs to keep the use of these devices in perspective and not lose sight of the primary focus, which should be outcome. Compliance is the process or a means to the end.[3,30] We cannot become fixated on the numbers indicating levels of compliance but rather use these data to help us achieve improved adherence and outcomes. With this in mind, the cost and effort involved in the use of these devices will be paid off in improved health.

References

1. Urquhart, J. Pharmacoeconomic consequences of variable patient compliance with prescribed drug regimens. *Pharmacoeconomics* 1999;15(3):217–228.
2. Cramer, JA. Microelectronic systems for monitoring and enhancing patient compliance with medication regimens. *Drugs* 1995;49:321–327.
3. Urquhart, J. The electronic medication event monitor: Lessons for pharmacotherapy. *Clin Pharmacokinet* 1997;32:345–356.
4. Blackwell, B. From compliance to alliance—a quarter century of research. *Netherlands J of Med* 1996;48:140–149.
5. Straka RJ, Fish JT, Benson SR, et al. Patient self-reporting of compliance does not correspond with electronic monitoring: An evaluation using isosorbide dinitrate as a model drug. *Pharmacother* 1997;17:126–132.
6. Dunbar-Jacob J, Burke LE, Rohay JM, et al. How comparable are self-report, pill count, and electronically monitored adherence data? *Circ* 1997;96(8), Suppl I-734.
7. Berg J, Dunbar-Jacob, J, Rohay JM. Compliance with inhaled medications: The relationship between diary and electronic monitor. *Ann of Behav Med* 1998;20(1):36–38.
8. Tashkin DP, Rand C, Nides M, et al. A nebulizer chronolog to monitor compliance with inhaler use. *Am J Med* 1991;911:33s–36s.

9. Urquhart J. Role of patient compliance in clinical pharmacokinetics—A review of recent research. *Clin Pharmacokinet* 1994;27(3):202–215.
10. Cramer JA, Spilker B. Patient Compliance in Medical Practice and Clinical Trials. New York: Raven Press, 1991;3–10.
11. Urquhart J, Chevalley C. Impact of unrecognized dosing errors on the cost and effectiveness of pharmaceuticals. *Drug Inf J*, 1988;22:363–378.
12. Cramer JA, Scheyer RD, Mattson RH. Compliance declines between clinic visits. *Arch Int Med*, 1990;150:1509–1510.
13. Rudd P, Ahmed S, Zachary V, et al. Improved compliance measures: Applications in an ambulatory hypertensive drug trial. *Clin Pharmcol Ther* 1990; 48:676–685.
14. Kruse, W, Eggert-Kruse W, Rampmaier J, et al. Compliance and adverse drug reactions: A prospective study with ethinylestradiol using continuous compliance monitoring. *Clin Investig* 1993;71:483–487.
15. DeKlerk, E, van der Linden SJ. Compliance monitoring of NSAID drug-therapy in ankylosing spondylitis, experiences with an electronic monitoring device. *Br J Rheuematol* 1996;35:60–65.
16. Burke LE, Dunbar-Jacob J, Hill MN. Compliance with cardiovascular disease prevention strategies: A review of the research. *Ann Behav Med* 1997; 19(3):239–263.
17. Dunbar-Jacob J, Burke LE, Puczynski S. Clinical assessment and management of adherence to medical regimens. In Nicassio PM, Smith TW (eds): Managing Chronic Illness—A Biopsychosocial Perspective. Washington, DC: American Psychological Association, 1995:313–349.
18. Mueller JK, Gossard D, Adams FR, et al. Assessment of prescribed increases in physical activity: Application of a new method for microprocessor analysis of heart rate. *Am J Cardiol* 1986;57:441–445.
19. Roger F, Juneau M, Taylor CB, et al. Assessment by a microprocessor of adherence to home-based moderate-intensity exercise training in healthy, sedentary middle-aged men and women. *Am J Cardiol* 1987;60:71–75.
20. Pambianco G, Wing RR, Robertson R. Accuracy and reliability of the Caltrac accelerometer for estimating energy expenditure. *Med Sci Sports Exerc* 1990; 22(6):858–862.
21. Bouten CV, Westerterp KR, Verduin M, et al. Assessment of energy expenditure for physical activity using a triaxial accelerometer. *Med Sci Sports Exerc* 1994;26(12):1516–1523.
22. Schlenk EA, Okifuji A, Dunbar-Jacob J, et al. Exercise adherence promotion in fibromyalgia: Baseline results. Poster presented at the Ninth Annual Scientific Sessions of the Eastern Nursing Research Society, Philadelphia, PA, April 1990.
23. Jakicic JM, Wing RR, Butler BA, et al. Prescribing exercise in multiple short bouts versus one continuous bout: Effects on adherence, cardiorespiratory fitness, and weight loss in overweight women. *Internat J Obes* 1995;19: 893–901.
24. Jakicic JM, Winters C, Lang W, et al. Effects of intermittent exercise and use of home exercise equipment on adherence, weight loss, and fitness in overweight women. *JAMA* 1999;282:1554–1560.
25. Patterson SM, Krantz DS, Montgomery LC, et al. Automated physical activity monitoring: Validation and comparison with physiological and self-report measures. *Psychophsiolog* 1993;30: 296–305.

26. Tyron WW, Williams R. Fully proportional actigraphy: A new instrument. *Behavior Res Methods, Instruments, and Computers* 1996;28(3):392–403.
27. Herman C, Peters ML, Blanchard EB. Use of hand-held computers for symptoms-monitoring: The case of chronic headache. *Mind & Body Med* 1995;1(2):59–71.
28. Donovan S, Miller J, Goulder MA, et al. Electronic patient diaries: A pilot study. *Applied Clin Trials* 1996;40–48.
29. Shiffman S, Hufford M, Hickcox M, et al. Remember that? A comparison of real-time versus retrospective recall of smoking lapses. *J Consul & Clin Psych* 1997;65(2):292–300.
30. Norell SE. Methods in assessing drug compliance. *Acta Med Scand Suppl* 1984;683:35–40.

Chapter 9

Analysis of Electronic Event Monitored Adherence

Susan M. Sereika, PhD and
Jacqueline Dunbar-Jacob, PhD, RN, FAAN

Introduction

The evaluation of adherence, or compliance, to treatment regimen is of major importance whether conducted for use in the management of and interpretation of findings from a large-scale multi-center clinical trial or in the appraisal of an individual patient's therapeutic response in a clinical practice setting. In each situation, nonadherence with treatment can lead to the underestimation of both therapeutic and adverse effects.[1,2] As discussed by Rand et al.,[3] health care providers often tend to underreport the degree of patient nonadherence and fail to identify patients who have problems with adherence to their prescribed regimen. Thus, for the individual being treated in a clinical practice, the lack of a treatment response due to nonadherence that is undetected by the clinician may lead to the occurrence of toxic side effects when the regimen is increased to elicit the desired effect and adherence is resumed, or it may lead to the abandonment of an otherwise efficacious treatment. In the context of a clinical trial, nonadherence can seriously undermine even the most well designed study, biasing estimates of the treatment effect and eroding statistical power when testing hypotheses. Hence, the monitoring of adherence is critical to the valid interpretation of therapeutic outcomes as intra-individual variability in adherence to

Acknowledgements: The authors wish to thank Elizabeth Schlenk for her invaluable editorial assistance and useful feedback.
This paper was supported in part by the National Heart, Lung, and Blood Institute (U01-HL48992), the National Institute of Nursing Research (P30-NR03924), and the University of Pittsburgh Central Research Development Fund.

From: Burke LE, Ockene IS (eds). *Compliance in Healthcare and Research.* Armonk, NY: Futura Publishing Company, Inc.; © 2001.

a prescribed regimen may contribute substantially to the variability observed in treatment response, both in clinical research and practice.[4,5]

In an effort to measure adherence to prescribed regimens a multitude of methods have been proposed.[3,6] Conventional approaches, such as patient self-reports and pill counts, have well-recognized limitations, which compromise their validity and reliability as adherence measures.[7] Even the more regarded direct approaches—biochemical analysis or directly observed therapy—have their disadvantages, which restrict their usefulness, especially with ambulatory patients.[3] During the past two decades, advances have been made to more precisely measure regimen adherence through the use of electronic event monitoring (EEM).[3,8] With the advent of electronic monitoring technology, the measurement of patient adherence to treatment—oral and inhaled medications as well as exercise—has become even more comprehensive, recording vast quantities of information on the occurrence of behaviors that can produce indirect objective assessments of adherence chronicled in real time.[9–13]

Along with this increased precision in measurement, however, has come the added complexity of the adherence data.[14,15] Rather than a single index such as a pill count or level of byproduct or chemical marker, each individual's adherence to a regimen may now be represented longitudinally as a time series of behavioral "events."[16] Recently, efforts have been made toward the analysis of adherence information based on electronic event monitoring.[15–21] This report seeks to discuss some of these statistical methods and how the results obtained from their application can aid in the understanding of treatment adherence for the individual patient as well as a group's adherence experience as in a clinical trial. Hence, the intent of this report is several-fold: 1) to highlight issues to consider when managing EEM data; 2) to review methods that have been proposed to summarize and visualize adherence information collected via EEM; and 3) to discuss the merits of cross-sectional and longitudinal analytic strategies for the analysis of EEM data.

Empirical Example—Adherence in Clinical Trials: Induction Strategies

For illustrative purposes in this report, electronically monitored adherence data obtained from a subgroup of subjects who participated in a study entitled "Adherence in Clinical Trials: Induction Strategies" (U01–HL48992) was evaluated using some of the methods presented. The purpose of this ancillary clinical trial was to examine the efficacy of two induction approaches—habit training alone and habit training with problem solving—in an effort to enhance the medication adherence in subjects newly diagnosed with hyperlipidemia who were enrolled in a larger randomized, double-blind clinical trial designed to investigate the behavioral effects of lipid-lowering. In the parent study, subjects were recruited from the community throughout southwestern Pennsylvania. To be eligible, persons had to be between 25 and 60 years of age; have fasting low density lipoprotein (LDL) values greater than 160 mg/dL; be able to read and write English; and have no personal history of hepatic or renal insufficiency, marked hypertriglyceridemia, hypertension, cancer, diabetes, or untreated hypothyroidism. Following informed consent, subjects were randomly assigned to either a 20 mg dose of lovastatin or a placebo to be taken once daily in the evening and then observed for 24 weeks to examine the behavioral effects of lipid lowering. Key assessment points during follow-up included baseline (B), 8 weeks (M1), 16 weeks (M2), and 24 weeks (F2) after the baseline evaluation.

For the ancillary adherence study, all participating, eligible subjects were randomized within the treatment arms of the parent study to the control condition (usual care) (UC), habit training alone (HT), or habit training plus problem solving (HT + PS). Subjects were then followed for 24 weeks for their medication adherence using APREX MEMS electronic medication monitoring devices (APREX Corporation, Fremont, CA), self-report, and pill counts. For this report, adherence based on the first 16 weeks of electronic medication monitoring event data was evaluated.

Managing EEM Data

As presented in an earlier chapter on the electronic measures for adherence, there are a number of electronic monitoring devices that can be used to objectively track behaviors and provide indirect measures of adherence to prescribed treatment recommendations. Each of these devices conveys, at a minimum, information concerning the timing of "events," whether they be related to the administration of oral or inhaled regimens, the monitoring of peak flow, or the occurrence of physical activity. When tracking medication-taking behaviors to oral regimens, the typical monitoring device consists of a medication vial cap, which discretely houses a microprocessor chip. As a patient or subject opens and closes his or her medication bottle when dispensing prescribed medication, the microprocessor chip records the date and time of the dosing event. The information stored summarizes the paired openings and closings of the bottle in time and hence the presumptive timing of medication administrations over the period of observation.

The medication monitoring devices that are designed for use with inhaled medications are even more informative than those used for oral medications since the date and time of a metered dose is recorded, thus yielding information on the amount and pattern of dosing at a particular administration. Likewise, activity monitors, which measure acceleration or movement, record a patient's activity in one or more dimensions on a minute-by-minute basis.

Electronic monitoring devices yield a wealth of information concerning either the occurrence of events or activity levels in time. For instance, in the randomized clinical trial previously described where subjects were tracked for their medication-taking behavior of a once daily oral medication regimen for lipid-lowering using MEMS monitor, more than 25,000 records containing information as to the date and time of the event were generated for 165 subjects over a 24-week observation period.[22] In a small-scale feasibility study, where a TriTrac R3D activity monitor (Reining International, Ltd., Madison, WI) was used to validate the frequency and duration of physical activity documented in a daily diary and to estimate energy expenditure, more than 4,000 entries recording three-dimensional acceleration, total kilocalories, and kilocalories expended on activity were accrued on each subject over a 3-day observation period.[23]

Fortunately, software and additional hardware developed by the manufacturer are available for most electronic monitoring devices to support a variety of functions, including the downloading of data from the monitor to a computer, the browsing and editing of event files, the calculation of descriptive statistics over user-specified time intervals, the generation of reports, and the output of raw data for additional data analysis. Although frequently viewed as one of the most informative measures of adherence and a "near" gold standard for monitoring medication intake in ambulatory patients,[15] more than 10 years of past experience using commercially available electronic monitors recommends that additional steps be taken to facilitate the processing of EEM information once accumulated to enhance its accuracy. While improvements in design have made today's electronic monitors more durable than past models, verbal and written instructions to patients on the handling and care of the monitors prior to use during the observation period may further obviate device failures attributable to patient misuse (eg., wearing activity monitors while swimming, placing medication monitors in dishwashers) and lessen the inaccuracy of recorded data due to improper handling by the patient (eg., removing multiple doses for later administration, leaving the monitor cap off the medication vial, storing additional medications with the medication to be monitored, variable placement of the activity monitor, not wearing the activity monitor during waking hours). Nonetheless, information should be collected concurrently with the use of the monitor regarding the period of time the subject was to be monitored (eg., start and stop dates and times), the time intervals of monitor usage, and, if monitoring medication-taking behavior, the comprehensive history of the medications to be monitored. In particular, subjects should be queried on monitor usage to insure that instructions are being followed. This should be accomplished periodically, rather than at the end of observation, to avoid recall errors and to correct instances of improper use before the conclusion of observation. Periods of time when the monitor is not in use should be documented along with their rationale (eg., hospitalizations, physician-scheduled regimen holidays, physical activity during bathing or other water activities when the monitor could not be worn). To prevent data loss in the event of the failure or loss of the monitor, devices should be downloaded intermittently during the period of observation. For example, in the clinical trial presented earlier, medication monitors were downloaded at each visit to the project office at the key assessment times at which point a project nurse conducted a pill count. In medical studies where the subject is responsible for refilling the vial with the medication being tracked, subjects should be instructed to either make note of the date and time of the refill, or to replenish when administering the last dose of the previous refill, to avoid additional erroneous actuations. For those studies tracking medication regimens that are prescribed by the subject's personal physician, changes in the treatment being monitored, either in the number of administrations to be taken or a change from current treatment to an alternative regimen, should be recorded. Using such supplementary information, amendments may be made to the event listing to enhance the accuracy of the EEM data to correct for the invalid recordings through the substantiated filtering of events and for changes in prescriptions and nonuse of the monitor by updating the values of the denominator of adherence indices (eg., number of prescribed administrations, number of days prescribed).

Describing Treatment Adherence Using EEM Data

Once properly structured for statistical analysis, EEM data can be examined using any number of graphical and statistical methods that have been proposed to describe adherence for the individual patient or group of patients.[14,15,19] To date, much of the work pertaining to the analysis of EEM adherence data has been developed with medication monitors in mind; however, most of these methodological developments may be straightforwardly extended to handle other types of EEM data, such as physical activity recordings from accelerometers. Indeed, many of these methods can also be applied to data obtained from daily self-report measures where the date and time of an event are recorded (eg., daily diaries, recalls). Some of the approaches may be readily implemented using the software available from the monitor's manufacturer, while other methods require programming capabilities on the user's part.

Adherence Indices

A variety of simple summary measures, typically reported as percentages or proportions, have been proposed to help capture the adherence information contained in EEM data.[14,19,24] Some of these adherence indices emphasize the *number of events*, while others try to incorporate information concerning the actual *timing of events*. Regardless of the index constructed, critical to the retention of information contained in the electronic event data is the length of the time period used for summarization. Aggregating over long periods of time may result in a loss of information related to differences in medication-taking behavior due to the time of day, day of the week, as well as the seasons of the year.[17,19]

Percentage of Prescribed Administration Taken

One of the most popular indices used to summarize medication-taking behavior is to count the number of prescribed administrations or "doses" that were taken in a defined period of observation (ie, pill count).[2,10,14,19,24,25] In a similar vein, one can use electronic event monitoring data to summarize the percentage of prescribed administrations that were taken by a subject over a defined monitoring period of M_i days as

$$A_{1,i} = \frac{\sum_{j=1}^{m_i} a_{ij}}{\sum_{j=1}^{m_i} f_{ij}} \times 100 = \frac{K_i}{(f_i \times M_i)} \times 100 = \frac{K_i}{P_i} \times 100, \qquad [1]$$

where i indexes a particular subject ($i = 1, \ldots, N$), j indexes a specific day of observation for a subject ($j = 1, \ldots, M_i$), a_{ij} is the number of administrations taken by the i-th subject on the j-th day, f_{ij} is the prescribed daily frequency of administration for the i-th subject on the j-th day (and if the frequency of daily administration is fixed throughout the period of monitoring, then $f_{ij} = f_i$), K_i is the total number of administrations taken (ie, the total number of events recorded during the observation period), and P_i is the number of administrations prescribed during the observation period (ie, the product of the prescribed fixed daily frequency, f_i, and the total number of days in the observation period, M_i). Multiplication by 100 places an index formulated as a proportion on a percentage scale. Values for [1] may range from 0 to $+\infty$ (positive infinity), where values near 0% suggest underdosing, those approaching 100% indicate good adherence, and those greater than 100% point to overdosing.

Vrijens et al.[19] highlighted the advantages and disadvantages of this summary measure. In particular, [1] provides an estimate of subject's average daily adherence. Although [1] can signal a general tendency toward underdosing or overdosing during the observation period, it fails to capture any information on precise timing of administrations (ie, time recorded for cap openings/closings). For example, a subject who registers all his or her prescribed administrations for the time interval in a single day would be viewed as perfectly adherent to the regimen, having a value of 100% for [1], as would a subject who consistently overdoses and then underdoses from day to day.

Percentage of Days with the Prescribed Number of Administrations

In an attempt to improve upon [1], researchers have considered the evaluation of adherence on a daily basis.[10,14,15,19,24] Each day a subject is classified as either adherent ($=1$) or not ($=0$) given the number of prescribed administrations taken. The resulting series of binary variables is summed and a ratio is formed of the total number of days with the prescribed intake (D_i) to the total number of days monitored (M_i) as

$$A_{2,i} = \frac{\sum_{j=1}^{N_i} I\{a_{ij} = f_{ij}\}}{M_i} \times 100 = \frac{D_i}{M_i} \times 100, \qquad [2]$$

where $I\{\cdot\}$ is an indicator function taking on the values of 1, if the condition is satisfied, or 0 if the condition is not met. The definition of beginning of day is traditionally set at 12:00:00 a.m. and ends at 11:59:59 p.m. local time; however, when monitoring adherence on a daily basis, this definition is typically modified to accommodate subjects having nighttime schedules. In particular, the 24-hour dosing day is often defined, relative to the patient's local time, as starting at 3:00:00 a.m. and ending at 2:59:59 a.m. the following day, since 3:00:00 a.m. represents a time of low dosing or activity for the typical subject, thus minimizing aliasing errors.[15,26] When expressed as a percentage, this summary statistic ranges from 0% to 100%, with values near 0% indicating no adherence and values near 100% suggesting perfect adherence. This summary statistic [2] attempts to depict some aspects of timing in terms of days, but fails to incorporate the actual timing of administrations within the day. Furthermore, [2] treats the days of underdosing and overdosing similarly, giving each zero weight.

Percentage of Drug Holidays and Days of Underdosings and Overdosings

In an effort to reflect the occurrence of drug holidays (ie, no administrations recorded for one or more consecutive days) and days of underdosings and overdosings, variations on [2] have been proposed[10,15,19] as

$$
A_{3a,i} = \frac{\sum_{j=1}^{N_i} I\{a_{ij} = 0\}}{M_i} \times 100 = \frac{H_i}{M_i} \times 100 \tag{3}
$$

$$
A_{3b,i} = \frac{\sum_{j=1}^{N_i} I\{a_{ij} < f_{ij}\}}{M_i} \times 100 = \frac{U_i}{M_i} \times 100 \tag{4}
$$

$$
A_{3c,i} = \frac{\sum_{j=1}^{N_i} I\{a_{ij} > f_{ij}\}}{M_i} \times 100 = \frac{O_i}{M_i} \times 100 \tag{5}
$$

where the binary variables indicate whether either no administrations were recorded on the j-th day (ie, a drug holiday occurred) ($=1$), whether underdosing occurred on day j (ie, less than the correct number of administrations were recorded) ($=1$), or whether overdosing occurred on day j (ie, more than the correct number of administrations were recorded) ($=1$); or for each of these cases the correct number of administrations were recorded ($=0$); and H_i, U_i, and O_i represent the total number of days of medication holidays, underdosing, and overdosing during the observation period, respectively. For regimens taken once daily, [3] will equal [4] if drug holidays are enumerated on a daily basis. When expressed as percentages, values near 100% indicate poor adherence for each of these summary statistics.

Each of these measures overlooks the exact timing of administrations, but takes into account the extent of different protocol deviations with respect to adherence. Vrijens et al.[19] noted that the numerator of [3] can be modified to consider drug holidays of a particular length. de Klerk et al.[15] combined [2] and [5] to reflect the "percentage of days on which at least the prescribed dosage was taken."

Percentage of Administrations with Correct Timing and Percentage of Days with Correct Number of Administrations and Timing

The previously described summary statistics focus on the number of medication events and more or less ignore information concerning the timing of the medication events. Modified versions of [1] and [2] have been proposed,[14,24,25] where the numerators also take into account the timing of administrations by considering the relative timing of adjacent medication events, ie, the inter-administration, or inter-dose, interval. Let t_{ik} be the time of the k-th administration for the i-th subject and set the lower (L_i^*) and upper (U_i^*) values for the dosing window, then define

$$A_{4,i} = \frac{\sum_{k=1}^{K_i} I\{L_i^* \le (t_{i,k+1} - t_{ik}) \le U_i^*\}}{K_i - 1} \times 100 = \frac{T_i}{K_i - 1} \times 100, \quad [6]$$

$$A_{5,i} = \frac{\sum_{j=1}^{N_i} I\{a_{ij} = f_{ij} \cap I_j[L_i^* \le (t_{i,k+1}) \le U_i^*]\}}{M_i} \times 100 = \frac{G_i}{M_i} \times 100, \quad [7]$$

where the binary variables, $I\{\cdot\}$ and $I_j\{\cdot\}$, denote respectively whether the k-th inter-administration interval is optimal ($=1$), whether the correct number of administrations occurred on the j-th day, each having near optimal inter-administration intervals ($=1$), or not ($=0$); T_i is the total number of administrations having near optimal inter-administration intervals during the observation period; and G_i is the total number of days with correct number of administrations, each having near optimal inter-administration interval. A variation on [6] uses the number of prescribed inter-administration intervals (i.e., $\sum_{j=1}^{N_i} f_{ij} - 1 = P_i - 1$) to yield the "percentage of prescribed administrations taken on schedule." The determination of a "near" optimal interval between administrations is based on the prescribed daily frequency of administration with a clinically reasonable window of medication-taking about the targeted time of administration. A standard convention is to set the dosing window within 20% to 25% of the prescribed interval;[14,19,27,28] however, more conservative grace periods are sometimes used in cardiovascular research and practice. For example, Rudd et al.[24] used a window of 10 to 14 hours for anti-hypertensive regimens prescribed twice daily, and Kruse et al.[25] specified a window 24 ± 15% hours for either a cardiac glycoside or diuretic regimen prescribed once a day. When expressed as percentages, values for [6] and [7] range from 0% to 100%, with values near 100% indicating adherence.

Although these adherence measures [6, 7] incorporate information on timing when evaluating correctness of intake and its regularity, each summary statistic fails to distinguish between underdosing and overdosing. Additionally, the determination of the optimal inter-administration interval may be problematic.

Percentage of Short and Long Inter-Administration Intervals

Using the information contained in the inter-administration intervals, Vrijens et al.[19] derived indices, which address the issues of underdosing and overdosing defined as

$$A_{6a,i} = \frac{\sum_{k=1}^{K_i} I\{(t_{i,k+1} - t_{ik}) < L_i^*\}}{K_i - 1} \times 100 \qquad [8]$$

$$A_{6b,i} = \frac{\sum_{k=1}^{K_i} I\{(t_{i,k+1} - t_{ik}) > U_i^*\}}{K_i - 1} \times 100 \qquad [9]$$

Percentage values of [8] and [9] range from 0% to 100%, where values near 0% point to overdosing and underdosing, respectively.

Unlike [6], [8] and [9] together provide information on the extent of underdosing and overdosing based on the exact timing of administrations. However, like [6], both require the determination of clinically meaningful lower and upper bounds for the identification of inter-administration intervals that are excessively short or long.

Variability in the Time of Administration

To capture information about the precise timing of medication administrations, Vrijens et al.[19] proposed a summary statistic for adherence to a once-daily regimen as the ratio of the sum of the absolute deviations between the median administration time based on a 24-hour clock and the timing of administrations to the number of prescribed days. This index may be generalized for more complex regimens (ie, regimens taken more than once daily) as

$$A_{7l,i} = \frac{\sum_{l=1}^{f_{ij}} \sum_{k=1}^{K_i} |t_{ikl} - median(i,l)|}{P_i}, \qquad [10]$$

where l indexes the number of times per day the medication was prescribed ($l = 1, \ldots, f_{ij}$), $median(i,l)$ is the median time for the l-th daily administration based on a 24-hour clock for the i-th subject, and k indexes the l-th administrations that happened at time t_{ikl}. For medications prescribed once daily, Vrijens et al.[19] recommended that $t_{ikl} - median(i,l)$ should be set to 12 hours if no administrations occurred on a day. In like fashion, to capture the variability in timing pattern related to underdosing for more complex regimens, t_{ikl} may be fixed at $24/(l+1)$ hours when underdosing occurs. Values of [10] near zero are suggestive of good adherence.

Unlike summary measures described in [1] through [5], [10] uses information about the exact timing of administrations. Underdosing and overdosing are considered in [10] and are reflected by additional variability in administration timing about median timing(s). Vrijens et al.[19] cited key disadvantages to this summary statistic that lessen the merit of this index: it is not proportional to the number of administrations taken and the absolute deviation is symmetric about zero.

Percentiles of Inter-Administration Intervals

Intra-subject percentiles can also be used to summarize the variability of inter-administration intervals among subjects prescribed the same frequency of administration.[19] Based on the length of the inter-administration interval, various percentiles may be calculated as

$$A_{8,i} = P_x(t_{i,k+1} - t_{ik}), \qquad [11]$$

where $P_x(\cdot)$ denotes the x-th percentile. If the frequency of administration varies from between subjects as well as within subjects as in medical studies where the subject's personal physician controls the prescription for the medication being monitored, then subjects should be stratified by their daily administration frequency before examining percentiles.

Vrijens et al.[19] found in their empirical work for a once daily regimen that the extreme percentiles, $P_5(\cdot)$ and $P_{95}(\cdot)$, tended to identify different individuals, ie, the subjects having small inter-administration intervals at the 5th percentiles were not the same as those having large intervals at the 95th percentiles. This suggests that extreme percentiles may provide additional information concerning adherence. On the other hand, the median inter-administration interval, $P_{50}(\cdot)$, tended to have low inter-subject variability, making it a poor candidate for portraying adherence.

Therapeutic Coverage

By taking into account the duration of action of a medication, the percentage of time a subject was receiving therapeutic benefit from the medication may be determined.[14,29,30] The *duration of action* estimates the interval of time that a medication was active in an individual. Information concerning a medication's duration is available in the literature from the manufacturer or listed in the Physician's Desk Reference and is approximately inversely related to the frequency of administration (eg, 12 hours would be the approximate duration of action for a medication prescribed twice per day). Once taken, a medication provides therapeutic coverage for a patient throughout the medication's duration of action. Periods of uncovered time result when there is a delay in medication-taking. Intervals of time preceding the first administration in the period of time being considered for analysis that are larger than the duration of action are treated as uncovered time, while initial periods that are shorter that the duration of action are assumed to be covered. Overlaps in coverage are counted as covered time. The therapeutic coverage is calculated as

$$A_{9,i} = \frac{C_i}{AP_i} \times 100, \qquad [12]$$

where C_i is total time therapeutically covered in the period of analysis for i-th subject and AP_i is the total time in the defined "analysis period." When expressed as a percentage, values of [12] range from 0% to 100%, where percentages approaching 0% suggest poor therapeutic coverage (ie, gaps in medication coverage).

Therapeutic coverage takes into account both the duration of action of a drug and timing of administrations and thus translates adherence data to pharmacodynamic scaling.[29] The above definition [12], however, does not take into consideration periods of overlap, where overdosing may be occurring. Variations on this definition of therapeutic coverage have been proposed, which penalize both undercoverage and overcoverage,[18] counting only periods of medication coverage with no overlap. Additionally, in a manner analogous to [4] and [5], individual measures, which distinguish between undercoverage, and overcoverage, may be formulated.

Graphical Displays

In general, graphs can serve as excellent visual summaries of medication-taking behavior.[14] For a single individual, time plots, long used in time series analysis, can be extremely effective at depicting behaviors over time. The event time, or "chronology", plot, where medication events are charted as a function of the time of event occurrence based on a 24-hour clock over the days or dates of monitoring, can illuminate patterns in the timing of events that may signal problems with medication-taking, which may not always be apparent from summary indices computed for the individual. Plotting symbols or marks, distinguishing the specific days of the week, can further help to identify whether specific adherence problems (eg., unscheduled holidays, underdosing, overdosing) occur on particular days of the week. Calendar-style charts, where the number of daily administrations or administrations with correct inter-administration intervals is recorded in calendar format, can also be informative for individual patterns over time and may more clearly display gross adherence problems over longer periods of observation than chronology plots, although information about the exact timing of administrations is lost.

For groups of subjects, each of the adherence indices described in the previous section can be displayed using conventional graphical displays (eg., histograms, box plots, quantile-quantile plots) to discern trends univariately in EEM adherence data. Scatterplots and scatterplot matrices, where bivariate scatterplots are displayed side-by-side in a matrix format, may be utilized to visualize multidimensional EEM adherence data. Loess plots may be used to nonparametrically assess the functional form of the bivariate relationship between adherence measures, outcomes, and covariates. For large groups of individuals, de Klerk et al.[15] devised a spread-sheet method of tabulating selected features of each subject's medication-taking behavior (eg., prescribed medication being monitored, frequency counts for duration of unscheduled medication holidays, duration of monitoring), with the subject rows being rank-ordered on a variable reflecting the degree of correspondence with prescribed regimen (eg., percentage of days with prescribed intake). This method, which compactly structures an individual's adherence history relative to other subjects being monitored, can greatly "facilitate the identification of dosing correlates of clinically important events."[15]

To illustrate the utility of these descriptive methods, especially when used in conjunction, EEM data from the adherence clinical trial previously described was examined, considering an entire observation period of 16 weeks (B to M2). Programs were written using standard statistical software (SAS for Windows, version 8.1, SAS Institute, Inc.,

Cary, NC) to derive the selected adherence indices considered in this empirical study. Plots were generated using graphics facilities supported within statistical packages (S-PLUS 2000 Professional, MathSoft, Inc., Seattle, WA; SPSS for Windows, version 10.0.5, SPSS, Inc., Chicago, IL). (Sample programs are available for download at *http://curly.nursing.pitt.edu*.) Since medication was to be taken once daily, the expected number of prescribed days or administrations was 112, and a dosing window of 24 ± 4 hours between subsequent administrations was chosen (ideal time ± 15%). The choice of this dosing window is supported by Schwed et al.,[31] who established a dosing window of 24 ± 4 hours for lipid-lowering therapy prescribed once per day. Inter-administra-

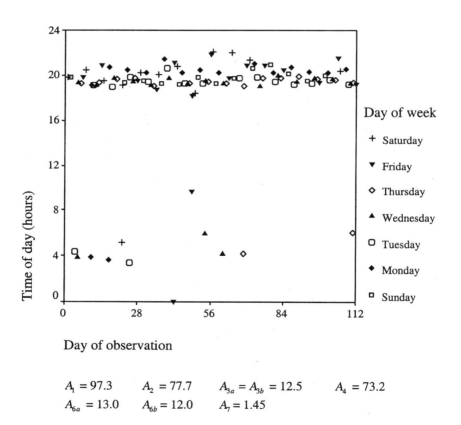

$$A_1 = 97.3 \qquad A_2 = 77.7 \qquad A_{3a} = A_{3b} = 12.5 \qquad A_4 = 73.2$$
$$A_{6a} = 13.0 \qquad A_{6b} = 12.0 \qquad A_7 = 1.45$$

Figure 1. Event time plot of medication-taking behavior over a 16-week period of observation for an oral medication regimen prescribed once per day to be taken in the evening and values for selected summary measures for EEM measured adherence. (Note that the time of day axis has been shifted 3 hours to accommodate nighttime schedules.)

tion intervals that were less than 20 hours were defined as "too short", while inter-administration intervals greater than 28 hours were considered as "too long."

Figure 1 shows an event time plot of the oral medication-taking behavior of an individual subject over the 112-day observation period. Although not always apparent given the density of the events displayed, some variability in the timing of events and possible instances of overdosing on certain days of the week can be observed. Figure 2 illustrates more clearly the actual variability in the timing of the administrations. Based on this histogram, it is evident that medication-taking by this subject tends to cluster around 20:00 hours (or in reality 17:00 hours, since the time of day is shifted by 3 hours to better accommodate nighttime schedules), with relatively few administrations occurring at earlier times of the day. Examination of the adherence indices reported

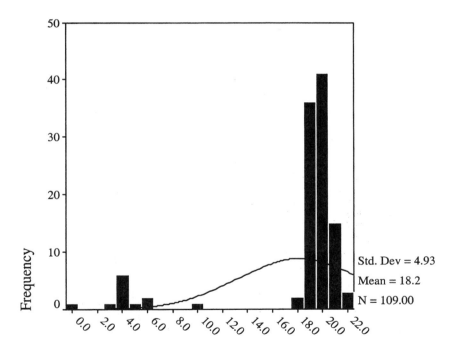

Time of administration (in hours)

Figure 2. Histogram of administration times over a 16-week period of observation for an oral medication regimen prescribed once per day to be taken in the evening. (Note that the time of day axis has been shifted 3 hours to accommodate nighttime schedules.)

in Figure 1 lends further support to this conclusion, but provides additional insight as to the extent of errors in dosing.

Exploratory data analysis conducted on each of the summary statistics considered revealed significantly skewed distributions as typified by the percentage of days with the prescribed number of administrations (A_2) shown in Figure 3. Examination of the descriptive statistics for the selected indices reported in Table 1 confirms this finding when comparing the estimated means and medians. These findings suggest that, based on EEM adherence data, subjects appear to be fairly adherent over the 12-week period of observation with almost half the sample (49.7%) having between 80% to 100% of days with the prescribed number of administrations (skewness $= -1.42$, kurtosis $= 1.28$). Application of base 10 logarithmic transformation to the reflected data resulted in an empirical distribution which more closely approximates a normal distribution. In general, data transformations can in many cases improve the distributional properties sufficiently to permit the reliable use of standard parametric methods for estimation and hypothesis testing. In this context, the geometric mean [ie, anti-logarithm (mean of log transformed variables)] is a good substitute for the arithmetic mean.[32]

If data are not amenable to transformation (ie, do not "normalize"), then nonparametric methods may be used, or alternatively, cutpoints may be considered. Attention must be given when choosing cutpoints to categorize or group individuals on "similar" adherence behavior. As a general rule, clinically meaningful cutoffs should be applied rather than values that are suggested *post hoc*. Data-driven cutpoints can be

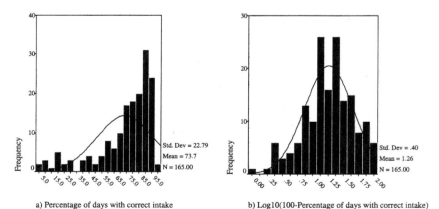

a) Percentage of days with correct intake   b) Log10(100-Percentage of days with correct intake)

Figure 3. Histograms of the frequency distribution of the percentage of days with correct intake with superimposed normal curve based on sample statistics: a) Original scaling ($A_{2,i}$); b) Log-transformed after reflecting adherence values [ie, $\log_{10}(100 - A_{2,i})$].

Table 1

Descriptive Statistics for Selected Summary Measures for Adherence

Adherence Index	Mean	SD	Median	Interquartile Range
Percentage of prescribed administrations taken ($A_{1,i}$)	83.8	23.2	92.0	19.2
Percentage of days with the prescribed number of administrations ($A_{2,i}$)	73.7	22.8	80.4	23.7
Percentage of drug holidays ($A_{3a,i}$)	21.5	22.6	14.3	19.6
Percentage of prescribed administrations taken with correct time ($A_{4,i}$)	64.5	25.2	72.3	33.9
Percentage of short inter-administration intervals ($A_{6a,i}$)	11.3	8.8	8.7	9.3
Percentage of long inter-administration intervals ($A_{6b,i}$)	16.4	16.2	12.0	14.7
Variability of the time of administration ($A_{7l,i}$)	1.7	1.2	1.4	1.2

SD = standard deviation.

misleading, yielding statistically significant findings where differences really do not exist.[33] From the standpoint of adherence management in a clinical practice, Insull[34] recommended three graded categories of adherence, empirically supported by the observation of common frequency distributions for EEM measured adherence across five treatment modalities: adherent ($\geq$80%), partially adherent (20%—79%), and nonadherent (<20%).[35] Application of these cutpoints to A_2 yields the marginal percentages of 5%, 43%, and 52%, as adherent, partially adherent, and nonadherent, respectively, comparable to Rudd's[35] findings.

When expressed in terms of their absolute values or magnitude of the relationship, the bivariate correlation coefficients among the summary measures ranged from 0.10 to 0.97, with the strongest correlations being observed among those indices that give greater emphasis to the number rather than timing of events. Closer examination of the scatterplot for A_2 versus A_1 reveals that although highly correlated (r = 0.79, P < 0.001) A_1 is almost always consistently higher than A_2, suggesting a possible overestimation of adherence when only the counts of events are considered. Somewhat smaller correlations were found

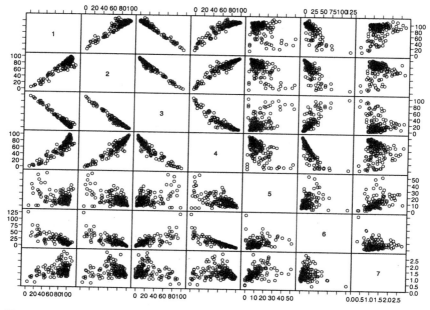

Figure 4. Scatterplot matrix of selected summary statistics for adherence aggregated over a 16-week observation period: 1) A_1, 2) A_2, 3) $A_{3a} = A_{3b}$, 4) A_4, 5) A_{6a}, 6) A_{6b}, and 7) A_7.

between summary measures focusing on numbers of events with those emphasizing timing of events as well as among only those indices targeting timing. This finding suggests that less shared variance between these types of measures and that additional information concerning adherence (ie, number of events versus timing) is being brought to light (See Figure 4).

Modeling EEM Adherence Data

Besides yielding indices suitable for characterizing medication-taking history for a single patient and groups of subjects, these derived variables can be used as dependent variables when statistically modeling adherence behavior for groups of subjects to assess adherence to treatments in clinical research. Such modeling techniques allow the researcher to compactly summarize the relationship between adherence as an outcome of random and fixed patient factors, as well as providing a framework for statistical inference. When contrasting groups and ignoring the change of adherence over time, standard comparative procedures, such as analysis of variance (ANOVA) procedures (eg., ANOVA, ANCOVA, MANOVA) may be used. A key assumption underlying all analysis of variance methods is that the data are normally distributed (ie, the model errors have a normal distribution), or are amenable to normalizing transformations. If summary measures cannot be transformed, then analogous nonparametric approaches could be considered. Or alternatively, clinically meaningful cutpoints may be used, avoiding data-based values. If data are transformed this way, either binary, or ordinal, logistic regression may be used to model the binary or graded adherence categories.[36] Furthermore when using any of these statistical methods, data are assumed to be complete with no missing data for either the dependent or independent variables. If data are missing, imputation (single or multiple) or the more ad hoc methods of handling missing data (eg., listwise deletion, pairwise deletion) that are available in most statistical packages may be used.[37,38] Before implementing either of these techniques, a thorough assessment of patterns of missing data should be undertaken to try to elucidate the underlying missing data mechanism (eg., missing completely at random [MCAR], missing at random [MAR], and non-ignorable missingness).

Although easy to use and familiar, the cross-sectional view of the data produced by the analysis of global adherence indices fails to capture adherence patterns over time. Several studies have investigated the impact of the aggregation of adherence data and method of summarization.[17–19] Their results indicated that summary measures that account for the relative timing of doses tend to be more informative than measures that consider only the number of daily doses. Nevertheless, both Rohay et al.[18] and Vrijens et al.[19] concluded that the summarization of data may lead to a substantial loss of information on adherence patterns over time and a subsequent loss of power when investigating time effects for adherence.

Extensions of ANOVA methods have been considered which attempt to capture the within-subject variation lost through aggregation. Diggle et al.[39] presented a number of ANOVA strategies that have been adapted to model longitudinal data (eg., time-by-time ANOVA, derived variables, and repeated measure ANOVA). Although more informative about the evolution of adherence over time, these more longitudinal ANOVA based strategies still possess many of the same limitations as the standard one-way ANOVA approach (eg., normality, complete data). In particular, repeated measures ANOVA has restrictive assumptions regarding the structure of the covariance matrix of the repeated measures, which limits its utility for the longitudinal analysis of EEM adherence data. Covariance pattern models are parametric repeated measures models that allow for different covariance structures among the repeated measures.[40] With this approach, investigators can fit competing models with a variety of covariance structures and then choose that model which best fits the adherence data. Unlike the ANOVA methods, covariance pattern models can handle missing data due to its underpinnings in mixed modeling methodology. These methods have also been extended to include other members of the class of generalized linear models allowing for the modeling of categorical outcomes.

Of late, these and other longitudinal data analytic methods (ie, marginal modeling, random effects modeling) have been utilized to better capture the temporal evolution of adherence.[16,19,20,41] To model binary adherence data of a once daily regimen of anti-hypertensive medication, Vrijens et al.[19] fitted conditional and marginal models and tested for differences in adherence measured by EEM between subjects randomized to one of two adherence-enhancing strategies: home blood pressure monitoring versus no monitoring. Results of the conditional model suggested that current adherence behavior was dependent on past adherence behavior and that adherence was lower in the no home monitoring group. To better depict the effect of randomized assignment, Vrijens et al.[19] next used marginal modeling with generalized estimating equations[42] and found similar, albeit more interpretable, results. A limitation to the generalized estimating equations approach is that it cannot handle long time series of repeated measurements. To address this limitation, Smith et al.[16] modeled binary adherence data assuming a subject's likelihood to adhere at any given time is governed by the value of an underlying latent stationary continuous process and covariates at that time.

To illustrate the use of various modeling strategies one might use when analyzing EEM data, consider again the EEM data collected from the adherence clinical trial. Comparisons using summary measures aggregating over the 16 weeks of EEM data (B to M2) revealed no statistically significant differences ($P > 0.05$) among adherence treatment groups (UC, HT, HT + PS), similar to what Vrijens et al.[19] found in their application. When comparisons were made using standard repeated measures ANOVA analysis using 2 week summary measures about the key assessment points of B, M1, and M2, significant time effects ($P < 0.05$) for all summary measures were found; however no significant interactions were detected ($P > 0.05$). Use of covariance pattern models, where models were fitted assuming different patterns of correlational structure between equally spaced repeated assessments of EEM adherence, indicated that the correlation or covariance between adherence assessments tended to decay within increasing time between assessments, indicative of first-order autoregressive structure for EEM adherence. Because of the length of the time series, longitudinal data analytic models based on daily measures of adherence were unfeasible. However, the longitudinal modeling of weekly summary measures showed significant effects for time ($P < 0.05$) and marginally significant effects for the interaction of time and ACT group ($P < 0.10$) using either marginal and random effects modeling.

Summary

In conclusion, a myriad of data analytic methods for adherence data, and more recently EEM data, have been proposed in the literature, some of which have been reviewed and expanded upon here. For descriptive purposes, summary statistics can provide easy to understand measures of adherence with respect to the number of administration events and timing of events. These indices may be modified to incorporate dosage taken at each administration (ie, Nebulizer Chronlog for inhaled medications) or the level of physical activity (ie, accelerometers) and can also be applied to data collection using self-report formats (ie, diaries, recalls). Those adherence indices, which integrate the number and timing of events, tend to be more sensitive to instances of nonadherence and correlate more strongly with clinical outcome (than those that emphasize only the number of events). Unfortunately, as Vrijens et al.[19] pointed out, no one summary statistic sufficiently captures the information contained in longitudinally measured electronic event data. However, as an examination of the formulas for the adherence indices would indicate and as Vrijens et al.[19] observed, there may be a large amount of shared variance between some adherence indices, pointing to instances of near redundancy with little new information being contributed. These issues indicate a need for using summary measures jointly, giving judicious consideration for which to include based on the study's research aims and treatment's properties, and/ or for refining the level of aggregation to capture the variability of adherence over time.

Time-based graphical displays, such as chronology plots and calendar-type charts, can be utilized for describing an individual patient's dosing pattern over time. To visually portray a group's adherence behavior, exploratory plots (eg., histograms, box plots, scatterplots) of derived adherence indices can be used. In fact, when descriptive methods are used in tandem (eg., graphs accompanied by reports of adherence indices as either an individual's values or a group's descriptive statistics), problems with adherence can typically be uncovered.

As mentioned, aggregating EEM data over time simplifies the structure of data, but removes information related to time effects. Hence, the researcher must balance the parsimony of data structure with the retention of possibly valuable information. If the evaluation of change in adherence over time is of interest, then repeated measures, or longitudinal data analytic, methods are required. Each of these approaches was developed in light of certain assumptions that affect the conduct of data screening and ultimately the validity of results. Conventional repeated measure approaches (ie, repeated measures ANOVA) tend to be very limited, while longitudinal methods tend to be more flexible and can better accommodate the complex structure of EEM data (ie, missing data due to subject attrition, intermittent missing data due to nonuse or failure of the monitor, correlated measurement errors, nonnormal error distributions). So long as the individual time series of events are not too long, longitudinal models (eg., marginal modeling, random effects modeling) are good candidates for capturing the temporal variability of adherence. Indeed, these approaches are generally more informative than standard repeated measures methods, can be viable with some forms of missing data (MCAR and MAR), can incorporate time-varying covariates, can handle both continuous and categorical dependent variables, and can allow for error distributions other than normal (eg., binomial, Poisson).

References

1. Feinstein A. Clinical Biostatistics: Biostatistical problems in "compliance bias." *Clin Pharmacol Ther* 1974;16:846–857.
2. Goldsmith CH. The effect of compliance distributions on therapeutic trials. In Hayes RB, Taylor DW, Sackett DL (eds): Compliance in Health Care. Baltimore: The Johns Hopkins University Press, 1979;297–308.
3. Rand CS, Weeks K. Measuring adherence with medication regimens in clinical care and research. In Shumaker SA, Schron EB, Ockene JK, et al. (eds): The Handbook of Health Behavior Change (2nd ed.) New York: Springer Publishing Co, Inc, 1998;114–132.
4. Freedman LS. The effect of partial noncompliance on the power of a clinical trial. *Control Clin Trials* 1990;11:157–168.
5. Kastrissios H, Flowers NT, Blaschke TF. Introducing medical students to medication compliance. *Clin Pharmacol Ther* 1996;59:577–582.
6. Dunbar J. Adherence measures and their utility. *Control Clin Trials* 1984;5: 515–521.
7. Gordis L. Conceptual and methodologic problems in measuring patient compliance In Hayes RB, Taylor DW, Sackett DL (eds): Compliance in Health Care. Baltimore: The Johns Hopkins University Press, 1979;23–45.
8. Dunbar-Jacob J, Sereika S, Rohay JM, et al. Electronic methods in assessing adherence to medical regimens. In Krantz DS, Baum A (eds): Technology and Methods in Behaviroral Medicine. Mahwah, NJ: Lawrence Erlbaum Associates Inc, 1998;95–113.
9. Cramer JA, Mattson RH, Prevey ML, et al. How often is medication taken as prescribed? A novel assessment technique. *JAMA* 1989;261:3273–3277.
10. Kruse W, Weber E. Dynamics of drug regimen compliance—its assessment by microprocessor-based monitoring. *Eur J Clin Pharmacol* 1990;38:561–565.

11. Pullar T, Feely M. Problems of compliance with drug treatment: New solutions? *Pharm J* 1990; 245:213–215.
12. Urquhart J. Clinical impact of partial patient compliance. *Cardiovasc Rev Rep* 1990;11:11–15.
13. Matthews CE, Freedson PS. Field trial of a three-dimensional activity monitor: Comparison with self report. *Med Sci Sports Exerc* 1995;27(7):1071–1078.
14. Kastrissios H, Blaschke TF. Medication compliance as a feature in drug development. *Annu Rev Toxicol* 1997;37:451–475.
15. de Klerk E, van der Linden S, van der Heijde D, et al. Facilitated analysis of data on drug regimen compliance. *Stat Med* 1997;1653–1664.
16. Smith D, Diggle PJ. Compliance in an anti-hypertension trial: A latent process model for binary longitudinal data. *Statistics in Medicine* 1998;17:357–370.
17. Rohay JM, Marsh G, Sereika S, et al. The effects of aggregation on medication compliance history in repeated measures ANOVA: A simulation study. *Control Clin Trials* 1994;15(3S):98S.
18. Rohay JM, Dunbar-Jacob J, Sereika S, et al. The impact of method of calculation of electronically monitored adherence data. *Control Clin Trials* 1996; 17(2S):82S-83S.
19. Vrijens B, Goetghebeur E. Comparing compliance patterns between randomized treatments. *Control Clin Trials* 1997;18:187–203.
20. Girard P, Blaschke TF, Kastrissios H, et al. A Markov mixed effect regression model for drug compliance. *Stat Med* 1998;17:2313–2333.
21. Vrijens B, Goetghebeur E. The impact of compliance in pharmacokinetic studies. *Stat Methods Med Res* 1999;8:247–262.
22. Sereika S, Dunbar-Jacob J, Rand C, et al. Adherence in clinical trials: A collaborative investigation of self-reported and electronically monitored adherence. Paper presented at the 19th annual meeting of the Society for Clinical Trials, 1998, Atlanta, Georgia.
23. Schlenk EA, Dunbar-Jacob J, Sereika S, et al. Comparability of daily diaries and accelerometers in exercise adherence in fibromyalgia syndrome. *Measurement in Physical Education and Exercise Science* 2000;4:133.
24. Rudd P, Ahmed S, Zachary V, et al. Antihypertensive drug trials: Contributions from medication monitors. In Cramer JA, Spilker B (eds): Patient Compliance in Medical Practice and Clinical Trials. New York: Raven Press Ltd, 1991;283–299.
25. Kruse W, Koch-Gwinner P, Nikolaus T, et al. Measurement of drug compliance by continuous electronic monitoring: A pilot study in elderly patients discharged from hospital. *J Am Geriatr Soc* 1992;40:1151–1155.
26. Norell SE, Granstrom PA, Wassen R. A medication monitor and flurorescein techniques designed to study medication behavior. *Acta Ophthalmology* 1980;58,459.
27. Lee JY, Kusek JW, Green PG, et al. Assessing medication adherence by pill count and electronic monitoring in the African American Study of Kidney Disease and Hypertension (AASK) Pilot Study. *Am J Hypertens* 1996;9: 719–725.
28. Paes AHP, Bakker A, Soe-Agnie CJ. Impact of dosage frequency on patient compliance. *Diabetes Care* 1997;20(10):1512–1517.
29. Urquhart J. Therapeutic coverage: A parameter for analyzing the pharmacodynamic impact of partial patient compliance. Program and Abstracts, Society for Clinical Trials/International Society for Clinical Biostatistics, Joint Meeting, Brussels, 1991, 12.

30. APREX Corporation, 1993. MEMS View℠ User's Guide. Fremont, CA, APREX Corporation, pp C-1.
31. Schwed A, Fallab CL, Burnier M, et al. Electronic monitoring of compliance to lipid-lowering therapy in clinical practice. *J Clin Pharmacol* 1999;39: 402–409.
32. Pocock SJ. Clinical Trials: A Practical Approach. New York: John Wiley & Sons Ltd, 1983.
33. Friedman LM, Furberg CD, Demets DL. Fundamentals of Clinical Trials (3rd ed.) St. Louis: Mosby-Year Book Inc, 1996.
34. Insull W. The problem of compliance to cholesterol altering therapy. *J Intern Med* 1997;241:317–325.
35. Rudd P. Compliance with antihypertensive therapy: A shifting paradigm. *Cardiol Rev* 1994;2(5):230–240.
36. Hosmer DW, Lemeshow S. Applied Logistic Regression (2nd ed.) New York: John Wiley & Sons, Inc, 2000.
37. Little RJA, Rubin DB. Statistical Analysis with Missing Data. New York: John Wiley & Sons Inc, 1987.
38. Schafer JL. Analysis of Incomplete Multivariate Data. London, England: Chapman & Hall, 1997.
39. Diggle PJ, Liang KL, Zeger SL. Analysis of Longitudinal Data. Oxford, England: Oxford University Press, 1994.
40. Brown H, Prescott R. Applied Mixed Models in Medicine. Chichester, England: John Wiley and Sons, Ltd, 1999
41. Dunbar-Jacob J, Erlen JA, Schlenk ES, et al. Adherence in chronic disease. In Goepingher J (ed): Volume 18 of Annual Review of Nursing Research: Chronic Illness. New York, NY, Springer: 2000;48–90.
42. Liang KL, Zeger SL. Longitudinal data analysis using generalized linear models. *Biometrika* 1986;73:13–22.

Chapter 10

Self-Report Data

James R. Hebert, ScD, Yunsheng Ma, MD, MPH, Cara B. Ebbeling, PhD, Charles E. Matthews, PhD, and Ira S. Ockene, MD

Introduction

Although issues regarding biases and random errors in individuals' reports of health-related behaviors pertain to just about any self-report measure, we will be using diet as an example for this chapter. We have chosen to do so because various dietary factors are widely thought to be important in cardiovascular disease, and in other conditions that are important causes of morbidity and mortality. Additionally, diet represents a set of ubiquitous "exposures" that may affect health—virtually everybody eats, and most people consume a wide variety of foods. Finally, diet is one of the areas where we have the possibility of using "construct validators" to get a better sense of how well we have measured what we have intended to measure. By "construct validators," we mean phenomena that behave according to physical or biological laws. These would include constructs as simple as the second law of thermodynamics (ie, if caloric intake increases without a compensatory increase in energy expenditure, a person gains weight), or the more complex relationship between changes in consumption of dietary fatty acids and changes in serum lipids.[1–3]

Nearly all epidemiologic research pertaining to diet relies on data obtained from structured questionnaires. By far, the most commonly used of these are food frequency questionnaires (FFQs). FFQs are grid-like instruments in which a list of foods and beverages, usually between

This work was supported by National Institute of Diabetes and Digestive and Kidney Diseases grant DK 52079-02 and National Heart, Lung and Blood Institute, Grant HL 44492.

From: Burke LE, Ockene IS (eds). *Compliance in Healthcare and Research.* Armonk, NY: Futura Publishing Company, Inc.; © 2001.

60 and 120 items, comprise the rows. Columns consist of a defined set of options for selecting the frequency with which the item was consumed over some moderate to long period of time (usually 3 months to a year). Often, additional columns are available for the subject to select the typical portion size of the food that (s)he consumed. Usually, this consists of three columns representing an average "comparison" size, one half as large, and another twice as large. Because of their focus on relatively long time periods, they rely on generic (ie, habitual, long-term) memory of intake patterns rather than memory of specific food encounters. Although originally designed for use in observational studies and validated only in that context,[4–8] FFQs are sometimes used in clinical intervention studies.[9,10]

In addition to FFQs, there are other types of structured questionnaires, including a 7-day dietary recall (7DDR) developed at the University of Massachusetts Medical School specifically for use in dietary intervention trials for individuals with hyperlipidemia.[6] Due to its focus on a relatively short time frame, it relies somewhat on episodic (food encounter-specific) memory rather than exclusively on generic memory. Because the 7DDR was designed specifically to evaluate a dietary intervention to lower serum lipids, this instrument was validated under conditions of an intervention trial.[6]

Besides being list-limited, structured questionnaires such as FFQs or the 7DDR ask about diet over a period during which the respondent cannot be expected to remember all, or even most, of the content of specific food encounters.[11–14] In a typical 3-month period this could easily exceed 500 total encounters, including snacks. Given the perceptions that many people in the United States have with regard to what constitutes a "healthful" diet, certain foods are widely recognized as either "good for you" or "bad for you." Consequently, it is now widely held that some foods, such as fruits and vegetables, are "healthy," whereas other foods, such as those rich in saturated fat, are "unhealthy." By listing these foods, structured questionnaires contain answers that can be construed as "right" ("healthy") or "wrong" ("unhealthy"). The last characteristic of these structured questionnaires that is important to consider is the time frame for establishing intake. By focusing on relatively long time periods, the instruments query diet as a "trait." By trait, we mean a personality characteristic that does not vary greatly over time. When an FFQ asks questions about dietary intake over a period of 3 months or longer, it is calling upon the respondent to report on diet as a basic "component of her/his being." This is in contrast to reporting on a much shorter period that the individual may specify as an atypical diversion from an otherwise "healthy" diet.

In order to assess the utility of these structured questionnaires aiming to establish long-term dietary intake, a limited set of comparison methods typically are used. These include the 24-hour diet recall interview (24HR) and food diaries. These comparison methods tend to be costly, are time intensive, and require a high level of literacy and commitment from the study participant. In contrast to structured questionnaires, these comparison methods are open-ended (ie, they do not specify a particular food list). They also minimize reporting errors due to memory by focusing on very short time intervals, where minimal memory is involved (eg, in keeping food diaries), or where memory is limited to very short-term episodic recall (eg, in completing a 24HR). Rather than a trait, these methods query diet as a "state" (ie, a short-term, temporary "condition of being"). This gives the participant the opportunity to report on having "misbehaved" on a particular day without indicting her- or himself as a person who generally eats an "unhealthy" diet. These characteristics of the short-term comparison methods are in contrast to those of structured questionnaires in which a person is asked to select from a relatively short list of items so as to respond about how s(he) typically eats over a relatively long period of time.

When comparing discrepancies between structured questionnaires and reasonable estimates of metabolic requirements: women tend to underestimate relative to men[15-17]; pregnant women tend to overestimate relative to nonpregnant women[18]; and obese subjects tend to underestimate relative to individuals of normal weight.[19-24] Reporting errors in each of these population subgroups reflect either explicit health messages such as eating to feed one's baby, or implicit ones such as restraining caloric intake to remain thin or lose weight.

The underlying reasons for these differences fall generally into two related categories. The first is social. Eating is a behavior often done in social groups, and the consequences of eating may be readily apparent, including weight gain in violation of an implicit societal censure of obesity, especially in women.[25] The second category is psychological, deriving from the strong emotional attachments that people have to their food.[26] Both social and psychological correlates of reporting errors are conditioned by "cultural" influences, including culture of origin, cultural beliefs pertaining to gender, educational status, and professional affiliation.

A general pattern of consistent underreporting on the structured questionnaires relative to criterion measures, especially by women, constitutes *prima facie* evidence of non-random error, or "bias," in the data. Response sets, representing personality "traits" characteristic of the subject, constitute a particular set of reporting biases that are very well known to psychologists. They express one's reaction to social influences, and are evident in situations that people perceive to be tests.[27-31] The kinds of biases seen in dietary data are consistent with well-known response sets, including social desirability and social approval.[27-31] Social desirability reflects the defensive tendency to respond in such a way as to present oneself more in keeping with socially acceptable modes of behavior and to avoid criticism in a situation perceived to be a test.[27,32] Social approval is a response set which reflects the tendency to actively seek approval in a situation perceived to be a test.[31,33,34] Because of their format, structured questionnaires such as the FFQ and 7DDR often are perceived as tests. Their focus on moderate to long time periods makes the response concerning diet more consistent with reporting diet as a trait.[16,35] Subjects are not asked simply to report on certain episodes of eating that may depart, temporarily, from some ideal. Rather, the report of habitual diet may be perceived as a "test" of their general behavior and therefore may be subject to biases such as those due to social desirability and social approval that are evident in such circumstances.

In order to assess whether or not self-report measures obtained from a structured questionnaire are subject to response set biases such as social desirability or social approval, it is necessary to compare them to some reference standard, such as the 24HR or food diary. The analysis would follow along the lines of a conventional validation study, using regression analysis, and would take the general form described here: the nutrient score derived from the instrument to be tested is fit as the dependent variable; independent variables include the corresponding nutrient score from the comparison method, social approval and social desirability scores, plus any other covariates (eg, measures of body habitus). This modeling approach provides results that are identical to fitting the response set bias measure to the difference derived from subtracting the instrument's nutrient score from the criterion measure. Because comparison methods relying on self-report are not really "gold standards," we will refer to them here as "relative criteria." Therefore, such studies are able only to assess "relative validity." Other studies, employing a biologic measure of some aspect of diet, may assess "true validity."

In previous relative validity studies, comparing data from the 7DDR with the 24HR, we found that social desirability was related to a downward bias in 7DDR-derived energy and fat intakes in women.[16,35] Social approval was found to be associated with upward biases in men.[16] When we used construct validators as a check on the self-reported dietary data, we found that statistical control for social desirability, but not social approval, improved agreement between the measures.[36] This finding has very important implications for intervention studies, because it indicates potential both for refining our ability to assess the effect of an intervention, and for measuring compliance of study subjects. In order to shed light on this important issue, we have examined data from one new study and have re-examined data from one previous study. In addition, we briefly refer to results from other published studies that help put these results into context.

Methods and Results from Selected Studies

The Energy Study

The Energy Study, conducted in Worcester, MA, from June to October 1997, represents the first time that an estimate of total energy expenditure (TEE) based on stable isotope methodology was used as the criterion measure in a study designed to test for specific response set biases. In this study, TEE was measured during a 14-day metabolic period. Subjects completed a 7DDR at baseline and again at day 14. Seven 24HRs were administered during the study.

TEE is almost perfectly correlated with energy intake (EI)[17,37] among individuals who are in energy balance, an assumption that holds extremely well in the vast majority of the population. For example, in the US, despite our relatively high rate of obesity, body weight is extremely well regulated over moderate to long periods, with average weight gains among US adults amounting to less than a half kilogram per year.[38,39,40] For this reason, TEE has been used extensively as a criterion by which to evaluate the validity of EI data in studies relying on self-report methodology.[17,22,23,41,42] The doubly labeled water (DLW) method provides an estimate of TEE over a moderate time period (14 days in this study). It relies on the carbonic anhydrase reaction, which is responsible for equilibrium between oxygen atoms in exhaled carbon dioxide and body water ($CO_2 + H_2O \leftrightarrow H_2CO_3 \leftrightarrow H^+ + HCO_3^-$). As such, it provides a biochemical basis for the use of DLW to measure average daily TEE over a 14-day metabolic period based on the principles of indirect calorimetry. Following oral administration of DLW ($^2H_2{}^{18}O$), the ^{18}O label is eliminated from the body as both carbon dioxide and water, and the deuterium label is excreted exclusively as water. Thus, the difference between the urinary elimination rates of ^{18}O and deuterium provides a measure of carbon dioxide production (rCO_2). TEE can be calculated from rCO_2 using an estimate of respiratory quotient (RQ).[43,44]

Social desirability was measured using the Marlowe-Crowne Social Desirability (MCSD) Scale.[32] This consists of 33 true/false questions that quantify a tendency to avoid criticism and to defend one's social image in a testing situation. Respondents are asked to react to extreme statements about how they would react in a variety of situations; for example: "I never hesitate to go out of my way to help someone in trouble." Eighteen questions (including this example) are scored one point on a "true" response and 15 are scored one point on a "false." In general, individuals scoring high on social desirability are far more acquiescent to perceived situational demands in experimental settings,[27] and thus are more likely to portray themselves as conforming to societal expectations.

By contrast, social approval is less focused on defensiveness.[33] It correlates negatively with self-esteem and positively with social self-consciousness and an intolerance of ambiguity.[45] The 20 questions on the Martin-Larsen Approval Motivation (MLAM) Scale are less extreme (eg, "I am willing to argue only if I know that my friends will back me up") and provide five-level Likert scale responses rather than the simple dichotomies of the MCSD. Individuals with a high social approval score are more likely to seek a positive response in testing situations.[33]

Selected demographic and other variables for the 73 women with complete data for these analyses are shown in Table 1 (for categorical variables) and Table 2 (for continuous variables). These women were middle-aged and of about average body weight. Their TEE from DLW (Table 2) averaged about 2100 kcal/day, which was higher than either the 24HR- or the 7DDR-derived energy intake values, results consistent with other research studies.[17,22,23,37,46-49] Inspection of the ranges from the 25th to the 75th percentile values for TEE and EI derived from the 24HRs and 7DDR (day 0) indicated smallest total error in the TEE and largest error in the 7DDR. There was no weight change over the 14-day period (mean change = -0.04 kg, standard error = 0.10 kg). Therefore, it appears that the assumption that TEE_{DLW} approximates EI is valid.

Table 1

Description of the Energy Study Population (n = 73):
Categorical Variables

	N	%
Married	47	64.4
White, Non-Hispanic	72	98.6
Postmenopausal	32	43.8
College or More Education	33	45.2
Employed Full Time	44	60.3
Currently Smoking*	7	9.6
Sedentary†	38	52.1

* Current smoking was defined as use of cigarettes, cigars, cigarillos, or pipes in the past year.

† Reported no leisure-time physical activity in the 30 days preceding study entry.[51]

Table 2

Description of the Energy Study Population: Continuous Variables

	Mean	Standard deviation	Minimum	25th percentile	75th percentile	Maximum
Age (years)	49.0	6.8	40	44	53	65
Body Mass (kg)*	70.0	10.4	43.9	62.1	76.9	90.5
Height (cm)	160.9	6.4	146.8	156.3	164.7	176.5
BMI (kg/m²)†	27.1	4.1	18.7	24.5	29.8	38.2
TEE from DLW (kcal/d)‡, §	2102	380	1378	1830	2318	3337
24-Hour Recall-Derived Data (7-day average)¶						
Energy Intake (kcal/d)§	1820	464	1147	1494	2002	3566
7DDR Energy (kcal/d)§						
Day-0 Administration	2066	964	784	1444	2410	7048
Day-14 Administration	1888	809	710	1387	2209	5777
Social Desirability Score	17.4	5.9	4.0	15.0	22.0	29.0
Social Approval Score	50.2	8.3	32.0	44.0	56.0	72.0

* Based on the average of 4 measurements at days 0, 1, 7, and 14.

† BMI = body mass index as weight (kg)/height(m)².

‡ Total energy expenditure as derived from the 14-day DLW method.

§ The conversion to SI units for energy is as follows: 1 kJ = 0.239 kcal.

¶ The seven 24-hour diet recall interviews were administered over the 14-day study period.

At baseline, across all education levels, there was a -55.9 kcal/day underestimate per point on the social desirability scale (95% Confidence Interval (CI) = -91.4, -20.4) at baseline (ie, day 0 of the metabolic period). The bias was confined to women with college or more education in whom the bias was -86.0 kcal per point (95% CI = -159.1, -12.9). However, at the end of the metabolic period, social desirability bias was not apparent in the entire group (-23.6 kcal/day per point; 95% CI = -57.5, 10.3); nor was it apparent in women with college or more education (-32.0 kcal/day per point; 95% CI = -103.3, 39.3).

Because the focus of this monograph is on compliance, we include all dietary data, even some that would fall outside of the normal conventional range for an epidemiologic investigation (ie, 600 to 4,000 kcal/day). Were those values excluded, we find that the picture of the bias changes; with differential social approval biases by education (ie, -16.0 kcal/day per point on the social approval scale in the highly educated group (95% CI = -41.2, -9.2) and +26.50 kcal/day per point on the scale in the group with less than a college education (95% CI = 0.6, 52.5)). Excluding outliers, there was only a suggestion of a bias due to social desirability (ie, -19.5 kcal/day per point on the social desirability scale in the entire group (95% CI = -44.8, 5.8)). In the day-14 data, the bias was attenuated in the entire data. For example, in women with college or more education, it was -32.0 kcal/day per point (95% CI = -103.3, 39.3). It is interesting to note that the bias was expressed to the largest degree in the well-educated women at baseline. Both the bias and the out-of-range values attenuated in the measurements at the end of the metabolic period.

The results of this study are broadly consistent with what we had observed in our first examination of response set biases in women, in the Worcester Area Trial for Counseling in Hyperlipidemia (WATCH) External Validation Study.[35] That was the original validation study for the 7DDR and the context in which we first tested the hypothesis that a structured questionnaire would evince a social desirability bias relative to multiple days of 24HRs. The bias observed there was -68.1 kcal/day per point on the social desirability scale, but fell to -47.3 kcal on the second 7DDR measured at the end of the three-week study period (and after 7 days of 24HRs had been administered). Both the Energy Study and WATCH External Validation Study were conducted in the absence of an intervention. A very important question in terms of assessing compliance would be: "How might the bias change after an intervention?" Although most validation studies are not conducted in the context of interventions, clearly there is an imperative regarding how biases might be affected under such conditions.

The Worcester Area Trial for Counseling in Hyperlipidemia (WATCH)

The Worcester Area Trial for Counseling in Hyperlipidemia (WATCH) is one study in which we could investigate the possibility of biases changing with an intervention. The WATCH study actually consisted of two interventions: one physician-delivered intervention that was randomized by physician practice,[50] and a second dietitian-led protocol consisting of two 1-hour individual sessions and two 2-hour group sessions to which any WATCH participant could be referred.[36] In the WATCH, a single 24HR and a single 7DDR were administered prior to the intervention and a second one of each was administered exactly one year later, after any intervention had been completed. A description of the individuals is contained in Table 3 (for categorical variables) and Table 4 (for continuous variables). In general, this hyperlipidemic group had less formal education, had a higher rate of smoking, weighed more and had a higher rate of obesity, and tended to under-report their dietary intake to a greater extent in comparison to both WATCH External Validation Study[35] and Energy Study (Tables 1 and 2) subjects.

As in the Energy Study, we observed that the bias due to social desirability was confined to women with college or more education (Table 5). Though there was a suggestion of a bias in less educated women, it was about 64% higher in the well-educated subset. However,

Table 3

Description of the WATCH Study Population at Baseline: Categorical Variables

	Female (n = 284)		Male (n = 220)	
	n	%	n	%
Married	202	71.4	178	81.3
White, Non-Hispanic	278	98.9	209	99.1
College or More Education	64	22.5	70	31.8
Employed Full Time	133	46.8	139	63.2
Currently Smoking*	51	18.0	34	15.5
Sedentary	150	53.0	118	53.9

* Current smoking was defined as use of cigarettes, cigars, cigarillos, or pipes in the past year.

† Reported no leisure-time physical activity in the year preceding study entry.[58]

Table 4

Description of the WATCH Study Population at Baseline: Continuous Variables

	Female		Male	
	Mean	Standard deviation	Mean	Standard deviation
Age (years)	49.2	10.5	51.3	10.3
Body Mass (kg)*	75.0	16.1	87.0	14.2
Height (cm)	161.3	7.6	174.2	8.0
BMI (kg/m^2)†	28.9	4.2	28.7	4.2
24-Hour Recall Data‡				
Baseline Energy Intake (kcal/d)§	1542.6	588.0	2091.1	730.5
Energy Intake (kcal/d) at 1 year§	1506.4	563.5	2016.3	807.5
Baseline Fat Intake (g/day)	56.5	31.9	72.2	38.0
Fat Intake at 1 year (g/day)	52.7	30.1	66.1	36.3
Baseline SFA (g/day)¶	19.2	11.8	25.6	15.2
SFA at 1 year (g/day)¶	17.7	11.6	23.6	15.3
7DDR-Derived Data‡				
Baseline Energy Intake (kcal/d)§	1795.0	711.6	2033.5	885.0
Energy Intake (kcal/d) at 1 year§	1692.7	748.1	1889.2	788.5
Baseline Fat Intake (g/day)	78.1	39.6	85.4	48.9
Fat Intake (g/day) at 1 year	69.9	42.5	76.4	40.2
Baseline SFA (g/day)¶	25.4	12.8	28.5	17.1
SFA at 1 year (g/day)¶	22.8	13.7	25.0	13.3
Social Desirability Score‖	18.7	5.4	18.5	5.6
Social Approval Score**	38.6	9.4	36.5	7.6

* Based on a single measurement taken at baseline.
† BMI = body mass index as weight (kg)/height(m)^2.
‡ This is based on a single administration at baseline and at 1 year.
§ The conversion to SI units for energy is as follows: 1 kJ = 0.239 kcal.
¶ SFA are the sum of all saturated fatty acids.
‖ Based on the Marlowe-Crowne Social Desirability Scale.[29]
** Based on the Martin-Larsen Approval Motivation Scale.[30]

the overall size of the bias was much smaller than in either the WATCH External Validation Study[35] or the Energy Study (at least when we examined all of the data). The bias was proportionally largest for saturated fatty acids at baseline, but was absent for any dietary variable at the 1-year measurement point. In contrast to women, in men there was a social approval bias that was confined to individuals with less than college education (Table 6). Also in contrast to women, the bias appeared to persist at the 1-year measurement point. There appeared to be no difference in the bias according to physician intervention condi-

Table 5

Social Approval and Social Desirability Bias in Females in the WATCH* Study, by Education and Study Period†

Study period	< College (n = 220)		≥ College (n = 64)	
	Social approval score	Social desirability score	Social approval score	Social desirability score
Baseline				
Total Energy (kcal/day)	−0.2 (−10.5, 10.2)	−14.8 (−34.7, 5.12)	−2.9 (−19.0, 13.3)	−24.3 (−47.7, −0.9)
Total Fat (g/day)	−0.02 (−0.59, 0.55)	−0.53 (−1.62, 0.56)	−0.34 (−1.30, 0.62)	−1.28 (−2.68, 0.12)
Total SFA (g/day)‡	0.03 (−0.15, 0.21)	−0.14 (−0.50, 0.22)	−0.10 (−0.40, 0.20)	−0.53 (−0.95, −0.11)
One-year	< College (n = 196)		≥ College (n = 63)	
Total Energy (kcal/day)	8.5 (−1.8, 18.7)	−8.5 (−29.1, 12.1)	−8.9 (−28.2, 10.4)	−2.7 (−30.7, 25.2)
Total Fat (g/day)	0.31 (−0.30, 0.92)	−0.81 (−2.03, 0.41)	−0.43 (−1.41, 0.55)	−0.04 (−1.46, 1.38)
Total SFA (g/day)‡	0.10 (−0.10, 0.30)	−0.26 (−0.63, 0.11)	−0.11 (−0.45, 0.23)	0.11 (−0.59, 0.37)

* WATCH = Worcester Area Trial for Counseling in Hyperlipidemia.

† All models were fit with the 7DDR-derived nutrient as dependent variable, corresponding 24-hour-derived nutrient, social approval score, body mass index (kg/m²), interval, in days, between mailing and receipt of the questionnaires, and incentive (subjects who were late in responding were given an incentive of $5 after one month or $10 after two months), as independent variables. Tabulated values are the regression coefficient and the (95% confidence interval).

‡ SFA = saturated fatty acids.

Table 6

Social Approval and Social Desirability Bias in Males in the WATCH*, by Education and Study Period†

Study period	< College (n = 150)		≥ College (n = 70)	
	Social approval score	Social desirability score	Social approval score	Social desirability score
Baseline				
Total Energy (kcal/day)	29.8 (10.2, 49.4)	12.2 (−13.6, 38.0)	8.6 (−16.2, 33.3)	10.3 (−27.2, 47.8)
Total Fat (g/day)	1.63 (0.55, 2.71)	0.93 (−0.51, 2.37)	0.58 (−0.76, 1.92)	0.47 (−1.54, 2.48)
Total SFA (g/day)‡	0.59 (0.22, 0.96)	0.33 (−0.18, 0.84)	0.26 (−0.20, 0.72)	0.17 (−0.53, 0.87)
One-year	< College (n = 128)		≥ College (n = 61)	
Total Energy (kcal/day)	22.2 (3.4, 41.0)	−12.3 (−35.1, 10.4)	18.2 (−5.1, 41.5)	0.3 (−29.4, 30.1)
Total Fat (g/day)	1.11 (0.18, 2.04)	0.02 (−1.11, 1.15)	1.35 (0.13, 2.57)	−1.02 (−2.56, 0.52)
Total SFA (g/day)‡	0.25 (−0.07, 0.57)	−0.03 (−0.43, 0.37)	0.33 (−0.01, 0.67)	−0.10 (−0.52, 0.32)

* WATCH = Worcester Area Trial for Counseling in Hyperlipidemia.

† All models were fit with the 7-day diet recall-derived nutrient as dependent variable, corresponding 24-hour-derived nutrient, social desirability score, social approval score, body mass index (kg/m²), interval, in days, between mailing and receipt of the questionnaires, and incentive as independent variables. Tabulated values are the regression coefficient and the (95% confidence interval).

‡ SFA = saturated fatty acids.

tion, in either women or men. However, there was an apparent increase in the social approval bias in men attending any of the dietitian-led sessions. Because of the small numbers, it was not possible to stratify by educational status in these analyses, and confidence limits tended to be very wide. Despite this, there was an interesting increase in social approval bias in attendees after 1 year; increasing to 147.0 kcal/day per point on the scale (95% CI = 92.9, 201.2) from 43.7 kcal/day per point (95% CI = -41.6, 129.0).

Practical Implications

Knowledge regarding observed biases can be used in a variety of ways. For example, psychologists delete bias-prone questions on study instruments.[51] However, this is not possible for a dietary assessment instrument because foods must be included due to their nutrient contribution to the diet, irrespective of any bias entailed in eliciting responses. Another option is to "filter" data from individuals with extreme social desirability scores. The risk of this "filtering" strategy is that it may result in discarding much useful information that can be made even more valuable if large sources of bias can be identified and controlled. For example, using this technique in the Energy Study would have excluded two individuals who had very low social desirability scores (4 and 8) *and* the highest estimates of EI (4812 and 7048 kcal/day). However, three individuals with social desirability scores of 4, 5, and 7 had within-range estimates of EI. A third approach is to statistically adjust the nutrient score for the bias. However, until there is compelling reason to believe that the bias is very predictable, this may be inadvisable. The final option is to fit the biaser (eg, social desirability score) as a covariate in analyses. This requires no specific model to be postulated, does not peremptorily exclude observations, and allows for querying food items no matter how biased the responses. This is the strategy we employed in the analysis of the 7DDR-derived data from the WATCH.[36]

In the WATCH, we found that social desirability was a significant covariate in the regression models in which total and saturated fat intake were fit as the dependent variables. A one-unit increase in the social desirability score was associated with decreases of 0.22% and 0.05% of energy as total and saturated fat, respectively.[36] However, social desirability did not significantly affect changes in serum lipids (ie, TC, LDL-C) or body weight. Social approval was not a significant covariate in any of the models. In approaching this issue, we had considered that both social desirability and social approval could be related to personality traits, such as acquiescence[27] or social self-consciousness.[45] Such characteristics could modify the effect of the intervention directly.[27,31,52] Given that the effects appear to be confined to self-report measures, it appears that inclusion of social desirability as a covariate in the specified analyses was controlling for bias in self-report rather than for personality traits that may affect responses to the intervention. The finding that social approval bias was not a significant covariate may be related to the fact that it was uniformly unrelated to the discrepancy (ie, it remained about the same at baseline and at 1 year) in women and that the bias tended to be more constant in men than social desirability was in women. The large increase in social approval bias in the small set of men attending the dietitian-led intervention is interesting and could be of great importance if it were to persist in a larger study group, though it did not change the overall conclusion regarding the social approval bias remaining relatively constant.

As we consider ways in which we can improve dietary assessments to reflect levels of compliance, we may need to broaden our conceptualization of validity to include constructs such as body weight or serum cholesterol measurements. These parameters relate changes in overall energy balance or specific nutrient exposures according to well-established physical or biological laws (or both).[3,53–55] If our dietary assessment instruments are measuring what we intend, then results obtained from these instruments should reconcile against such parameters, at least on a group level (eg, for cholesterol).[56] Our studies have shown that self-reported dietary changes in energy intake are concordant with changes in body weight and that agreement improves when we control for social desirability[36] as well as the agreement between group-level changes in dietary fatty acids and changes in serum lipids.[6]

Conclusion

In summary, we have shown that structured questionnaires are susceptible to biases. These biases are consistent with theoretical concepts and societal norms (ie, those differing by gender, education, and intervention status). The biasers that appear most prominent in distorting estimates of dietary intake from structured questionnaires are social desirability and social approval, both of which can be easily measured. Finally, statistical control for bias improves assessment of compliance with study recommendations and prediction of health effects due to the intervention. Such control also provides an improved fit between self-report data and relevant constructs (eg, weight and cholesterol change).

References

1. Keys A, Anderson JT, Grande F. Prediction of serum-cholesterol response of man to changes in fats in the diet. *Lancet* 1957;7003:959–966.
2. Keys A. Serum cholesterol response to dietary cholesterol. *Am J Clin Nutr* 1984;40:351–359.
3. Hegsted DM, McGandy RB, Myers ML, et al. Quantitative effects of dietary fat on serum cholesterol in man. *Am J Clin Nutr* 1965;17:281–295.
4. Block G, Woods M, Potosky A, et al. Validation of a self-administered diet history questionnaire using multiple diet records. *J Clin Epidemiol* 1990;43: 1327–1335.
5. Block G, Thompson FE, Hartman AM, et al. Comparison of two dietary questionnaires validated against multiple dietary records collected during a 1-year period. *J Am Diet Assoc* 1992;92:686–693.
6. Hebert JR, Ockene IS, Hurley TG, et al. Development and testing of a seven-day dietary recall. *J Clin Epidemiol* 1997;50:925–937.
7. Willett WC, Sampson L, Stampfer MJ, et al. Reproducibility and validity of a semiquantitative food frequency questionnaire. *Am J Epidemiol* 1985; 122:51–65.
8. Willett W. *Nutritional Epidemiology—Second Edition*. Monographs in Epidemiology and Biostatistics. Vol. 30. New York: Oxford University Press, 1998.
9. Sorensen G, Morris DH, Hunt MK, et al. Worksite nutrition intervention and employees' dietary habits: The Treatwell Program. *Am J Public Health* 1992;82:877–880.
10. Kristal AR, Shattuck AL, Williams A. Food frequency questionnaires for diet intervention research., 17th National Nutrient Databank Conference—Baltimore, MD, June 7–9, 1992., Washington, DC, 1994. Vol. 17. International Life Sciences Institute.
11. Dwyer JT, Gardner J, Halvorsen K, et al. Memory of food intake in the distant past. *Am J Epidemiol* 1989;130:1033–1046.
12. Smith AF. Cognitive psychological issues of relevance to the validity of dietary reports. *Eur J Clin Nutr* 1993;47:S6-S18.
13. Smith AF. Cognitive processes in long-term dietary recall. [DHHS Publication No. PHS92–1079]. Vital Health Stat. Vol. 6. Washington, DC: US Government Printing Office, 1991.
14. Fraser GE, Lindsted KD, Knutsen SF, et al. Validity of dietary recall over 20 years among California Seventh-day Adventists. *Am J Epidemiol* 1998; 148:810–818.
15. Larkin FE, Metzner HL, Thompson FE, et al. Comparison of estimated nutrient intakes by food frequency and dietary records in adults. *J Am Diet Assoc* 1989;89:215–223.
16. Hebert JR, Ma Y, Clemow L, et al. Gender differences in social desirability and social approval bias in dietary self report. *Am J Epidemiol* 1997;146: 1046–1055.
17. Seale JL. Energy expenditure measurements in relation to energy requirements. *Am J Clin Nutr* 1995;62:1042–1046.
18. Suitor CJW, Gardner J, Willett WC. A comparison of food frequency and diet recall methods in studies of nutrient intake of low-income pregnant women. *J Am Diet Assoc* 1989;89:1786–1794.
19. Bandini LG, Schoeller DA, Cyr HN, et al. Validity of reported energy intake in obese and nonobese adolescents. *Am J Clin Nutr* 1990;52:421–425.

20. Heitmann BL, Lissner L. Dietary underreporting by obese individuals—is it specific or non-specific. *BMJ* 1995;311:986–989.
21. Katzel LI, Coon PJ, Dengel J, et al. Effects of American Heart Association Step 1 diet and weight loss on lipoprotein lipid levels in obese men with silent myocardial ischemia and reduced high-density lipoprotein cholesterol. *Metabolism* 1995;44:307–314.
22. Black AE, Bingham SA, Johansson G, et al. Validation of dietary intakes of protein and energy against 24 hour urinary N and DLW energy expenditure in middle-aged women, retired men and post-obese subjects: comparisons with validation against presumed energy requirements. *Eur J Clin Nutr* 1997;51:405–413.
23. Schoeller DA. Limitations in the assessment of dietary energy intake by self-report. *Metabolism* 1995;44:18–22.
24. Lichtman SW, Pisarska K, Berman ER, et al. Discrepancy between self-reported and actual caloric intake and exercise in obese subjects. *N Engl J Med* 1992;327:1893–1898.
25. Sobal J, Devine CM. Social aspects of obesity: Influences, consequences, assessments, and interventions. In: Dalton S, ed. *Overweight and weight management*. Gaithersburg, MD: Aspen Publishers, 1997, pp. 312–331.
26. Bancroft J, Cook A, Williamson L. Food craving, mood and the menstrual cycle. *Psychol Med* 1988;18:855–860.
27. Marlowe D, Crowne DP. Social desirability and responses to perceived situational demands. *J Consult Clin Psychol* 1961;25:109–115.
28. Crowne DP. *The experimental study of personality*. Hillsdale NJ: Erlbaum, 1979.
29. Edwards AL. *The social desirability variable in personality assessment and research*. New York: Dryden, 1957.
30. Edwards AL. *The measurement of personality traits by scales and inventories*. New York: Holt, 1970.
31. Martin HJ. A revised measure of approval motivation and its relationship to social desirability. *J Pers Assess* 1984;48:508–516.
32. Crowne DP, Marlowe D. A new scale of social desirability independent of psychopathology. *J Consult Clin Psychol* 1960;24:349–354.
33. Larsen KS, Martin HJ, Ettinger RH, et al. Approval seeking, social cost, and agression: A scale and some dynamics. *J Psychol* 1976;94:3–11.
34. Shulman A, Silverman I. Social desirability and need approval: Some paradoxical data and a conceptual reevaluation. *Br J Soc Clin Psychol* 1974;13:27–32.
35. Hebert JR, Clemow L, Pbert L, et al. Social desirability bias in dietary self-report may compromise the validity of dietary intake measures. *Int J Epidemiol* 1995;24:389–398.
36. Hebert JR, Ebbeling CB, Ockene IS, et al. A dietitian-delivered group nutrition program leads to reductions in dietary fat, serum cholesterol, and body weight: findings from the Worcester Area Trial for Counseling in Hyperlipidemia (WATCH). *J Am Diet Assoc* 1999;99:544–552.
37. Seale JL, Rumpler WV, Conway JM, et al. Comparison of doubly labeled water, intake-balance, and direct- and indirect-calorimetry methods for measuring energy expenditure in adult men. *Am J Clin Nutr* 1990;52:66–71.
38. Kuczmarski RJ. Prevalence of overweight and weight gain in the United States. *Am J Clin Nutr* 1992;55:495S–502S.
39. Ravussin E, Danforth E. Beyond sloth—Physical activity and weight gain. *Science* 1999;283:184.

40. Jeffery RW. Prevention of Obesity. In: Bray GA, Bouchard C, James WPT, (eds). *Handbook of Obesity*. New York: Marcel Dekker, Inc., 1998, pp. 819–829.
41. Bingham SA. The use of 24hr urine samples and energy expenditure to validate dietary assessments. *Am J Clin Nutr* 1994;59:227S-231S.
42. Black AE, Coward WA, Cole TJ, et al. Human energy expenditure in affluent societies: An analysis of 574 doubly-labeled water measurements. *Eur J Clin Nutr* 1996;50:72–92.
43. Black AE, Prentice AM, Coward WA. Use of food quotients to predict respiratory quotients for the doubly-labeled water method of measuring energy expenditure. *Hum Nutr:Clin Nutr* 1986;40C:381–391.
44. Surrao J, Sawaya AL, Dallal GE, et al. Use of food quotients in human doubly labeled water studies: Comparable results obtained with 4 widely used food intake methods. *J Am Diet Assoc* 1998;98:1015–1020.
45. Thaw J, Efran J. The relationship of the Marlowe-Crowne Scale and its components to defensive preferences. *J Pers Assess* 1967;43:406–410.
46. Anonymous. Errors in reporting habitual energy intake. *Nutr Rev* 1991;49: 215–217.
47. Black AE, Goldberg GR, Jebb SA, et al. Critical evaluation of energy intake data using fundamental principles of energy physiology: 2. evaluating the results of published surveys. *Eur J Clin Nutr* 1991;45:583–599.
48. Champagne CM, Baker NB, DeLany JP, et al. Assessment of energy intake underreporting by doubly labeled water and observations on reported nutrient intakes in children. *J Am Diet Assoc* 1998;98:426–433.
49. Martin LJ, Su W, Jones PJ, et al. Comparison of energy intakes determined by food records and doubly labeled water in women participating in a dietary-intervention trial. *Am J Clin Nutr* 1996;63:483–490.
50. Ockene IS, Hebert JR, Ockene JK, et al. Effect of physician-delivered nutrition counseling training and an office support system on saturated fat intake, weight, and serum lipid measurements in a hyperlipidemic population: The Worcester-Area Trial for Counseling in Hyperlipidemia (WATCH). *Arch Intern Med* 1999;159:725–731.
51. Anastasi A. *Psychological Testing*. New York: MacMillan Publ. Co., 1988.
52. Edwards AL. Social desirability or acquiescence in the MMPI? A case study with the SD scale. *J Abnorm Soc Psychol* 1961;63:351–359.
53. Keys A, Anderson JT, Grande F. Serum cholesterol response to changes in the diet-III. Differences among individuals. *Metabolism* 1965;14:766–775.
54. Flatt JP. Dietary fat, carbohydrate balance, and weight maintenance: Effects of exercise. *Am J Clin Nutr* 1987;45:296–306.
55. Romieu I, Willett WC, Stampfer MJ, et al. Energy intake and other determinants of relative weight. *Am J Clin Nutr* 1988;47:406–412.
56. Jacobs DJ, Anderson J, Blackburn H. Diet and serum cholesterol: Do zero correlations negate the relationship? *Am J Epidemiol* 1979;110:77–87.
57. Casperson CJ. A collection of physical activity questionnaires for health-related research: Behavioral Risk Factor Surveillance System. *Med Sci Sports Exerc* 1997;29:S146-S152.
58. Matthews CE, Hebert JR, Ockene IS, et al. The relationship between leisure-time physical activity and selected dietary variables in the Worcester Area Trial for Counseling in Hyperlipidemia. *Med Sci Sports Exerc* 1997;29: 1199–1207.

Section V

Issues In Special Populations

Chapter 11

Chronic Disease Prevention Among Children

Tom Baranowski, PhD,
Janice C. Baranowski, MPH, RD, LD, and
Karen Cullen DrPH, RD, LD

Introduction

Dietary and physical activity behaviors have been shown to be protective of several chronic diseases. Establishing these healthy habits in childhood should protect the person from the initiation and progression of these chronic diseases. Many studies have attempted to promote health-related behavior change among children. Most studies reported modest changes. A mediating variable analysis of these programs reveals three limits on the effectiveness of interventions: the low predictiveness of the theoretical frameworks upon which the interventions were designed; a significant impact on less than half of the proposed mediating variables; and the low level of implementation of some interventions. When moderators were assessed, the interventions appeared to work with girls, but not boys. Future research must a) increase the predictiveness of fruit juice and vegetables (FJV) consumption, b) identify methods to enhance change in the mediating variables, and c) enhance the delivery of the intervention to participants.

Background

Wouldn't it be wonderful if we could totally prevent, substantially delay, or minimize all the events associated with chronic disease: dis-

The authors were supported during the writing of this paper by grants from the National Cancer Institute (CA73503, CA75614), the U.S. Department of Agriculture (97–35200–4233) and the Cancer Research Foundation of America (Private Foundation).

From: Burke LE, Ockene IS (eds). *Compliance in Healthcare and Research.* Armonk, NY: Futura Publishing Company, Inc.; © 2001.

ruption of the patient's and family's lives, loss of income and productivity, pain, discomfort, emotional upset, etc., etc.? People who practice a healthier lifestyle are less likely to develop chronic disease at any particular age.[1,2] Not smoking is considered by many to be the most important lifestyle issue in preventing chronic disease.[3] Many believe that diet and physical activity are at least a close second as lifestyle factors in chronic disease prevention.[1,2] Fruit, juice and vegetable (FJV) consumption, in particular, has recently taken an eminent role in cardiovascular disease (CVD)[4–6] and cancer[2] initiation and progression. One review reported a 15% reduction in CVD risk[7], while another related FJV consumption to CVD risk factors.[8] While the operative agents and mechanisms need to be delineated, FJV consumption in general protects against CVD and most cancers.

Some of the earliest manifestations of CVD appear in childhood and adolescence, including arterial plaque[9,10] and elevated CVD risk factors.[11] There is some evidence that cancers initiate with puberty.[12] Dietary factors have been shown to be inversely correlated with CVD risk factors among children,[11] thereby suggesting some early protective effects. CVD risk factors track from childhood into the adult years,[11,13,14] with some weaker evidence that dietary practices track, as well.[15,16] Thus, there is a growing interest in dietary change interventions with children in order to obtain both an immediate health protection from CVD and its risk factors in childhood[11] and to establish positive health practices in childhood to help defend against the onset of chronic diseases in the adult years.[17] In addition, it has been suggested that childhood is a time when behavior is more malleable and thereby easier to establish healthful practices.[18] (All these issues deserve substantially more research.)

While the idea of "children's compliance with public health recommendations" could be used to describe this phenomenon, the term compliance tends to emphasize inadequacies and limitations on the part of the child. Public health professionals tend to pose the question, instead, as "Why aren't our interventions working to help children change as much as we would like them to?"

Interventions effect change in behavior through mediating variables[19,20] (see Figure 1), ie, changes are effected in the mediating variables which in turn change the behavior. The mediating variables are the theoretical variables that have been developed and used to understand and predict behavior.[19,20] Mediating variables that have higher predictiveness of the target behavior should provide a stronger handle or wedge for change. The mediating variable model thus imposes several limits on the effectiveness of an intervention: the predictiveness of the mediating variables; the impact of the intervention on the mediators; and the quantity and quality of the implementation of the intended

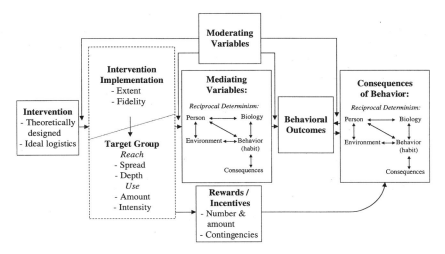

Figure 1. Mediating variable model of behavior change interventions.

intervention.[21] Interventions may also impact behavior through the application of rewards (or incentives) to behavior, but there has been some concern that when the rewards are removed the behavior may revert to its original levels.[22] Sometimes interventions work with subgroups (eg, just girls)[23] in a target population. The variables on which there is differential success are called moderating variables.

We have conducted several recent reviews of the literature on the effectiveness of interventions to help children and their families to make diet and physical activity behavior changes[19,20,24,25] and to assess psychosocial predictors of dietary behavior.[26] This chapter will briefly overview these publications concerning children and adolescents. The issues addressed will be: 1) what levels of behavior change were obtained? 2) what mediating variables were changed and by how much? 3) what rewards were used and how did they relate to outcome? 4) what was the level of program implementation? and 5) were any moderating effects detected?

Description of Studies

The lifestyle behavior change literature is diverse, using many channels for reaching children and their families, many theoretical perspectives, and many different kinds of interventions. The channels for reaching children have included elementary schools, middle schools, high schools, after-school programs, public housing projects, churches,

Boy Scout and Girl Scout troops, literacy classes, and many others. The target groups varied from primarily Euro-American, to multicultural, to primarily African-American or Hispanic. While most interventions use social cognitive theory[27] in one way or another, behavioral choice theory,[28] social systems,[29] Piagetian developmental theory,[30] Deweyan educational theory,[31] resiliency theory,[31,32] and the PRECEDE[31,32] and transtheoretical[31-33] models have all been used to guide the design of interventions. There has also been substantial variability in who provided the intervention including the investigators themselves,[34,35] existing elementary school teachers,[30,36-40] specially trained elementary school teachers,[41] dietitians trained in use of the curriculum,[30,36] Girl Scout troop leaders,[34] and major media.[31,32] The intervention components also varied across projects including combinations of classroom or troop meeting curricula with various learning activities,[28-32,34-45] home assignments,[30,34,36-38,42-44] videotapes sent home to parents,[37] newsletters sent home to parents,[36-38] packets sent home to parents,[39,40] point-of-purchase education at grocery stores near the participating schools,[37] weekend camping food competitions,[34,36] marketing stations on specific FJV,[33] modification of school food services practices,[33,39-41] activities at Parent Teacher Organization (PTO) meetings[33] or Family Fun Nights,[31,32,40] industry involvement,[31-33,39] comic books,[36,39,40] team competition,[37-39] and in-class recipe preparation and taste testings.[28-32,34-45]

Substantial creativity has been evidenced in the diversity of interventions designed and implemented as part of these projects. Most of the interventions used multiple components attempting to directly affect the students (eg, through classroom curricula and home activities), the parents of the students (through newsletters, videos, point-of-purchase education, and home activities), the school food services, the physical education program and other components of the children's environments.

Levels of Behavior Change

Changes have been obtained at different levels and at different times. For example, in FJV change, the documented levels of dietary change varied across studies with most showing increases of 0.2 to 0.6 servings per day, but several showing no statistically significant evidence of change in FJV consumption, to increases as high as 0.8[36] to 1.58 servings.[24] Some projects obtained more change in fruit, while others obtained more change in vegetables. All changes were documented either during the intervention or immediately afterward. None maintained changes at 3- or 6-month intervals after the end of the intervention.[33,34] With few exceptions, physical activity interventions with children had similar modest outcomes, except in changing the Physical Education program (an environmental intervention).[19] Interventions have shown few incremental outcome effects from involving families, except with highly motivated populations.[25]

The study with the largest FJV change (+ 1.68 servings) was obtained from 24-hour dietary recalls, but detected no change using observations at school lunch.[41] This pattern is in stark contrast to the other elementary school-based interventions that showed most changes occurred at school lunch.[37,39,43] The reasons for these inconsistencies are not clear. The studies with the two largest dietary changes[36,41] hired and trained their own staff to deliver the interventions. Other literature has demonstrated a substantial lack of fidelity to intervention protocols when usual classroom teachers or other service providers are used to implement interventions.[46] This suggests that our interventions have potentially powerful frameworks but need to be implemented with higher fidelity.

Two papers[37,45] revealed that regression to the mean occurred from baseline to post-assessments, with only 7% more participants in treatment than in control making positive changes. Some authors have argued that even these small levels of change have important public health implications.[47] The fact that these changes have not usually been maintained beyond the end of the intervention[33,34] suggests continuing interventions throughout childhood and adolescence. The fact that some of these interventions worked at the earlier grade levels, but not later grades,[33,37] suggests that either the interventions need to be very different across years to maintain student interest, or greater attention needs to be given to even minor nuances in child development to be more effective.

Mediating Variables Related to Outcome

Not all studies used or reported changes in mediating variables and the mediating variables have varied across studies. The mediating variable model (Figure 1) inserts concerns for theory into the design of effective interventions[19,20] similar to intervention mapping procedures.[48] Based on a mediating variable analysis (Figure 1)[19,20] of intervention program outcomes, attention must be drawn to the predictiveness of the mediating variables used and targeted in these studies. Most studies have used social cognitive theory (SCT) as one basis for program design. Yet, the four published studies predicting FJV consumption among children revealed that SCT constructs accounted for less than 15% of the variability in children's FJV consumption.[24] The results are only slightly improved among adults.[24] While we believe that many of the important variables for understanding dietary behavior are captured in SCT, perhaps we need to employ even more comprehensive models,[49] or we need to more narrowly focus our research on influences on more limited food groups (eg, fruit). FJV consumption varies substantially by specific meals and days of the week, which suggests they are under different influences,[50] and thereby require different interventions.

Impacting Mediators

Interventions have been inconsistent in impacting mediators, and relatively small changes have been obtained in mediating variables.[19,20,24,25] This suggests that our techniques for impacting mediating variables are not very strong. Most of what we do is based on common sense or experience with no strong empirical database.

The primary philosophy behind dietary intervention research strategy to date has been to design comprehensive interventions that have a maximum likelihood of producing change, and once demonstrated to work, decompose them to test which were the efficacious components.[51] Since our comprehensive interventions have not had enormous success there has been little work on decomposition to identify the effective components. Perhaps we need to change our philosophy and build toward comprehensive interventions by first identifying effective components for specific targets, and then progressively aggregating these effective components into more comprehensive interventions. Research that systematically varies and tests alternative ways of impacting mediators based on theory should be pursued.

Most of these interventions used goal setting and problem solving procedures. Unfortunately, very little is known about naturally occurring goal setting or problem solving among children, and very little is known about the optimal design of goal setting or problem solving procedures with children.[52] Much work needs to be done to remedy these limitations of our knowledge base.

Focus group discussions revealed that parents are reluctant to enhance accessibility of FJV for their children.[42] Natural motivators (outcome expectancies) need to be identified that would make parents want to take these simple steps, eg, "eating more FJV will lead to your child being more well-behaved at home," rather than perceiving them as additional burdens in an already complicated and overworked day.

Use of Rewards/Incentives

Many of these projects used rewards or incentives in one way or another as a part of the intervention program, but the contingencies varied across studies (eg, completing home assignments vs. attending evening sessions) or were not clearly reported or not reported at all. The designs did not allow the investigators to separate the effects of the rewards or incentives. Health promotion practitioners have extolled the use of incentives for many purposes.[53] However, there has been some concern that contingencies make projects more expensive and thereby not generalizeable. Alternatively, there has been some concern that once incentives are removed, the behavior will revert to pre-intervention levels or worse.[22] Incentives have not been systematically varied in the children's dietary or physical activity intervention arena nor their contribution to change assessed. In part, this reflects a tension between those trained primarily in behavioral learning theory (wherein rewards are considered the primary mechanism by which learning and thereby behavior change occurs)[54] and those trained in more cognitive perspectives (who believe in social incentives and intrinsic rewards).[22] Research needs to be conducted that tests how incentives affect behavior in order to provide better guidance on when, how, and how much incentive to use.

Moderating Effects

Few projects tested for moderating effects. There has been some evidence that programs work with some subgroups in the population (eg, girls), but not others.[23,25] Most frequently, only gender substantially moderated project outcomes (ie, the programs attained change among the girls only). Conceptually it is possible to have moderators of each relationship in the progression from intervention to outcome (see Figure 1). As far as we know, no one has tested for these effects earlier in the chain.

Quantity and Quality of Implementation, Reach and Use

Process evaluation has been conceptualized as having three components: assessment of implementation of the program, receipt by the participants (program reach), and use by the participants.[55] There has been inconsistency in use of terms and in measures used. The one measure obtained by all seven FJV intervention studies, percent of curriculum implemented, varied substantially across studies from < 50% to 95%. A problem with these findings is that the measure of implementation varied from in-class observations of teacher performance of specific tasks to teacher completed checklists. One recent article revealed that three methods used in the same study showed the same variability in implementation, suggesting severe measurement problems in the teacher checklist measure.[46] Methodological research needs to be conducted on optimal procedures for measuring curriculum implementation.

In one process evaluation of an elementary school program, only about 50% of the curriculum was implemented in classrooms, only about 50% of parents saw one or more of the videos, and approximately 10% of families attended one of the point-of-purchase education events.[37] This modest level of implementation by classroom teachers suggests that we either need to find ways to enhance the teachers' fidelity to the curriculum or we need to find ways to more directly deliver the curriculum. Teachers are expected to provide basic education plus many other classroom activities and are not extensively trained in behavior change and health education. Potential leads to encourage greater teacher involvement in nutrition education would be demonstrating (through research) that better student dietary practices results in better student performance in reading, writing and arithmetic.

Significance

While the goal of primary prevention is enormously attractive and potentially very important to the health of the nation, it has been elusive. Our programs have had modest effects for the most part. To enable us to achieve the goal of primary prevention for large numbers of people, we need to learn more about: 1) the influences on childrens' diet and physical activity behaviors (basic social and behavioral science research); 2) more effective methods for promoting change in these influences (impacting mediating variables); 3) more effective ways to ensure that interventions are delivered in ways they are most likely to be effective (program implementation, reach and use); 4) when and how best to employ incentives, if at all; and 5) how to modify our interventions for substantial effectiveness in all groups (moderators, eg, gender, ethnic, etc.). This research agenda including both basic and more applied research is not very different from the commitment the NIH has made to the biomedical sciences, which at least conceptually can be easily expanded to the behavioral and social sciences. We need to make that expansion.

References

1. Physical Activity and Health: A Report of the Surgeon General. Atlanta, GA: U.S. Department of Health and Human Services. Centers for Disease

Control and Prevention, National Center for Chronic Disease Prevention and Health Promotion; 1996.

2. Potter JD. Food, Nutrition and the Prevention of Cancer: A Global Perspective. Washington DC: World Cancer Research Fund and American Institute for Cancer Research; 1997.

3. Shopland DR. Changes in cigarette-related disease risks and their implications for prevention and control. *Smoking and Tobacco Control Monograph 8. NIH Publication Number 97–4213.* Bethesda, MD: National Cancer Institute; 1997.

4. Gale CR, Martyn CN, Winter PD, et al. Vitamin C and risk of death from stroke and coronary heart disease in cohort of elderly people. *Br Med J* 1995;310:1563–1566.

5. Ness AR, Powles JW, Khaw KT. Vitamin C and cardiovascular disease: A systematic review. *J Cardiovasc Risk* 1996;3:513–521.

6. Rimm EB, Ascherio A, Giovannucci E, et al. Vegetable, fruit, and cereal fiber intake and risk of coronary heart disease among men. *JAMA* 1996; 275:447–451.

7. Law MR, Morris JK. By how much does fruit and vegetable consumption reduce the risk of ischaemic heart disease? *Eur J Clin Nutr* 1998;52:549–556.

8. Zino S, Skeaff M, Williams S, et al. Randomised controlled trial of effect of fruit and vegetable consumption on plasma concentrations of lipids and antioxidants. *Br Med J* 1997;314:1787–1791.

9. Newman WP, III, Freedman DS, Berenson G. Relation of serum lipoprotein levels and systolic blood pressure to early atherosclerosis. The Bogalusa Heart Study. *N Engl J Med* 1986;314:138–144.

10. Stary HC. Evaluation and progression of atherosclerotic lesions in coronary arteries of children and young adults. *Ateriosclerosis* 1989;9:119–132.

11. Nicklas TA, Webber LS, Johnson CC, et al. Foundations for health promotion with youth: A review of observations from the Bogalusa Heart Study. *J Health Educ* 1995;26:S18-S26.

12. Colditz G, Frazier AL. Models of breast cancer show that risk is set by events of early life: Prevention efforts must shift focus. *Cancer Epidemiol Biomarkers Prev* 1995;4:567–571.

13. Lauer RM, Clarke WR, Mahoney LT, et al. Childhood predictors for high adult blood pressure. *Pediatr Clin North Am* 1993;40:23–40.

14. Rolland-Cachera M-F, Deheeger M, Guillond-Bataille M, et al. Tracking the development of adiposity from one month of age to adulthood. *Ann Hum Biol* 1987;14:219–229.

15. Resnicow K, Smith M, Baranowski T, et al. Two year tracking of children's fruit and vegetable intake. *J Am Diet Assoc* 1998;98:785–789.

16. Kelder SD, Perry CL, Klepp KI, et al. Longitudinal tracking of adolescent smoking, physical activity, and food choice behaviors. *Am J Public Health* 1994;84:1121–1126.

17. Gillman MW, Ellison RC. Childhood prevention of essential hypertension. *Pediatr Clin North Am* 1993;40:179–194.

18. Cashdan E. A sensitive period for learning about food. *Hum Nature* 1994; 5:279–291.

19. Baranowski T, Lin LS, Wetter DW, et al. Theory as mediating variables: Why aren't community interventions working as desired? *Ann Epidemiol* 1997;7:S89-S95.

20. Baranowski T, Anderson C, Carmack C. Mediating variable framework in physical activity interventions. How are we doing? How might we do better? *Am J Prev Med* 1998;15:266–297.

21. McGraw SA, Sellers DE, Stone EJ, et al. Measuring implementation of programs and policy to promote healthy eating and physical activity among youth. *Prev Med* 2000;31(2):586–597.
22. Lepper MR, Greene D. *The hidden costs of reward: New perspectives on the psychology of human motivation.* Hillsdale, NJ: Lawrence Earlbaum; 1978.
23. Stone EJ, Baranowski T, Sallis JF, et al. Review of behavioral research for cardiopulmonary health: Emphasis on youth, gender, and ethnicity. *J Health Educ* 1995;26:S9-S17.
24. Ciliska D, Miles E, O'Brien MA, et al. Effectiveness of community-based interventions to increase fruit & vegetable consumption. *J Nut Educ* 2000; 32(6):341–352.
25. Baranowski T, Hearn MD. Health behavior interventions with families. In Gochman DS (ed): *Handbook of Health Behavior Research.* New York: Plenum Press; 1997:303–323.
26. Baranowski T, Cullen KW, Baranowski J. Psychosocial correlates of dietary intake: Advancing intervention. *Annu Rev Public Health* 1999;19:17–40.
27. Baranowski T, Perry CL, Parcel G. How individuals, environments, and health behaviors interact: Social cognitive theory. In Glanz K, Lewis FM, Rimer B (eds): *Health Behavior and Health Education: Theory, Research and Practice.* 2nd ed. San Francisco: Jossey-Bass; 1996:246–279.
28. Gortmaker SL, Peterson K, Wiecha J, et al. Reducing obesity via a school-based interdisciplinary intervention among youth. *Arch Pediatr Adolesc Med* 1999;153:409–418.
29. Trevino RP, Pugh JA, Hernandez AE, et al. Bienestar: A diabetes risk-factor prevention program. *J Sch Health* 1998;68:62–67.
30. Auld GW, Romaniello C, Heimendinger J, et al. Outcomes from a school-based nutrition education program using resource teachers and cross-disciplinary models. *J Nutr Educ* 1998;30:268–280.
31. Foerster SB, Gregson J, Beall DL, et al. The California Children's 5 A Day Power Play! Campaign. (unpublished manuscript).
32. Foerster SB, Gregson J, Wu S, et al. 1997 California Dietary Practices Survey: Focus on Fruits and Vegetables, Trends Among Adults, 1989–1997, A Call to Action. Sacramento, CA, California Department of Health Services. 1998.
33. Nicklas TA, Johnson CC, Myers L, et al. Outcomes of a high school program to increase fruit and vegetable consumption: Gimme 5—a fresh nutrition concept for students. *J Sch Health* 1998;68:248–253.
34. Cullen KW, Bartholomew LK, Parcel GS. Girl Scouting: An effective channel for nutrition education. *J Nutr Educ* 1997;29:86–91.
35. Resnicow K, Yaroch AL, Davis A, et al. GO GIRLS!: Results from a pilot nutrition and physical activity program for low-income overweight African American adolescent females. *Health Educ Behav* 2000;27(5):616–631.
36. Baranowski T, Baranowski J, Cullen K. Results of 5 A Day Achievement Badge for African-American Boy Scouts. *Prevent Med* (submitted).
37. Baranowski T, Davis Hearn M, Resnicow K, et al. Gimme 5 fruit and vegetables for fun and health: Outcome evaluation. *Health Educ Behav* 2000;27(1): 96–11.
38. Baranowski T, Hearn M, Baranowski JC, et al. Teach Well: The relation of teacher wellness to elementary student health and behavior outcomes: Baseline subgroup comparisons. *J Health Educ* 1995;26:S61–S71.
39. Perry CL, Bishop DB, Taylor G, et al. Changing fruit and vegetable consumption among children: The 5-a-Day Power Plus program in St. Paul, Minnesota. *Am J Public Health* 1998;88:603–609.

40. Perry CL, Lytle LA, Feldman H, et al. Effects of the Child and Adolescent Trial for Cardiovascular Health (CATCH) on fruit and vegetable intake. *J Nutr Educ* 1998;30:354–360.

41. Reynolds KD, Franklin FA, Binkley D, et al. Increasing the fruit and vegetable consumption of 4th graders: Results from the High 5 project. *Prev Med* 2000;30:309–319.

42. Cullen KW, Baranowski T, Nwachokor A, et al. 5 A Day Achievement badge for urban boy scouts: Formative evaluation results. *J Cancer Educ* 1998;13:162–168.

43. Domel S, Baranowski T, Davis H, et al. Development and evaluation of a school intervention to increase fruit and vegetable consumption among 4th and 5th grade students. *J Nutr Educ* 1993;25:345–349.

44. Fitzgibbon ML, Stolley MR, Avellone ME, et al. Involving parents in cancer risk reduction: A program for Hispanic American families. *Health Psychol* 1996;15:413–422.

45. Resnicow K, Davis M, Smith M, et al. Results of the Teach Well Worksite Wellness Program. *Am J Public Health* 1998;88:250–257.

46. Resnicow K, Davis M, Smith M, et al. How best to measure implementation of health curricula: A comparison of three measures. *Health Educ Res* 1998; 13:239–250.

47. Colditz G, Frazier A. Population approaches to cancer prevention: How much change do we need to achieve substantial reductions in cancer rates? (unpublished manuscript).

48. Cullen KW, Bartholomew LK, Parcel GS, et al. Intervention Mapping: Use of theory and data in the development of a nutrition program to increase fruit and vegetable intake in girls ages 9–12. *J Nutr Educ* 1998;30:188–195.

49. Baranowski T. Beliefs as motivational influences at stages in behavior change. *Int'l Quart Comm Health Educ* 1992–1993;13:3–29.

50. Baranowski T, Smith M, Hearn MD, et al. Patterns in children's fruit and vegetable consumption by meal and day of the week. *J Am Coll Nutr* 1997; 16:216–223.

51. West SG, Aiken LS. Toward understanding individual effects in multicomponent prevention programs: Design and analysis strategies. In Bryant KJ, Windle M, West SG (eds): *The Science of Prevention, Methodological Advances from Alcohol and Substance Abuse Research*. Washington, DC: American Psychological Association; 1997.

52. Cullen KW, Baranowski T, Smith SP. Goal setting for dietary change. *JADA* (in press).

53. Chapman LS. The role of incentives in health promotion. *The Art of Health Promotion* 1998;2:1–4.

54. Elder JP, Geller ES, Hovell MF, et al. *Motivating Health Behavior*. Albany, NY: Delmar Publishers; 1994.

55. Baranowski T, Stables G. Process evaluation in the 5 A Day Studies. *Health Educ Behav* 2000;27(2):157–166.

Chapter 12

Minority Populations

Shiriki K. Kumanyika, PhD, MPH, RD

The collective experience of a people (the culture) prepares them to deal with and sometimes subvert and transform oppressive conditions in ways unknown to the oppressor. Such experiences and their resultant wisdom transcend levels of income, age, and generation. We must never assume that because a group is economically poor its members are also cerebrally, philosophically, and practically poor, nor should we assume that wisdom in and of itself will overcome economic oppression. Programmatic efforts must, therefore, be directed towards synchronizing the philosophy of the people with their practices. C. Airhihenbuwa, 1995. *

Introduction

The influence of being an African American, Hispanic American, American Indian/Alaska Native, or Asian/Pacific Islander American, that is having "minority" status, on morbidity and mortality has become an increasing focus of health research and policy during the past decade.[1-4] The striking contribution of minority status to several health disparities underlies this increased attention. Conditions for which disease or death rates in one or more minority populations are disproportionately high compared to whites of the same age and sex include cardiovascular and cerebrovascular diseases, certain types of cancer, and Type 2 diabetes.[1-4] Although some racial/ethnic differences in disease susceptibility exist, disparities in occurrence or progression of these common diseases are primarily due to modifiable factors.[5,6] Inadequate adherence to lifestyle change recommendations among those with diagnosed disease may be among the factors that contribute to high incidence or low survival rates.

---

* See Reference 17, page 123.

From: Burke LE, Ockene IS (eds). *Compliance in Healthcare and Research.* Armonk, NY: Futura Publishing Company, Inc.; © 2001.

This chapter highlights conceptual issues related to understanding and improving compliance or "adherence"—the more common term in the lifestyle change literature—in minority populations. Both societal and individual perspectives on determinants of adherence and intervention approaches are discussed. The focus is on dietary adherence—one of the most complex areas of lifestyle change.[7-9] However, the perspective herein may relate to a much broader set of health-related behaviors.

What is "Special" About Minority Populations in the US?

Current US Census Bureau minority group categories are shown in Table 1. Although race and ethnicity are separate categories (that is, "Hispanics" can be of any race), they are conceptually intertwined; operationally people are usually classified by either race or Hispanic ethnicity.[10] Individuals self-designate race/ethnicity, although this is within the context of the social constructions and policies of who is

Table 1
Race/Ethnicity Categories in the 1990 Census

Race	White
	Black or Negro
	Chinese
	Indian (Amer.)
	Japanese
	Filipino
	Asian Indian
	Korean
	Aleut
	Eskimo
	Hawaiian
	Vietnamese
	Guamanian
	Samoan
	Other Asian/Pacific Islander
	Other race
Hispanic ethnicity	Mexican, Mexican Amer., Chicano
	Puerto Rican
	Cuban
	Other Spanish/Hispanic/Latino
	Not Spanish/Hispanic/Latino

Source: from Pollard and O'Hare, 1999, reference 10

"black," "Hispanic," "American Indian," or "Asian American," and when this is relevant.

To understand why adherence might differ according to minority status or according to membership in one of the ethnic groups listed in Table 1 requires reflection on what it is that defines "special populations" in health care settings. One characteristic of ethnic minority populations is that they are non-white (in the sense that those who identify themselves as Hispanics are considered different from other white Americans). In this sense, they are outside of the mainstream, where "mainstream" can be thought of as the dominant expectation about cultural food habits, health beliefs, and about other aspects of life circumstances that affect adherence. Those who deviate from these expectations are usually labeled in stigmatizing ways, such as "hard to reach."[11]

Being small in number relative to the dominant societal group is also an implicit aspect of minority status in the United States. Being few in number and having different needs may mean "falling between the cracks" and having no "voice," if services are conceived with the majority in mind. The more distinct the needs, eg, with respect to literacy, language, content of educational materials, or logistics, the greater the implied need for special staffing or service design considerations. This might not be cost-effective when the number of those affected is small in relation to the white population or even in relation to another, larger minority population (Latinos is a predominantly black community, for example). There might also still be the perception, although it is probably less common currently than in past decades, that the minority should make every effort to align their perspectives with those of the majority.[12–14]

In the absence of a deliberate effort to be client-centered or culturally appropriate, expectations about what should be offered and how the client will, or should, respond to what is offered occurs in the form of taken-for-granted assumptions on the parts of those who are designing and providing services. These assumptions are influenced not only by the life experiences and cultural background of health professionals but also by the cultural assumptions and social constructions that are embedded within the core paradigms of the health disciplines.[14] In such a scenario, numerous variables may contribute to the specialness of minority populations with respect to the context for dietary adherence. Foremost among these are socioeconomic status (SES) factors including literacy levels, income, educational attainment, unemployment or type of employment, and health insurance. Minority populations, on average, are disadvantaged on these variables.[3,10] The entire experience with the health care system is, therefore, marginal for many individuals in these populations.[15] Paul Farmer has introduced the term "structural violence" to indicate how these SES factors impact on the experience of the disadvantaged minorities.[16] Furthermore, minority status may reflect a host of other cultural and lifestyle variables, including country of origin, language spoken at home, household composition (eg, female-headed households; multigeneration households), region of residence within the U.S., religion, and a variety of culturally-influenced beliefs, preferences, and practices related to food intake and to health.[3,10] These variables may interact with socio-demographic factors, with additional special considerations based on gender and life stage.

Theoretically, cultural influences on dietary behaviors and other aspects of health lifestyles could be positive, negative, or neutral.[17] However, to the extent that minority clients have adherence characteristics for which the health care system is unprepared, the overall effect of being different will probably be negative. The perception that populations are hard to reach or inconvenient to serve may be demotivating to staff and predispose to negative or intolerant views of client behaviors.[11,14] Even where what is offered or the way it is offered is positive and at least a partial match with what is needed, the effective "dose" will probably be somewhat diluted in proportion to the extent of inappropriateness.[18] Undoubtedly, the possibility of cultural inappropriateness or mismatch may also apply for white Americans, who are also diverse by SES, religion, ethnic reference culture, and health beliefs. In this sense, considerations about adherence issues for minority populations may open a window to improved understanding of the importance of social and cultural influences in adherence overall.

Societal Influences on Adherence and the Importance of Context

The importance of individual behavior in determining chronic disease has been a central theme in both general population and minority-focused health promotion within the US.[1,19] Concern has been raised about the tendency to "blame the victim" for health problems that are strongly determined by social structural factors, such as those that limit access to health care and limit choice of options.[19,20] Nevertheless, many have accepted the necessity of attempting to reach individuals in minority or socially disadvantaged communities with programs that address health promotion and adherence to medical regimens while avoiding the trap of victim-blaming.[19,21] However, as will be discussed, the feasibility of health promotion programs under circumstances where there are severe environmental constraints is unclear. Given the many aspects of our environment that are potentially damaging to health, eg, those that promote inactivity and overeating, environmental constraints on adherence are an issue for the general population.[22] However, these issues are especially relevant to communities with the most unfavorable conditions and least power to alter these conditions, eg, inner city communities where low-income African Americans or Hispanic Americans reside.[3,10]

Figure 1 shows a hypothetical "causal web" of societal level influences on levels of food intake and physical activity and, through these variables, on obesity.[22] This model was developed as a conceptual framework for analyzing determinants of the global increase in obesity prevalence and identifying possible points of leverage for effecting public health approaches to obesity prevention. The schema reminds us, for example, that food selections depend on variables in the work, school, or home environment, such as what foods are available, how they are prepared, when they are offered, and at what cost. Barriers to dietary adherence are often defined and addressed at this level by counseling patients to practice avoidance behaviors (eg, avoid high fat foods) or to relieve social pressures to eat in a certain way through negotiation with family members and coworkers.[8,23] Policy approaches that might decrease the presence of environmental factors that are counter to adherence are much less common[8,24] and may be considered

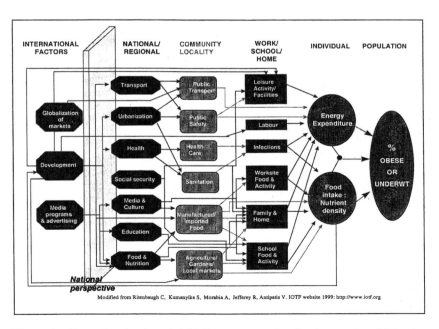

Figure 1.   Causal web of societal influences on obesity, International Obesity Task Force, www.iotf.org (adapted with permission from reference 22).

outside of the domain, or at least outside of the expertise, of health workers.[25]

Furthermore, the experience to date with community-level interventions that include interventions to address environmental barriers has been disappointing.[26] Figure 1 suggests that local community factors may be difficult to leverage without changes in policies at state, national, and even international levels.[22] For example, globalization of trade increases competition in many market sectors. Profit-driven marketing of food may skillfully promote consumption patterns that are counter to dietary recommendations, and the less healthful foods may become increasingly more affordable than healthful ones.[27] Regulatory policy and constitutional issues influence manufacturers' latitude in food advertising and related health claims. Governmental policies affect the content of school lunches. School fund raising policies may lead to vending of less healthful foods in competition with meals that meet dietary guidelines. Employment policies, urban transport systems, and education policies may influence lifestyles and daily routines in ways that increase the likelihood of consuming foods away from home with consequent influences on the amounts and kinds of foods consumed. Similar reasoning can be applied to how structural factors influence options for physical activity, eg, transportation, public safety, and urban design issues that determine where one cannot safely walk or ride a bicycle or whether children have active play during the school day.

Sociocultural Influences

Notwithstanding the importance of structural factors that act as enablers of or constraints on lifestyle behaviors, within any given set of constraints, individuals do maintain some behavioral latitude. Sociocultural factors impact directly on the choices that each individual makes among the available options. Sociocultural influences can be thought of as a set of invisible guidelines that shape institutions and that tell people how to view the world.[28] Cultural norms and values influence how we relate to other people and to our environments, and they vary with ethnic background(s), social class, gender, age, profession, and a host of other social stratification and social role variables. Cultural perspectives influence everyone. What stands out about the cultural perspectives of minority populations is—as suggested previously—that they may differ from those of the majority of health care providers and from the "mainstream" expectation, in ways that alter the likelihood of following our advice.[14] The greater the social distance between two cultures, the more apparent the differences will be to the respective participants in those cultures. This is especially true if the differences are manifest in tangible characteristics such as language or dress. In contrast, cultural differences among people who share many common experiences and characteristics (eg, African Americans and whites raised in the Southeastern US) may be much subtler. Furthermore, as reviewed elsewhere[18], culture—as such—is a societal or group level variable. How culture influences any given individual depends on numerous personal experiences and psychosocial characteristics.

The model in Figure 2 describes the relationship between societal-level cultural influences and individual attitudes and practices.[18] Figure 2 has been framed in terms of cultural influences on individual attitudes and practices related to weight status, but the general schema is potentially applicable to other aspects of lifestyle. Socialization is shown as the dynamic process in which individuals develop specific expectations, attitudes, beliefs, and behaviors based on their cultural participation and exposures. The US mainstream culture is a complex synthesis of multiple cultures.[13] The traditional cultures of English-speaking European countries are dominant but are blended with many others, including some that are unique to US history, social structure, and ethnic composition.

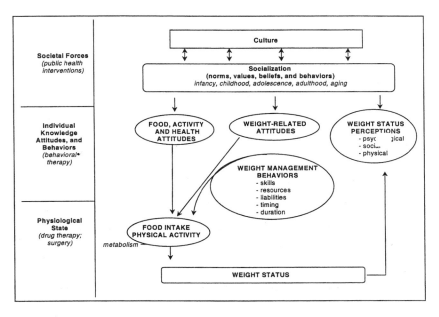

Figure 2. Levels and types of cultural influences on weight status (reprinted with permission from reference 18).

Figure 2 depicts cultural influences acting through both usual or underlying attitudes and behaviors and special health lifestyle attitudes and behaviors. Underlying or usual behaviors are obligatory or related to everyday functioning, survival, and well being. They endure for reasons that may be unrelated to specific health motivations and beliefs. In Figure 2, the underlying attitudes relate to health, food, activity, body weight, and to their interrelationships. Adherence issues encountered in modifying these behaviors must take into account the primary functions and anchors of these behaviors. For example, modifying the ways one interacts with one's family members about food will have sociocultural and psychosocial implications that extend far beyond weight maintenance or cholesterol reduction. These broader implications may drive the potential for long-term adherence. The less congruent the behavior modifications with the bigger picture, the less likely they are to be maintained. In this sense the individual's immediate sociocultural and family milieu can be viewed as imposing structural constraints—as discussed previously—at the microenvironmental level.

Health lifestyle attitudes and behaviors are superimposed onto this backdrop of usual behaviors. In Figure 2, these include weight-specific attitudes such as self-perceptions about one's own body size and shape and the reactions of others to it, as well as specific dieting and exercise knowledge and skills deliberately learned and undertaken for the purpose of weight maintenance: perceived need for weight control, perceived effectiveness, difficulty, and cost of various weight control strategies, and perceived contingencies related to adherence or nonadherence. More broadly, health lifestyle behaviors are driven by the person's specific attitudes, motivations, and role perceptions related to having a given health condition or problem.

Elements of African American cultural perspectives can be used to further illustrate how culture influences dietary and lifestyle change. Underlying food habits of African Americans are often influenced by direct or indirect exposure to the eating patterns in the US South.[29,30] Core foods that are frequently consumed and highly valued include chicken and pork, cooked green leafy vegetables, okra, tomatoes, legumes, corn, and yams. Fresh fruits and vegetables and dairy products are more peripheral and less frequently consumed.[29] Although individuals with a Southern dietary pattern will vary in their preferences for these foods, an awareness on the part of nutrition counselors of the high values for both meat and legumes may be helpful when attempting to foster substitutions of plant sources of protein for animal sources. Perceptions of African Americans about appropriate foods to eat may be strongly influenced by perceptions of the choices that are, or have been historically, available to African Americans, as suggested by the following comments from focus group interviews:[31]

> *"Blacks eat what they are accustomed to eat"*;
> *"But basically, I feel that we eat what our parents ate when they were growing up"*;
> *"Food practices are handed down from generation to generation."*

On the other hand, some extant opinions among African Americans are supportive of dietary modifications and diversity in food choices, eg:

> *"There are certain things in the black community that we as a black community need to stay away from. That fat, that grease, that oil, that living in America we basically become a society of fast food. Black people are not informed about healthy nutritional practices."*
> *"I don't care if Greeks make it, Chinese made it or whatever, if it's something I like, hey . . ."*[31]

These cultural themes can be addressed in interventions at the group or community level. For individual counseling it is helpful to recognize them as potential influences on what a person might perceive as the right type of eating pattern and how dietary modifications (eg, recommendations to switch to something that is not usually sold in the neighborhood stores) might be viewed.

Sidney Mintz, an anthropologist who has studied food culture in Caribbean societies has pointed out the potential importance of freedom of expression in preparing and flavoring food.[32] If the kitchen was the place where the slave could express herself, where food was relatively available, and where there were a lot of things to choose from in order to make a dish unique, then changing the method of preparing food may have a very deep impact on the sociocultural meanings. The individual in question might not be aware of these when attempting to make dietary changes. Once made aware she might prefer to find a different food to substitute for one that, if prepared differently, would violate cultural norms. Without assistance in recognizing the cultural issues, cultural attitudes about sick roles and responsibilities can be invoked to support such a change, ie, a belief that having a health problem changes the cultural expectation about what and how one should eat. Cultural food ideologies may influence dietary or medication adherence.[33,34] These underlying beliefs may negate adherence to advice that is perceived as contradictory. Other beliefs may have positive implications for adherence. It is important to work within both types of beliefs.

Family interactions are other aspects of day-to-day life and core survival patterns that differ across cultures and that affect health behaviors.[18] African American extended families are characterized as more interconnected, with less of a distinct nuclear unit of individuals compared to the prototypical American family. There are also demographic patterns, such as the high proportion of female-headed households in the African American community[10], that influence intra family interactions and social support networks. People who are more connected to and interdependent with others might experience less success with intervention programs that are oriented towards the individual client. In this respect, Kumanyika and Morssink[18] noted a finding of Wadden et al.[35] from their weight study in African American girls. The condition in which the mother and daughter were treated together was more animated, more fun, and more supportive than the conditions with the child alone or the child and mother separate. This was contrasted with Brownell's prior finding from a similar study in white girls in which the mother and child together condition was inhibiting.[36]

Much has been written about differences in body image norms among African Americans and whites, norms that are associated with generally less negative attitudes about overweight women in the black community.[18] These attitudes and the related fact that overweight or obesity is present in two-thirds of black women[37]impact on black women's weight control efforts. The obesity-tolerant attitudes co-exist with mainstream values for leanness and thinness, making weight management issues potentially more complicated for black women. There may be greater ambivalence or uncertainty about the trade-offs involved in losing weight and in overcoming the difficulties needed to maintain long permanent weight loss.

There are also mixed attitudes about physical activity that affect attempts of African Americans to become more active. A substantial amount of data suggest that usual physical activity levels are lower for blacks than whites.[18] Attitudes about physical activity in the black community may, however, be shaped by images of hard physical labor under conditions of slavery or low paying jobs. For example, both focus group data[38] and questionnaire data administered to African Americans enrolling in a dietary modification study (Kumanyika, unpublished data) indicated a common perception that rest is as or more important to health than exercise. The focus group data also suggested that beliefs about harmful effects of exercise (eg, as a stressor that raises blood pressure) were also common among African Americans.[38]

Although it is beyond the scope of this review to discuss the potential applicability of the conceptual framework in Figure 2 to other behaviors, a hypothetical example of adherence to a prescription to take antihypertensive medication may suffice to illustrate the general approach. Underlying attitudes and behaviors might involve the general concepts of preserving one's health, tolerating disease, remedies, how the body works, pill taking, following medical advice, and determinism. Relevant health lifestyle attitudes might include the personal perception of what it means to have high blood pressure, whether it is associated with having symptoms, how blood pressure is affected by medication on a daily and long-term basis, as well as learned routines for remembering to fill prescriptions, take medications, or check blood pressure at home for self-monitoring.

The main points to be gleaned from Figure 2 and from the foregoing examples are: 1) that cultural influences on adherence reflect individual's exposure to societal level processes that are not directly accessible for direct intervention in behavioral change programs; and 2) that many culturally-influenced behaviors are anchored to the rest of the person's life in ways that constrain the ability to or the appropriateness of modifying them. Societal level public health approaches may shift cultural norms and values over time—the change in cultural norms for cigarette smoking is a good example—perhaps in response to attitudinal and behavioral changes among influential groups in the population. Individual-level interventions must either take advantage of cultural influences that are consistent with what is being promoted or may work around those that are in opposition.

Within each ethnic group there are subgroup issues related to variables such as gender, age cohort (ie, generation), life stage, health status, religious beliefs, socioeconomic status, region, and urban-rural residence. This applies to ethnic minorities and to whites. There is also diversity on the cultural factors themselves. Members of any ethnic group identify with and participate in their ethnic cultures to varying degrees. Both qualitative and quantitative aspects of cultural identity may influence the adoption and maintenance of lifestyle changes promoted in the mainstream culture.

Comparisons of Dietary Adherence of African Americans and Whites

Within the available literature on adherence to dietary behavior change, comparisons of adherence across ethnicity or income status are difficult to identify in the literature. One reason for this is the relative lack of ethnic diversity among subjects in studies on relevant questions, particularly when considering the sample size needed to support formal subgroup comparisons. Where study populations include substantial proportions of individuals from more than one ethnic group, subgroup analyses by ethnicity may not be reported. When reported, such subgroup analyses must be interpreted with particular care. The primary deterrents to adherence may operate very early on in the pro-

Table 2

Studies Reporting Ethnic Differences in Direct or Indirect Measures of Dietary Adherence

Authors	Study objective	Study design	Findings
Mojonnier et al, 1980, reference 43	Evaluation of nutrition education approaches in preparation for a trial of cardiovascular disease risk reduction	Participants (199 whites and 84 blacks) with hypercholesterolemia were randomly assigned to one of four teaching formats or to no-education	Compared to whites, black participants had greater gains in knowledge at one month; at 6 to 9 month follow up black participants reported larger dietary changes and had greater reductions in serum cholesterol
Kumanyika et al, 1991, reference 41	Efficacy of weight reduction for the prevention of hypertension:	Analyses of sex and race-specific results from 2 separate, randomized, controlled multi-center studies, involving men and women ages 25–49 (HPT) or 30–54 (TOHP) who were not using antihypertensive medications and had diastolic blood pressures between 80 and 89 mmHg at baseline; follow up was 18 or 36 months	In both studies, mean overall weight change was less in blacks than whites; particularly among women.
Kiley et al, 1993, reference 44	Assessment of compliance with dietary and medication regimens post kidney transplant	Observational data on a series of 105 patients (27 white; 54 black; 21 Hispanic, and 3 Asian) who received a kidney transplant at an urban university hospital during a two year period; follow up was 18 to 55 months; mean 34.6 months.	Black patients were underrepresented among patients compliant to both diet and medication; Hispanic patients were compliant to both diet and medication or to neither

Wylle-Rosett et al, 1993, reference 45	Efficacy of low sodium/ high potassium diet or of weight reduction alone or in combination with medications for hypertension management	Ethnic comparison at 6 months of an intensive randomized trial of dietary intervention with 582 men and women (324 and 158 black); participants were mildly hypertensive (DBP 90 to 100 mmHg), overweight (110% to 160% of MLIC standard weight), and off antihypertensive medications for at least 2 weeks	Significantly fewer black participants achieved dietary goals for sodium and potassium
Kumanyika et al, 1993, reference 46	Efficacy of sodium reduction in preventing high blood pressure	Multicenter randomized controlled trial of sodium reduction in 30–54 year old men and women with DBP between 80 and 89 mmHg at baseline	Black participants were significantly less likely than white participants to achieve the sodium reduction goal
Wing and Anglin 1996, reference 47	Randomized comparison of weight loss in two different year long treatment programs	Treatments were a behavioral program with a low calorie diet throughout or which included two 12-week periods of a very low calorie diet, over 1 year.	Blacks lost less weight, reported smaller initial changes in calorie intake and had lower attendance than whites
Van Horn et al, 1997, reference 48	Cardiovascular disease risk reduction in high risk men	Analyses of direct and indirect adherence measures, including modeling of baseline factors as adherence predictors	Blacks had poorer dietary adherence and smaller decreases in serum cholesterol as whites, while the reverse was true for Asians.

TOHP = Trials of Hypertension Prevention; MLIC = Metropolitan Life Insurance Company cess of recruitment or enrollment into clinical or research programs. Study populations may, therefore, include only those individuals with a high motivation for participation. This factor—ie, selection into studies of highly motivated individuals—is commonly understood as a limitation on the external validity of data from randomized clinical trials.[39] However, the potential effect of self-selection on the validity of ethnic comparisons *within* studies may be less well recognized. As noted by Ness et al.,[40] *"minority participants for whom majority patterns of participation are comfortable may be different from minority participants for whom logistic and cultural influences are real barriers to participation"* (p. 476). They cited two relevant examples: 1) among women enrolled in the Trials of Hypertension Prevention, Phase 1, African Americans were much more likely to be college educated than the whites[41]; and 2) a worksite health program in which blacks were significantly less likely than whites to enroll but, once enrolled, equally likely to be successful in weight reduction.[42] Differential adherence across ethnicity may be reflected in differential drop out rates, which would distort ethnic comparisons of adherence among those remaining.

Table 2 summarizes relevant studies identified through an extensive search of published literature on cardiovascular diseases and diabetes. These studies[41,43–48] appeared to be the only ones with informative ethnic comparisons of dietary interventions. As shown, they primarily involve African American and white study populations. However, they do include varied dietary behaviors, counseling approaches, and settings, and both men and women. All of these studies indicate differences between African Americans and whites in either direct (eg, changes in dietary intake or urinary sodium and potassium excretion) or indirect measures (eg, change in weight or serum cholesterol) measures of adherence. The Mojonnier et al. report[43] suggests better adherence in blacks than whites. This study evaluated several counseling approaches (self-teaching, group teaching, individual teaching, and a multi-method approach involving all three methods). Which approaches were particularly effective with the African American participants was not reported. All of the other studies listed in Table 2 suggest that African American participants had more problems with dietary adherence than white participants did. If selection factors operating at enrollment tend to equalize motivation in study participants, true adherence differences in blacks and whites in the general population may be larger than those observed in these studies.

Examples of Studies Designed for Effectiveness with Minority Populations

The five studies in Table 3 were selected to illustrate recent approaches to the development and evaluation of lifestyle change programs specifically attuned to the social cultural and contextual issues of minority populations.[49–53] In contrast to the studies in Table 2, which permit relative effectiveness across ethnic groups, the studies in Table 3 relate to the absolute level of effectiveness within a particular group. Both perspectives are important and they have different strengths and limitations. The cross-ethnic comparisons help in determining different expectations of success (eg, smaller effects, longer time to achieve the effect, or preferences for different program elements) or possible problems (ie, less enrollment or more attrition among minority participants) that might ensue from using a general approach. Note that this assumes that the "general" approach is biased towards the mainstream culture. Studies within a single ethnic group are indispensable because they allow for evaluation of ways to achieve optimum results by matching the intervention as closely as possible to the relevant culturally defined norms, values, and preferences and to the lifestyle context.

The studies in Table 3 include three that were conducted with African American populations, one with a Mexican American population, and one with Pima Indians. Outcomes addressed included control of weight, high blood pressure, elevated cholesterol, and blood glucose. All of these programs indicate effectiveness at some level. Whether effect sizes are similar to or greater than those that would have been observed without the special culturally-relevant design features might be assessed indirectly by comparing results from each of these studies with results of more conventional studies on similar outcomes and of similar duration. The most appropriate evaluation of these studies is internal, based on results in the comparison groups. However, differences between intervention and control groups may be minimized when the control groups also receive an intervention. The CARDES results for women were similar for the intervention (full instruction) and control (self-help) groups at the end of the 1-year follow-up.[53] This points out that outcomes in control groups receiving low intensity interventions may be informative along with those in the treatment group. In any population, a little intervention (health monitoring and basic information) may go a long way with those who are highly motivated to change.[54]

Almost all of the interventions described in Table 3 can be viewed as "culturally-adapted" to varying degrees. That is, they are programs based on a pre-existing framework for which the content, format, and venue are modified to reflect the culture of the participants. For example, adaptations of *Cuidando el Corazon* related to language, foods, and family involvement.[49] CARDES adaptations included the use of familiar characters and family processes in a narrative format as well as presentation of nutrition information in a form that was nonquantitative and couched in broader cultural views of food and health.[53]

Table 3

Examples of Studies Designed for Effectiveness with Minority Populations

Authors and title	Program focus and population	Description	Evaluation
Cousins et al, 1992, reference 49 "Family Versus Individually Oriented Intervention for Weight Loss in Mexican American Women"	Weight reduction in Mexican American women (n = 168 overweight women, ages 18 to 45) who were married and had at least one pre-school aged child	A behavior change manual, "Cuidando el Corazon" and cookbook were developed to facilitate an eating plan low in total and saturated fat and weight reduction. The cookbook was based on typical Mexican American foods in Texas. Both Spanish and English versions of the materials were available. Individual treatment consisted of 24 weekly and then 6 monthly classes led by bilingual dietitians. Family treatment used the same approach but included information for partners, encouragement of spouses to attend, and separate classes for pre-school children.	Participants were stratified on weight and randomly assigned to receive the manual only (control) or to treatment on an individual versus family basis. A linear trend towards weight loss in all groups was observed, with the significant improvements in both the family and individual treatment groups (greater in the family group, but not significantly so) compared to the control group.

Turner et al, 1995 reference 50 *"Cardiovascular Health Promotion in North Florida African-American Churches"*	Church based CVD health promotion in a rural county in North Florida; annual participation at church-based health promotion activities was 294 in year 1 and 343 (89% of the year 1 participants plus 81 new participants); 68% women	A Health Advisory Council of local church leaders was formed and guided by staff in the development of a program; the HAC reviewed background information on successful health programs, conducted a needs assessment from vital statistics data and a survey of local health problems, and developed a model program. Staff conducted health promotion workshops to facilitate program development by church leaders. Programs involved medial publicity, a fashion show, cooking demonstrations, an exercise videotape to church music (Gospelsize), and nutrition and mental health awareness activities. The Council facilitated these activities, including development or identification of readily accessible resource materials.	High participant rates indicated achievement of the goal of increasing community; weekly exercise classes were among the most popular activities; systolic and diastolic blood pressure decreased in year 2 vs. year 1; improvements in dietary practices and physical activity were observed, although not all behavioral changes were statistically significant

(continued)

Table 3

(continued)

Authors and title	Program focus and population	Description	Evaluation
Flores 1995, reference 51, *"Dance for Health"*	Aerobic exercise program for low-income African American and Hispanic adolescents (n = 81; 54% female); 43% were Hispanic, 44% were African American, and 13% other ethnicity; 41% spoke Spanish at home; mean age was 12.6 years	Dance for Health was a dance-oriented physical activity curriculum developed to replace regular school physical education classes (mostly playground activities) for 7th grade students; attendance was mandatory, as for the regular class; students from each ethnic group were invited to recommend popular music; in addition, Dance for Health students attended health education classes (adapted from a cardiovascular disease education curriculum) twice a week and aerobics three times a week	Classes were randomized to Dance for Health or regular physical education over 12 weeks. Dance for Health was associated with lower BMI, heart rate, improved fitness, and these changes were statistically significant in the girls. Girls in Dance for Health also had improved attitudes towards physical activity, but boys' attitudes worsened.
Narayan KMV et al, 1998, reference 52 *"Randomized Clinical Trial of Lifestyle Interventions in Pima Indians: A Pilot Study"*	Lifestyle intervention for NIDDM prevention in Pima Indians in Arizona (n = 95) overweight, non-diabetic men and women ages 25–54 y)	Pima Pride emphasized self-directed learning and included monthly small group discussions of Pima culture, history, and current lifestyles. Written materials included a newsletter and basic nutrition and exercise information; Pima Action was a more conventional and more structured program with active encouragement to change diet and activity patterns through behaviorally-oriented weekly	Individuals were randomized to one of the two programs and re-examined at 6 and 12 months. Feedback on weight, glucose and serum cholesterol was provided at follow up visits. An additional observational group of individuals who had refused randomization was also followed; both interventions were associated with increases in physical activity, and starch intake decreased in those

Kumanyika et al, 1999, reference 53 *"Outcomes of a cardiovascular nutrition counseling program in African Americans with elevated blood pressure or cholesterol level?"*	Cardiovascular nutrition education for African Americans with diverse literacy skills (n = 244 women and 86 men; mean age 55y); all participants had high blood pressure or high cholesterol	The CARDES program Nutrition counseling materials were developed for use in outpatient settings; core items were a boxed deck of 100 food picture cards depicting typical servings of commonly eaten foods and including African American ethnic foods and an accompanying booklet with replicas of the cards and additional nutrition guidance. For a non-quantitative approach, cards were coded with symbols to indicate low, medium, or high content of fat, cholesterol, and sodium. A video and 12-program audioseries about an African American extended family were also developed to motivate behavior change and provide specific dietary change instructions in a vignette format	Individuals were randomized to receive the full CARDES package or only the food cards and booklet. All participants received brief counseling by a nutritionist and feedback on their blood pressure and serum cholesterol; full instruction participants attended one class each month for the first four months. Follow up at 12 months was complete for 77%. Both formats were associated with significant improvements in lipid profiles in women; men had better lipid results with full instruction; blood pressure improved for those with elevated blood pressure at baseline; outcomes did not differ by literacy level but were linked to the initial frequency of using the CARDES materials
		group meetings and home visits as warranted.	in Pride. Several clinical measures, including weight, worsened in Action compared to Pride; clinical indicators also worsened in the observational group; program satisfaction was greater for Pride

CARDES also used African American staff and was offered by an African American community institution (a black University Hospital). The Florida church program[55] implemented the concept of cultural adaptation at a more in-depth level, by involving members of the population being served in the development and conduct of the program. Thus, not only were the content and format of the program culturally congruent with that of church members, the ultimate program implementation was from within rather than from outside of the community.

The Narayan et al.[52] study in Pima Indians shows the distinction between cultural adaptation—Pima Action—and what might be termed "within-culture" programming—Pima Pride. Pima Pride was built upon cultural traditions and perceptions from the beginning and was the core ethic. The more distant the culture of the participants is from that of the programmers, the more important it is to allow programs to evolve from within the group. This risks, of course, the evolution of such a program along lines that are different from or broader than those that the health professionals (and sponsors) might have intended. However, the alternative approach risks evolution of the program as one with which participants can only interact in a relatively superficial and ultimately ineffective way. The difference in outcomes observed between Pima Action and Pima Pride are consistent with this interpretation. More exploration of within-culture approaches to lifestyle interventions is warranted.

Conclusions

The views expressed here are intended to provide a conceptual framework for understanding adherence to dietary and lifestyle changes in minority populations and help to explain some apparent contradictions between the motivations to adhere and the ability to adhere. The difficulty of long-term adherence to dietary or physical activity recommendations is much more than simply a matter of individual will. This has clear implications for the type of research needed to identify ways to improve adherence. Studies to document factors that are favorable or unfavorable to adherence should encompass not only individual psychosocial or perceived social support variables but also practical information about the range of adherence options and perceived and real constraints in the larger environment. An example of a relevant approach is that of Cheadle and coworkers[55], in which a relatively high correlation was observed between individual food selections and the shelf-space assigned to the respective type of food in the person's neighborhood supermarkets. Analytic approaches that nest variation in individual behavior (eg, fruit and vegetable consumption frequency) within group-level variables (eg, neighborhood characteristics) that describe the context for adherence may be informative.[56,57] Research has identified practices of targeted advertising of tobacco and alcohol in minority communities.[58] Studies are needed to determine whether this type of advertising also influences the food environments of minority populations.

The assumptions of the average clinician or health educator about underlying health attitudes and beliefs, day-to-day eating and activity habits, and what is important to day-to-day survival are less likely to be on target for populations who are "special," as defined here. The resources and strategies available for coping and overcoming obstacles in populations that have been socially disadvantaged may be underestimated by outsiders who primarily see the deficits.[17]

Studies designed to assess ethnic differences in adherence are relatively few. Related analyses tend to be ancillary to the main objectives of the study, and usually do not include individual, programmatic, or contextual variables that mediate observed differences. However, at least for African Americans, lower effectiveness of conventional programs compared to whites can be documented. Of the available approaches to culturally competent programming, those that build the program concept and implementation from within the culture of the participant group may be the most promising.

References

1. US Department of Health and Human Services. Report of the secretary's task force on black and minority health. Volume 1. Executive summary. Washington: US Government Printing Office, 1985.
2. Reynolds G. American College of Epidemiology Tenth Annual Scientific Meeting. *Ann Epidemiol* 1993;3(2):119–206.
3. Council of Economic Advisors for the President's Initiative on Race. Changing America. Indicators of Social and Economic Well-Being by Race and Hispanic Origin. September 1998. http://www.access.gpo.gov/eop/ca/index.html
4. Nickens HW. The role of race/ethnicity and social class in minority health status. *Health Serv Res* 1995;30:151–162
5. Kumanyika SK, Golden PM. Cross-sectional differences in health status in U.S. racial/ethnic minority groups. Potential influence of temporal changes, disease, and lifestyle transitions. *Ethnicity and Disease* 1991;1: 50–59.
6. Cooper R. A note on the biologic concept of race and its application in epidemiologic research. *Am Heart J* 1984;108:715–722.
7. Glanz K. Compliance with dietary regimens. Its magnitude, measurement and determinants. *Preventive Med* 1980;9:787–804.
8. Brownell KD, Cohen LR. Adherence to dietary regimens 2. Components of effective interventions. *Behavior Med* 1995;20:155–164.

9. Kumanyika SK, VanHorn L, Bowen D, et al. Maintenance of Dietary Behavior Change. *Health Psychology* (in press).
10. Pollard KM, O'Hare WP. America's racial and ethnic minorities. Population Bulletin 54.3 Washington DC: Population Reference Bureau, 1999.
11. Freimuth VS, Mettger W. Is there a hard-to-reach audience? *Public Health Reports* 1990 105;232–238.
12. Leininger M. Becoming aware of types of health practitioners and cultural imposition. *J Trancult Nurs* 1991;2:32–39.
13. Spain D. American diversity. On the edge of two centuries. *Population Reference Bureau Reports on America* 1999;1(2).
14. Kavanagh KH, Hennedy PH. Promoting cultural diversity. *Strategies for Health Care Professionals*. Newbury Park, CA: Sage Publications, Inc. 1992
15. King G. Institutional racism and the medical/health complex. A conceptual analysis. *Ethnicity Dis* 1996;6:30–46.
16. Farmer P. Social Scientists and the New Tuberculosis. *Soc Sci Med* 1997;44: 347–358.
17. Airhihenbuwa CO. *Health and Culture*. Beyond the western paradigm. Thousand Oaks, CA: Sage Publications, Inc., 1995
18. Kumanyika SK, Morssink CB. Cultural appropriateness of weight management programs. In Dalton S (ed): *Overweight and Weight Management*. Aspen Publisher, Gaithersburg, MD, pp. 69–106, 1997.
19. Dougherty CJ. Bad faith and victim-blaming. The limits of health promotion. *Health Care Analysis* 1993;1:111–119.
20. Allegrante JP, Green LW. Sounding Board. When health policy becomes victim blaming. *New Eng J Med* 1981;305:1528–1529.
21. Neighbors HW, Braithwaite RL, Thompson E. Health promotion and African-Americans. From personal empowerment to community action. *Am J Health Prom* 1995;9:281–287.
22. Ritenbaugh C, Kumanyika S, Antipatis V, et al. Caught in the causal web: A new perspective on social factors affecting obesity. *Healthy Weight Journal* November/December 1999 (in press).
23. El-Kebbi IM, Bacha GA, Ziemer DC, et al. Diabetes in urban African Americans V. Use of discussion groups to identify barriers to dietary therapy among low-income individuals with non-insulin dependent diabetes mellitus. *Diabetes Educator* 1996;22(5):488–492.
24. Morrison CM, Cassady D, Deeds S, et al. California is "ON THE MOVE". *J Health Education* Supplement 1999;30(2):S1-S71.
25. Antipatis V, Kumanyika S, Jeffery RW, Morabia A, Ritenbaugh C. from the Public Health Approaches to the Prevention of Obesity (PHAPO) Working Group of the International Obesity TaskForce (IOTF). Confidence of health professionals in public health approaches to obesity prevention. *Int J Obesity* 1999;23:1004–1006.
26. Winkleby MA, Feldman HA, Murray DM. Joint analysis of three U.S. community intervention trials for reduction of cardiovascular disease risk. *J Clin Epidemiol* 1997;50:645–658.
27. Drewnowski A, Popkin BM. The nutrition transition: New trends in the global diet. *Nutr Rev* 1997;55:31–43.
28. Helman CF. *Culture, Health, and Illness*. An introduction for health professionals. Boston, MA: Wright, 1990.
29. Veale Jones D, Darling M. *Ethnic Foodways in Minnesota*; St. Paul MN: University of Minnesota Press, 1996.
30. Kittler PG, Sucher KP. Food and culture in America. *A Nutrition Handbook*. Second Edition. Washington DC: West/Wadsworth, 1998.

31. Airhihenbuwa CO, Kumanyika S, Agurs TD, et al. Cultural aspects of African-American eating patterns. *Ethnicity and Health* 1996;1(3):245–260.
32. Mintz SW. *Tasting Food, Tasting Freedom.* Excursions into eating, culture, and the past. Boston: Beacon Press, 1997.
33. Matthews HF. Rootwork. Description of an ethnomedical system in the American South. *South Med J* 1987;80:885–891.
34. Brown CM, Segal R. The effects of health and treatment perceptions on the use of presecribed medication and home remedies among African American and white hypertensives. *Soc Sci Med* 1996;43:903–917.
35. Wadden TA, Stunkard AJ, Rich L, et al. Obesity in black adolescent girls. A controlled clinical trial of treatment by diet, behavior modification, and parental support. *Pediatrics* 1990;85:345–352.
36. Brownell KD, Kelman JH, Stunkard AJ. Treatment of obese children with and without their mothers. Changes in weight and blood pressure. *Pediatrics* 1983;71:515–523.
37. Flegal KM, Carroll MD, Kuczmarski RJ, et al. Overweight and obesity in the United States: Prevalence and trends, 1960–1994. *Int J Obes Relat Metab Disord* 1998;22:39–47
38. Airhihenbuwa CO, Kumanyika S, Agurs TD, et al. Perceptions and beliefs about exercise, rest, and health among African Americans. *Am J Health Prom* 1995;9:426–429.
39. Holmberg L, Baum M. Can results from clinical trials be generalized? *Nature Medicine* 1995;1:734–736.
40. Ness RB, Nelson DB, Kumanyika SK, et al. Evaluating minority recruitment into clinical studies: How good are the data? *Ann Epidemiol* 1997;7:472–478.
41. Kumanyika SK, Obarzanek E, Stevens VJ, et al. Weight-loss experience of black and white particiapants in NHBLI-sponsored clinical trials. *Am J Clin Nutr* 1991;53:1631S-1638S.
42. Brill PA, Kohl HW, Rogers T, et al. The relationship between sociodemographic characteristics, recruitment, and health improvements in a worksite health promotion program. *Am J Health Prom* 1991;5:215–221.
43. Mojonnier ML, Hall Y, Berkson DM, et al. Experience in changing food habits of hyperlipidemic men and women. *J Am Diet Assoc* 1980;77:140–148.
44. Kiley DJ, Lam CS, Pollack R. A study of treatment compliance following kidney transplantation. *Transplantation* 1993;55:51–56.
45. Wylie-Rosett J, Wassertheil-Smoller S, Blaufox MD, et al. Trial of Antihypertensive Interventions and Management. Greater efficacy with weight reduction than with a sodium-potassium intervention. *J Am Diet Assoc* 1993; 93:408–415.
46. Kumanyika SK, Hebert PR, Culter JA. Feasibility and efficacy of sodium reduction in the Trials of Hypertension Prevention, Phase I. *Hypertension* 1993;22:502–512.
47. Wing RR, Anglin K. Effectiveness of a behavioral weight control program for blacks and whites with NIDDM. *Diabetes Care* 1996;19(5):409–413.
48. Van Horn LV, Dolecek TA, Grandits GA, et al. Adherence to dietary recommendations in the special intervention group in the Multiple Risk Factor Intervention Trial. *Am J Clin Nutr* 1997;65:289S–294S.
49. Cousins JH, Rubovits DS, Dunn JK, et al. Family versus individually-oriented intervention for weight loss in Mexican American women. *Public Health Reports* 1992;107:549–555.
50. Turner LW, Sutherland M, Harris GJ, et al. Cardiovascular health promotion in North Florida African-American churches. *Health Values* 1995;19(2): 3–9.

51. Flores R. Dance for health . Improving fitness in African American and Hispanic adolescents. *Public Health Reports* 1995;110:189–193.
52. Narayan KMV, Hoskin M, Kozak D, et al. Randomized clinical trial of lifestyle interventions in Pima Indians. A pilot study. *Diabetic Medicine* 1998; 15:66–72.
53. Kumanyika SK, Adams-Campbell L, Van Horn B, et al. Outcomes of a cardiovascular nutrition counseling program in African Americans with elevated blood pressure or cholesterol level. *J Am Diet Assoc* 1999;99: 1380–1388,1391.
54. Grufferman S. Complexity and the Hawthorne effect in community trials. *Epidemiology* 1999;10:209–210.
56. Diez-Rouz AV, Nieto FJ, Caufield L, et al. Neighborhood differences in diet. The Atherosclerosis Risk in Communities Study. *J Epidemol Comm Health* 1999;53:55–63.
57. Van Korff M,Koepsell T,Curry S, Diehr P. Multi-level analysis in epidemiologic research on health behaviors and outcomes. *Am J Epidemiol* 1992;135: 1077–1082.
58. Moore DJ, Williams JD, Qualls WJ. Target marketing of tobacco and alcohol-related products to ethnic minority groups in the United States. *Ethnicity Dis* 1996;6:83–98.

Chapter 13

Obese Populations

Michael G. Perri, PhD

Improving Adherence in the Treatment of Obesity

Over the past two decades, the prevalence of obesity in the US has increased at an alarming rate,[1] and evidence continues to accumulate documenting the deleterious impact of excess weight on health and longevity.[2,3] Weight loss can reverse many of the disadvantages associated with obesity.[4,5] However, the effectiveness of obesity treatments is limited by poor adherence to the behavioral changes necessary to maintain weight loss.[6] In this chapter, I will review a variety of strategies designed to improve adherence to changes in diet and exercise in the treatment of obesity. The strategies examined include extended treatment, skills training, food provision, monetary incentives, telephone prompts, peer support, exercise, and multicomponent maintenance interventions.

Behavioral Treatment of Obesity

The use of behavioral strategies to produce changes in diet and exercise has become routine practice in dietary intervention programs and in pharmacological management of obesity.[7] Participants in behavioral or "lifestyle" interventions are taught to modify their eating and exercise patterns so as to produce a negative energy balance and thereby lose weight. The behavioral strategies typically used in lifestyle interventions include self-monitoring, goal setting, performance feedback, reinforcement, stimulus control, cognitive restructuring, and problem solving.

More than 150 studies have evaluated the effectiveness of behavior

From: Burke LE, Ockene IS (eds). *Compliance in Healthcare and Research.* Armonk, NY: Futura Publishing Company, Inc.; © 2001.

therapy for obesity. Reviews of recent randomized trials[8,9] show that behavioral treatment, typically delivered in 15 to 24 weekly group sessions, produces an average weight loss of approximately 8.5 kg (mean body weight reduction = 9%). This degree of weight loss is associated with significant improvements in health and psychological well being, but its clinical significance is determined by whether the weight loss is maintained over the long run. During the year following behavioral treatment, participants regain typically 30% to 40% of their lost weight. Moreover, follow-up studies conducted 2 to 5 years after behavioral treatment have documented a gradual but reliable return to baseline weights.[10,11]

A complex interaction of physiological, psychological, and environmental variables appears responsible for poor maintenance of weight loss. Physiological factors, such as low metabolic rate,[12] adaptive thermogenesis,[13] and increased adipose tissue lipoprotein lipase activity,[14] prime the obese person for a regaining of lost weight. Continuous exposure to an environment rich in fattening foods, combined with a dieting-induced heightened sensitivity to palatable foods, further disposes the individual to setbacks in dietary control.[15] Most obese persons cannot on their own sustain the substantial degree of psychological control needed to cope effectively with this unfriendly combination of environment and biology.

During the period following weight-loss treatment, fewer reinforcers are available to maintain adherence to intervention goals. Many, if not most, obese participants are motivated by a desire to improve their appearance, and most hold unrealistically high expectations about the amount of weight loss they can accomplish.[16] Thus, when they stop losing weight or fail to accomplish their expected losses, their motivation to adhere to prescribed changes in diet and exercise falters, thereby increasing the chances for regaining weight. As a consequence, many become discouraged by the difficulties they experience in trying to sustain their lower weights, and their negative psychological reactions to initial weight gains contribute further to poor adherence. Often, they ascribe their lack of success in weight-loss maintenance to personal failings.[17,18] Such attributions can trigger feelings of depression and guilt and precipitate a sense of hopelessness thereby leading to an abandonment of the weight-loss effort and ultimately to a total relapse.

What factors are associated with successful outcome in obesity treatment? Retrospective analyses typically show that weight loss is associated with treatment adherence.[19] Correlational studies show that attendance at treatment sessions, the use of written self-monitoring, and the completion of exercise are associated with weight loss.[20] In addition, good adherence during the first month of treatment is a reliable predictor of favorable treatment outcome.[20] However, caution is required in interpreting correlational findings such as these because participants with higher levels of motivation are more likely to show better adherence and better outcome. Consequently, it is difficult to determine whether it is the participant's adherence or motivation that is responsible for the better outcome. A clearer understanding of factors that promote long-term success can be derived from clinical trials that test the effects of various adherence strategies.

Strategies to Improve Long-term Adherence

Long-term success may be more likely to occur when obese participants are provided with programs or training specifically designed to enhance long-term adherence. A variety of such approaches have been examined, including: extended treatment, skills training, monetary incentives, food provision, telephone prompts, peer support, exercise, and multicomponent maintenance programs.

Extended Treatment

Over the past 20 years, the amounts of weight loss accomplished in behavioral treatment have doubled.[8] The increase appears to be due to increases in the length of treatment. The longer participants are in treatment, the longer they adhere to prescribed changes in eating and exercise behaviors. The effects of length of treatment on continued adherence and weight loss have been demonstrated experimentally. Perri and colleagues[21] compared the effects of standard length behavioral treatment (ie, 20 sessions) with extended treatment (ie, 40 sessions) and found that the extended treatment resulted in continued adherence and continued weight loss during the extended treatment from weeks 20 to 40 (see Figures 1 and 2). However, both adherence and weight loss deteriorated when the extended treatment ended after 40 weeks.

In a recent review,[6] seven studies[21-27] were examined that included behavior therapy with treatment extended beyond 6 months through the use of clinician contacts in weekly or biweekly sessions. Collectively, these studies provided 224 participants with a total of 35 to 65 group sessions ($M = 44.5$ sessions) over the course of 40 to 78 weeks ($M = 55.1$ weeks). Three of the studies[21,23,24] included control groups that received an initial course of behavioral treatment (20 weekly group sessions) but no additional contacts except for follow-up assessments. At the conclusion of the extended treatment period (approximately 12 months), those groups that received behavior therapy *with* extended contact demonstrated mean net weight losses of 11.3 kg and maintained

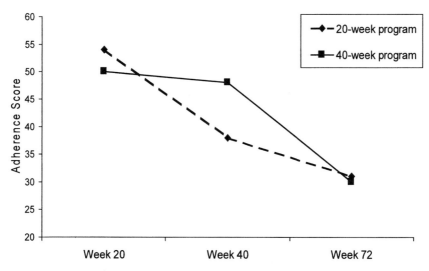

Figure 1. Effects of 20-week and 40-week treatment programs on adherence (adapted from Perri et al.[21]).

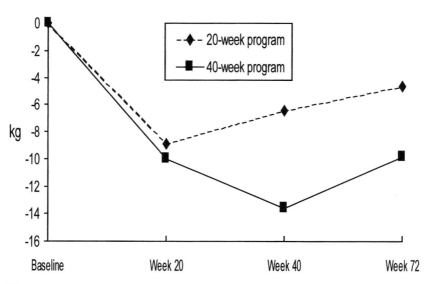

Figure 2. Effects of 20-week and 40-week treatment programs on weight loss (adapted from Perri et al.[21]).

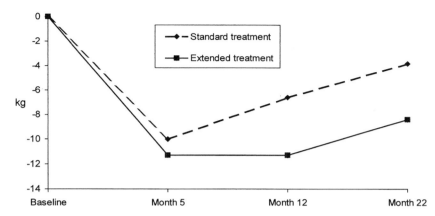

Figure 3. Summary of mean weight losses in seven studies with extended behavioral treatment (adapted from Perri[6]).

the entire amount (101.6%) of weight that they had lost in initial (or first 6 months of) treatment. Over approximately the same period of time, those groups that received behavior therapy *without* extended treatment had a mean net loss of 6.6 kg and maintained about two-thirds (66.5%) of their initial weight reduction (see Figure 3).

Five of the studies included additional follow-up periods without therapist contacts.[21-27] The results of these additional follow-ups conducted on average 21 months after the start of treatment showed that the extended treatment groups demonstrated mean net loss of 8.4 kg (73.2% of their initial reduction) compared to 3.8 kg (38.3% of their initial reduction) for the groups without extended contact. Collectively, these data show that providing participants with extended treatment fosters better maintenance of weight reductions compared to behavior therapy without extended contact. However, additional treatment does not result in additional weight loss.

While extended therapy seems effective in the maintenance of modest weight losses, it does not appear to be effective for the maintenance of large weight reductions such as those induced by very-low calorie diets. The large losses produced through severe energy restriction are poorly maintained even when initial treatment is extended through weekly or biweekly sessions.[27,28]

Skills Training

Several studies have tested relapse prevention training (RPT) in which participants are taught how to avoid or cope with slips and relapses as a means of maintaining long-term adherence.[29] Perri et al.[30] found that including RPT during the course of initial treatment was not effective, but combining RPT with a multicomponent program of patient-therapist contacts by mail and telephone significantly improved the maintenance of weight loss. Perri and Nezu[31] showed that the combination of RPT plus year-long posttreatment therapist contacts improved the maintenance of weight loss compared to initial treatment without follow-up care. Similarly, Baum et al.[32] showed that patients in a minimal contact maintenance condition experienced a significant regaining of weight while participants who received the combination of RPT and posttreatment contacts maintained their end-of-treatment weight losses.

Food Provision/Monetary Incentives/Telephone Prompts

As a means of promoting dietary adherence, Jeffery and colleagues[33] examined the effectiveness of providing participants with prepackaged, portion-controlled, low-calorie meals (10 per week at no cost) or with monetary incentives for weight loss, or with the combination of both. No significant effects were observed for monetary incentives, but participants in the food provision groups showed significantly greater weight losses than those without food provision both during initial treatment and during the 12-month maintenance period. However, the results of an additional 12-month follow-up showed poor maintenance of weight loss in all conditions.[34]

Wing et al.[35] tested the effectiveness of *optional* food provision as a means of promoting long-term dietary adherence. Participants who completed behavioral treatment were provided with the opportunity to purchase prepackaged, portion-controlled, low-calorie meals. The optional food provision strategy was not effective, largely because participants did not purchase the prepackaged meals. Wing et al.[35] also examined the effects of frequent telephone contacts designed to prompt adherence to self-monitoring. The telephone calls were made by interviewers who were unknown to the participants and who did not offer advice or counseling. The telephone prompts did not improve the maintenance of weight loss.

Peer Support

Can social support be marshaled to enhance adherence and weight loss? Perri et al.[23] examined the effects of a peer support program in which participants were taught how to run their own peer group support meetings. The participants were provided with a meeting place equipped with a scale, and biweekly meetings were scheduled over a 7-month period following initial treatment. Attendance at the peer group meetings was relatively high (67%), but no advantage versus a no-maintenance condition was observed in terms of adherence or weight change during the maintenance period. The results of a 48-week follow-up revealed significant regaining of weight in both conditions, but the peer support group had a greater mean net loss than the control condition (6.5 vs. 3.1 kg, respectively).

Wing and Jeffery[36] recently evaluated the benefits of recruiting participants with friends (versus alone) and providing enhanced social support for weight loss (versus standard behavioral treatment). Among participants recruited alone and given standard treatment, only 24% maintained their losses 6 months after treatment. However, among participants recruited with friends and provided with enhanced social support, 66% maintained their weight loss in full. These findings suggest that the benefits of peer support interventions may be limited to individuals who enter treatment with preexisting social ties to other group members.

Exercise

Correlational studies generally indicate that long-term weight loss is associated with increased physical activity.[19] Likewise, studies of obese persons who have achieved successful long-term weight losses show that exercise is associated with the maintenance of weight loss.[37] However, Wing[38] has recently documented that few controlled trials have shown that the combination of diet plus exercise produces significantly greater long-term weight loss than diet alone. A key limitation of many of the long-term studies of diet plus exercise versus diet alone is that often there is poor adherence to exercise. Thus, a key question is how to improve adherence to exercise by obese individuals. In a recent study, Perri et al.[22] examined the effects of group- versus home-based exercise regimens in the treatment of obesity. After 6 months, both conditions displayed significant improvements from baseline in exercise participation, cardiorespiratory fitness, eating patterns, and weight loss. At 12 months, however, the home-based program showed superior performance to the group condition in exercise participation and treatment adherence. Participants in the home condition completed

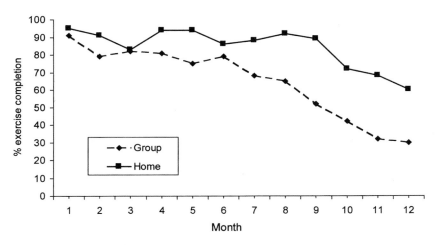

Figure 4. Effects of group-based and home-based exercise programs on exercise completion over 12 months (adapted from Perri et al.[22]).

a significantly higher percentage of prescribed exercise sessions than subjects in the group condition (83.3% vs. 62.1%, respectively, $P < 0.05$, see Figure 4). Moreover, the long-term superiority of the home-based program was also evident for weight loss.

Multicomponent Maintenance Programs

The majority of maintenance programs tested have entailed multiple components designed to enhance long-term adherence. Perri et al.[39] tested the effects a multicomponent maintenance program (conducted over a 65-week period) consisting of peer group meetings combined with ongoing patient-therapist contacts by mail and telephone. Patients were taught to run their own peer group meetings and were provided with preprinted sets of postcards designed for simplified self-monitoring of food intake and the use of key weight-loss strategies. The therapists in turn made brief phone calls to provide support and guidance during the maintenance phase. Compared to a comparison condition that received initial treatment plus 6 biweekly booster sessions, the multicomponent program demonstrated significantly better maintenance of weight loss both at the end of the maintenance phase and at additional follow-up six months later. These findings were replicated by Perri et al.[40] who used a longer initial treatment period (20 rather

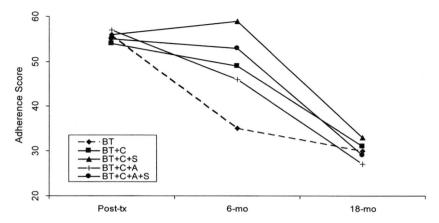

Figure 5. Effects of four maintenance programs on adherence (adapted from Perri et al.[24]). BT = behavior therapy; BT + C = behavior therapy plus extended contact; BT + C + S = behavior therapy plus extended contact plus social influence program; BT + C + A = behavior therapy plus extended contact plus aerobic exercise program; BT + C + A + S = behavior therapy plus extended contact plus aerobic exercise program plus social influence program.

than 14 weeks), included a group-based aerobic exercise program, and obtained larger weight losses at posttreatment and at follow-ups.

Perri et al.[24] tested the effects of adding increased exercise and a social influence program (or both) to a posttreatment therapist contact program consisting of 26 biweekly group sessions. At the conclusion of the posttreatment phase, all four programs produced significantly greater maintenance of weight losses than a comparison condition consisting of behavior therapy without posttreatment contact. The study showed no significant between-group effects for the exercise and social influence manipulations, but the group that received therapist contacts combined with both increased exercise and the social influence program was the only one to demonstrate a significant additional weight loss (4.1 kg—observed during the first 6 months of the maintenance period). The effectiveness of the therapist contact programs on adherence and on weight loss was most pronounced during the first half of the year-long maintenance phase. During the second half of the maintenance phase (which corresponded to the 11th through the 17th month of continuous treatment), adherence diminished in all maintenance groups (see Figure 5). Six months after the posttreatment programs ended, the four maintenance groups succeeded in sustaining 70% to

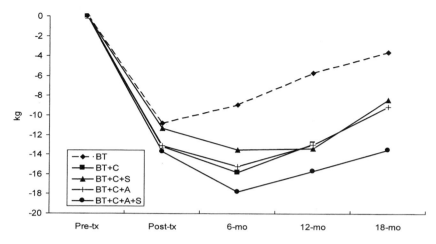

Figure 6. Effects of four maintenance programs on weight loss (adapted from Perri et al.[24]). BT = behavior therapy; BT + C = behavior therapy plus extended contact; BT + C + S = behavior therapy plus extended contact plus social influence program; BT + C + A = behavior therapy plus extended contact plus aerobic exercise program; BT + C + A + S = behavior therapy plus extended contact plus aerobic exercise program plus social influence program.

99% (M = 83%) of their initial weight losses compared to 33% for the group without posttreatment therapist contact (see Figure 6).

Implications

Support for the efficacy of extended treatment for obesity has been well-documented. Compared to obesity treatment without additional contact, extended treatment in the form of weekly or biweekly group therapy sessions improves the maintenance of treatment effects for as long as 1 year following initial therapy. Similarly, multicomponent approaches that combine ongoing patient-therapist contacts (whether in person or by telephone and mail) with relapse prevention training or social support programs have shown improved maintenance compared to behavioral treatment without such programs. Therapist contact appears to be the key ingredient in multifaceted programs. Strategies such as peer groups meetings, relapse prevention training without continued therapist contact, telephone prompts by nontherapists, monetary incentives, and the availability of portion-controlled meals, do not appear effective in enhancing the maintenance of treatment effects.

Continued adherence to the changes in eating and exercise patterns induced during the initial treatment phase appears to be the mechanism responsible for the better outcomes observed in extended treatments. Sustained adherence in extended treatments may be due in part to the social pressure of group treatment or the demand characteristics inherent in the therapy context. Weekly or biweekly therapy sessions also provide ongoing prompts of "appropriate" eating and exercise behaviors, combined with opportunities for therapists to reinforce adherence and to assist participants in problem solving to overcome obstacles to continued maintenance.[41] In addition, therapy contacts can boost participant morale during the period following the first 6 months of treatment. During this time, weight loss typically stops, and the motivation of participants begins to lag as the most reinforcing element of therapy (ie, weight loss) subsides.

Limitations of Extended Treatment

Extended treatment is not a panacea for the adherence problem in the treatment of obesity. Several factors require consideration in the evaluation of extended treatment. Continuing therapy is labor-intensive and expensive, yet the costs must be weighed against the alternative, namely, the invariant pattern of weight gain that occurs in therapy without posttreatment care. A second issue concerns the changes in the motivation of clients during extended therapy. As treatment duration approaches 1 year, session attendance becomes problematic, adherence falls off, and participants often begin to regain weight despite continued treatment. Participants often cling to unrealistic expectations about the amounts of weight loss that treatment can produce. Consequently, when their weight loss plateaus during the course of long-term treatment, many become disheartened and their participation in treatment flounders. Educating patients about realistic weight-loss expectations is essential to successful treatment, and special procedures may be needed to enhance motivation for participation in extended therapy. For example, Perri et al.[24] utilized an array of social influence tactics that increased adherence (but not weight loss) in maintenance sessions, including "bonus bucks" (ie, group contingencies with monetary incentives based on adherence), "learning by teaching" (ie, patient participation in preparing and delivering lectures on weight-loss maintenance strategies), and "telephone networking" (ie, planned peer support phone calls between sessions). In addition, recruiting participants with friends and providing enhanced social support may also improve long-term adherence.[36]

Extended therapy does not enhance the maintenance of large weight reductions induced by severe energy restriction. Extended therapy appears effective in helping patient to adhere to the energy intake level required to maintain the reductions of 6 to 12 kg typically accomplished in behavior therapy but not the losses of 15 kg or more produced with very-low calorie diets. The decreased energy intake required to sustain losses equivalent to 15% to 20% of body weight may require an unattainable degree of long-term dietary restraint.

Clinical Directions

Maintenance of "Behavior Change"

Because obese persons do not have direct control over how much weight they lose, treatment goals should be framed in terms of behaviors that they can control, such as the quantity and quality of food they consume and the amounts and types of physical activity they perform. Moreover, obese persons should be informed that significant health benefits can be derived from even modest amounts of weight loss.[42]

Comprehensive Assessment

The treatment of obesity should be preceded by a comprehensive assessment of the effects of obesity on the individual's health and emotional well-being. The impact of obesity on risk factors for disease (eg, hypertension, glucose tolerance, dyslipidemia etc.) and quality of life (eg, emotional state, body image, binge eating, etc.) should be assessed. A careful individualized assessment will often reveal important behavioral and emotional targets for intervention, such as binge eating, body image disparagement, and anxiety or depression—problems that need to be addressed regardless of whether weight loss itself becomes an objective of treatment.

Redefining Success

Successful outcome in the care of the obese person should not be viewed solely in terms of weight loss. Beneficial changes in risk factors for disease and improvements in quality of life represent important indicators of success in the care of the obese person. Improvements in the quality of diet should be a component of care independent of whether weight reduction is an identified objective of care. Reductions in amounts of dietary fats, particularly saturated fats, can improve health as well as assist in weight loss.[43] Similarly, increased physical activity and a decrease in sedentary lifestyle can represent beneficial components of long-term care irrespective of the impact of exercise on weight loss.[44]

Continuous Care Model

Finally, clinicians and patients alike must view obesity as a chronic condition requiring continuous care. Short-term treatments that strive to produce reduction to "ideal" weight are unlikely to succeed. A continuous-care approach focused on the achievement of realistic long-term objectives appears more appropriate for most obese patients. Although much work needs to be done in the development of long-term treatments for obesity, extended treatments have shown promise in promoting adherence to the behaviors required for the long-term maintenance of weight loss.

References

1. Flegal KM, Carroll MD, Kuczmarski RJ, et al. Overweight and obesity in the United States: Prevalence and trends. *Int J Obesity* 1998;22:39–47.
2. Pi-Sunyer FX. Medical hazards of obesity. *Ann Intern Med* 1996;119:655–660.
3. Sjöström LV. Mortality of severely obese subjects. *Am J Clin Nutr* 1992;55: 16S-23S.
4. Maggio CA, Pi-Sunyer FX. The prevention and treatment of obesity. *Diabetes Care* 1997;20:1744–1766.
5. Pi-Sunyer FX. Short-term medical benefits and adverse effects of weight loss. *Ann Intern Med* 1993;119:722–726.
6. Perri MG. The maintenance of treatment effects in the long-term management of obesity. *Clin Psychol Sci Pract* 1998;5:526–543.
7. Wadden TA, Van Itallie TB. *Treatment of the Seriously Obese Patient.* New York: Guilford, 1992.
8. Perri MG, Fuller PR. Success and failure in the treatment of obesity: Where do we go from here? *Med Exerc Nutri Health* 1995;4:255–272.
9. Sarwer DB, Wadden TA. The treatment of obesity: What's new, what's recommended. *J Womens Health Gend Based Med* 1999;8:483–493.
10. Kramer FM, Jeffery RW, Forster JL, et al. Long-term follow-up of behavioral treatment for obesity: Patterns of weight gain among men and women. *Int J Obes* 1989;13:124–136.
11. Wadden TA, Sternberg JA, Letizia KA, et al. Treatment of obesity by very low calorie diet, behavior therapy, and their combination: A five-year perspective. *Int J Obes* 1989, 13(Suppl. 2), 39–46.
12. Ravussin E, Swinburn BA. Energy metabolism. In Stunkard AJ, Wadden TA (eds): *Obesity: Theory and Therapy (2nd ed.).* New York: Raven Press, 1993:97–124.
13. Leibel RL, Rosenbaum M, Hirsch, J. Changes in energy expenditure resulting from altered body weight. *New Engl J Med* 1995;332:621–618.
14. Kern PA, Ong, JM, Saffari B, et al. The effects of weight loss on the activity and expression of adipose-tissue lipoprotein lipase in very obese humans. *New Engl J Med* 1990;322:1053–1059.

15. Rodin J, Schank D, Striegel-Moore R. Psychological features of obesity. *Med Clin N Amer* 1989;73:47–66.
16. Foster GD, Wadden,TA, Vogt, RA, et al. What is a reasonable weight loss? Patients' expectations and evaluations of obesity treatment outcomes. *J Consult Clin Psychol* 1997;65:79–85.
17. Jeffery RW, French SA, Schmid TL. Attributions for dietary failures: Problems reported by participants in the Hypertension Prevention Trial. *Health Psychol* 1990;9:315–329.
18. Goodrick GK, Raynaud AS, Pace PW, et al. Outcome attribution in a very low calorie diet program. *Int J Eat Dis* 1992;12:117–120.
19. Kayman S, Bruvold W, Stern JS. Maintenance and relapse after weight loss in women: Behavioral aspects. *Amer J Clin Nutr* 1990;52:800–807.
20. Wadden TA, Letizia KA. Predictors of attrition and weight loss in patients treated by moderate and severe caloric restriction. In Wadden TA, Van Itallie TB (eds): *Treatment of the Seriously Obese Patient*. New York: Guilford Press , 1992, pp. 383–410.
21. Perri MG, Nezu AM, Patti ET, et al. Effect of length of treatment on weight loss. *J Consult Clin Psycho* 1989;57:450–452.
22. Perri MG, Martin AD, Leermakers EA, et al. Effects of group- versus home-based exercise in the treatment of obesity. *J Consult Clin Psycho* 1997;65: 278–285.
23. Perri MG, McAdoo WG, McAllister DA, et al. Effects of peer support and therapist contact on long-term weight loss. *J Consult Clin Psychol* 1987;55: 615–617.
24. Perri MG, McAllister DA, Gange JJ, et al. Effects of four maintenance programs on the long-term management of obesity. *J Consult Clin Psychol* 1988; 56:529–534.
25. Viegener, BJ, Perri MG, Nezu AM, et al. Effects of an intermittent, low-fat, low-calorie diet in the behavioral treatment of obesity. *Behav Ther* 1990;21: 99–509.
26. Wadden TA, Vogt A, Andersen RE, et al. Exercise in the treatment of obesity: Effects of four interventions on body composition, resting energy expenditure, appetite, and mood. *J Consult Clin Psychol* 1997;65:269–277.
27. Wing, RR, Blair E, Marcus M, et al. Year-long weight loss treatment for obese patients with type II diabetes: Does including an intermittent very-low-calorie diet improve outcome? *Am J Med* 1994;97:354–362.
28. Wadden TA, Foster GD, Letizia KA. One-year behavioral treatment of obesity: Comparison of moderate and severe caloric restriction and the effects of weight maintenance therapy. *J Consult Clin Psychol* 1994;62:165–171.
29. Marlatt GA, Gordon JR. *Relapse Prevention*. New York: Guilford Press, 1985.
30. Perri MG, Shapiro RM, Ludwig WW, et al. Maintenance strategies for the treatment of obesity: An evaluation of relapse prevention training and post-treatment contact by mail and telephone. *J Consult Clin Psychol* 1984;52: 404–413.
31. Perri MG, Nezu AM: Can weight loss be maintained? The effects of post-treatment programs. *Ann Behav Med* 1998;20:S60.
32. Baum JG, Clark HB, Sandler J. Preventing relapse in obesity through post-treatment maintenance systems: Comparing the relative efficacy of two levels of therapist support. *J Behav Med* 1991;14:287–302.
33. Jeffery RW, Wing RR, Thorson C, et al. Strengthening behavioral interventions for weight loss: A randomized trial of food provision and monetary incentives. *J Consult Clin Psychol* 1993;61:1038–1045.

34. Jeffery RW, Wing RR. Long-term effects of interventions for weight loss using food provision and monetary incentives. *J Consult Clin Psychol* 1995; 63:793–796.

35. Wing RR, Jeffery RW, Hellerstedt WL, et al. Effect of frequent phone contacts and optional food provision on the maintenance of weight loss. *Ann Behav Med* 1996;18:172–176.

36. Wing RR, Jeffery RW. Benefits of recruiting participants with friends and increasing social support for weight loss and maintenance. *J Consult Clin Psychol*, 1999;67:132–138.

37. McGuire MT, Wing RR, Klem ML, et al. Long-term maintenance of weight loss: Do people who lose weight through various weight loss methods use different behaviors to maintain their weight? *Int J Obes* 1998;22:572–577.

38. Wing RR. Physical activity in the treatment of the adulthood overweight and obesity: Current evidence and research issues. *Med Sci Sports Exerc* 1999;31(11 Suppl):S547–S552.

39. Perri MG, McAdoo WG, Spevak PA, et al. Effect of a multi-component maintenance program on long-term weight loss. *J Consult Clin Psychol* 1984; 52:480–481.

40. Perri MG, McAdoo WG, McAllister DA, et al. Enhancing the efficacy of behavior therapy for obesity: Effects of aerobic exercise and a multicomponent maintenance program. *J Consult Clin Psychol* 1986;54:670–675.

41. Perri MG, Nezu AM, Viegener BJ. *Improving the long-term management of obesity: Theory, research, and clinical guidelines.* New York: John Wiley & Sons; 1992.

42. Wing RR, Jeffery RW. Effect of modest weight loss on changes in cardiovascular risk factors: Are there differences between men and women or between weight loss and maintenance? *Int J Obes* 1995;19:67–73.

43. Insull W, Henderson M, Prentice R, et al. Results of a feasibility study of a low-fat diet. *Arch Int Med* 1990;150:421–427.

44. Paffenbarger RS, Lee I-M. Physical activity and fitness for health and longevity. *Res Q Exerc Sport* 1996;67:11–28.

Section VI

Issues Across Settings

Chapter 14

Clinical Trials

Eleanor Schron, MS, RN and
Susan M.Czajkowski, PhD

Introduction

Adherence in clinical trials, like adherence in clinical care settings, is a critical element in ensuring that a treatment or therapeutic regimen produces the intended effect. In this chapter, we address four major issues regarding adherence in clinical trial settings: first, we discuss why adherence in clinical trials is important; secondly, we contrast the issues of adherence in clinical trials with those in clinical care settings, highlighting the methods used to optimize adherence in the clinical trial setting; thirdly, we discuss several of the strategies used in selected trials of cardiovascular interventions, both multicenter and single-site studies, to maintain high levels of adherence; and finally, we consider how what we learn about enhancing adherence in the clinical trial setting can help improve adherence in clinical practice. Although adherence is an important issue in all clinical trials, whether they involve medical or behavioral interventions, in this chapter we will focus on long-term trials of medications for cardiovascular diseases.

Why is Adherence in Clinical Trials Important?

Adherence has been defined as the extent to which a person's behavior in terms of taking medications, following diets, or executing lifestyle changes coincides with medical or health advice.[1] In clinical trials, adherence is a complex issue, involving a number of separate behaviors: participants are asked to adhere to study treatments—ie, take a particular dosage of medication at specific time intervals over a

From: Burke LE, Ockene IS (eds). *Compliance in Healthcare and Research.* Armonk, NY: Futura Publishing Company, Inc.; © 2001.

period of weeks, months or years, have various clinical procedures and blood draws for laboratory tests—in addition, they also must attend study appointments, meet study requirements such as filling out forms and questionnaires, participate in evaluations of quality of life or studies of cognitive function, and must provide self-reports of their medication consumption so that their adherence can be measured. Thus, participation in research protocols requires efforts beyond the mere act of taking the required amount of study medication. Adherence in trials can be assessed in several ways: as the number or percentage of pills taken by patients (as measured by pill counts at the time of clinic visits); by patients' self-reports of their medication-taking behavior; measurement of chemical markers, or by use of sophisticated electronic monitoring devices, which record the number and timing of patients' opening their pill bottles, for example.

The level of expected adherence is one of the critical elements to be considered when planning a trial, along with the expected event rates, and length of accrual and follow-up. Careful, realistic planning is essential because all of these factors will impact on the likelihood of successfully accomplishing the trial. While it is unreasonable to expect 100% compliance to an intervention, the investigators need to specify a level that is adequate to allow testing against a control or comparison treatment. Various levels of compliance will effect power, duration, and the sensitivity of the study to detect treatment effects.[2] For example, a 20% reduction in drug adherence may result in the need for a greater than 50% increase in sample size to maintain equivalent power. Obviously, if twice as many subjects are needed, the costs will be greater and/or the duration of the study will be longer. The interpretation of results will also be affected, and completion of the study may even be threatened as evidence may be presented or published sooner resulting in a lack of equipoise.[3]

Nonadherence to treatment regimens is a special problem in clinical trials. Trial data are generally analyzed by the "intent-to-treat" rule, which states that the data from a given particpant in a trial should be analyzed as belonging to the treatment group to which that participant was assigned, regardless of whether he or she actually received the assigned treatment.[4] Therefore, even a small amount of nonadherence has a large effect on the sample size needed to detect a difference between groups if one exists. Although adherence in clinical trials has been reported as better than that in the general population, with estimates of 80 percent and above, there is evidence that these rates overestimate actual adherence due to the use of measures that are easily manipulated by patients, such as pill count and self-report.

Trial results can be affected by nonadherence with the intervention. Nonadherence leads to underestimating possible therapeutic and toxic effects and can undermine even a properly designed study. High attrition rates will affect generalizability since the study's results may apply only to those patients who comply with the treatment regimens or do not experience side effects.[5]

Optimizing Adherence in Clinical Trials

The issue of compliance in research settings is different than that in clinical settings.[6] Some of these differences can be understood in terms of how the trial setting differs from the practice setting. In clinical trials, participants are volunteers who must meet eligibility criteria to be enrolled. These eligibility criteria often include exclusions (characteristics, behaviors or traits) that predict nonadherence, such as psychiatric disorders, drug use and alcohol abuse. In addition, a prerandomization "run-in" period is often used to determine whether participants will be good adherers and therefore eligible to be enrolled in the trial. During the "run-in," participants who cannot tolerate the intervention or do not take an acceptable amount of drug or placebo are identified and excluded from enrollment in the trial. Although the advisability of using a "run-in" period as a method of screening out nonadherers has been questioned, it is a widely used strategy for prescreening trial participants to select only those who are motivated or able to adhere in the clinical trial context.[2,7] In this situation we have a study of efficacy because the intervention is assessed in a group of highly compliant participants; whereas, a study of effectiveness is conducted in more generalizable circumstances.

Apart from the use of "run-in," individuals who volunteer to participate in a clinical trial are generally a highly selective group of patients who might be expected to demonstrate greater motivation and commitment to the treatment regimen than patients in a clinical care setting.[8] Enrolling in a trial also involves signing an informed consent document, which can create a sense of commitment on the part of the patient.

Finally, aspects of the trial and the study regimen are often designed to optimize adherence—eg, a single dose formulation may be used rather than multiple daily dosage, where feasible. Ideally, the intervention schedule is similar to clinical practice. Research personnel are specially trained to implement the protocol, using methods that are designed to ensure high levels of patient adherence.[9,10] These methods include frequent contact with the patient, providing incentives and reminders that promote patient participation, and working with patients to address logistical, transportation and other barriers that can impede adherence to the protocol. This level of patient contact and attention is the ideal in the clinical trial and standard clinical care settings.

There are many strategies used by staff to optimize adherence. Payment for transportation is offered, convenient hours are scheduled, including home visits for follow-up data collection, and reminders are routinely provided. It is common to use behavioral strategies, such as patient contracts, pill counts with tailoring and feedback, and diaries, to enhance adherence. In fact, the measurement of adherence itself as part of the trial may boost adherence.

Clinical trial staff go to great lengths to keep track of participants. Clinics are organized to provide continuity of contact with the trial team as well as access. In summary, problems with patient adherence can generally be prevented by identifying potential problems before enrollment and through the enhancement and monitoring of adherence after enrollment.[11]

Strategies for Enhancing Adherence: Some Examples in Selected Trials

These principles can be illustrated by considering some examples of adherence-enhancing activities from selected clinical trials of cardiovascular interventions. In both the Physicians Health Study (PHS), and the ongoing Women's Health Study (WHS), the populations were selected because investigators expected health professionals to be more adherent than other populations. PHS was a randomized, double-blind placebo-controlled trial designed to test aspirin and beta-carotene in over 22,000 US male physicians.[12] WHS involves almost 40,000 female health professionals in a study designed to evaluate the effects of vitamin E and low-dose aspirin in primary prevention of cardiovascular disease and cancer in apparently healthy women.[13] The investigators choose to conduct these studies among physicians and health professionals because of their knowledge, training and interest in health issues. The participants were considered prepared to understand the purpose of the clinical trial, to give truly informed consent, and to provide reliable information on any illnesses developing after enrollment. For these reasons, these studies were able to be conducted by mail rather than through clinic visits, thereby substantially reducing costs of conducting the studies.

In the PHS, the investigators also used a run-in to exclude individuals thought to be poor compliers, defined as those who took less than two-thirds of their study medication during a 3-month period.[14] The investigators excluded 11,000 otherwise eligible subjects through the run-in to get a compliant group. Adherence was further supported with the use of calendar packs for dispensing study medication. These were used to keep track of medication taken at a cost of $1.00 each, which added almost $3.5M to the trial. Adherence in the PHS was measured with blood levels and self-report. Compliance in the aspirin group was 85% after 5 years, with similar levels obtained for the placebo group.

The Systolic Hypertension in the Elderly Trial (SHEP), a trial of men and women over 60 years old, also recorded high levels of adherence. SHEP enrolled almost 5000 participants and involved a 5-year follow-up period.[15] Compliance for over 2300 participants on active drug was 89% at year 3 and 90% at year 5. The placebo group had similarly high levels of compliance. The SHEP regimen may have contributed to these high, sustained levels of adherence, since it was a relatively simple regimen, generally involving once-daily dosing. Nurse assessments were central to this trial. Referral procedures were established and there was no cost for study drug or visits. In addition, a variety of activities were planned to keep participants informed and involved, including a participant newsletter, periodic social events at the clinics, and the use of participants as clinic volunteers.

Unlike SHEP, which was organized as a traditional clinical center model, the Antihypertensive and Lipid Lowering Treatment to Prevent Heart Attack Trial (ALLHAT) is organized according to a practice-based model, therefore, it involves different kinds of issues regarding adherence. ALLHAT has enrolled over 42,000 participants in over 600 clinical settings. After the first year, participants are seen three times a year for an average of five years. The purpose of ALLHAT is to determine whether any of the newer antihypertensive medications—amlodipine, doxazosin or lisinopriil — provide significantly greater or lesser reduction of heart attacks or deaths from coronary heart disease compared to the diuretic, chlorthalidone.[16] A subset of these participants are enrolled in a cholesterol component that compares diet alone versus diet plus pravastatin to determine whether pravastatin reduces total mortality compared with diet alone in participants with moderately high LDL cholesterol.

Because long term adherence is a challenge, The ALLHAT Adherence Committee developed the Adherence Survival Kit (ASK).[17] The ASK notebook contains information and tools to help physicians and nurses keep track of their participants and study events, keep participants on the study drug, and keep blood pressure controlled. Reference materials are also provided. These materials have been introduced at dinner meetings which bring physicians together to discuss patient management.

A checklist included in the kit, labeled Red Flags, was adapted from work published by Probstfield, et al.[18] Sections of the checklist include a number of behavioral changes that might be observed from previously consistent behavior. For example, Burke[19] reports electronic event-monitoring data that shows a dramatic decrease in adherence, indicating that the patient is having difficulty. Areas covered include behavioral signs, medical signs, and clinic environment changes.

An ALLHAT Short Course provides tips for planning and managing adherence. Suggestions include developing a plan to ascertain outcomes at the end of the trial, think carefully about whom you enroll, understand that some participants have trouble so be ready to help, keep participants involved, provide information on study progress, and understand that good staff and a team approach make a difference. Although these activities are similar to what we have done in many multicenter trials over the years, the approach used in ALLHAT, which brings together information about enhancing adherence in an easy-to-use format, and involves a formal training program to reinforce adherence maintenance skills on an ongoing basis, is especially well-organized and comprehensive. (See Table 1.)

Prior to use of the ASK, ALLHAT visit adherence was 82% at 12 months, 79% at 24 months, and 76% at 36 months.[17] The ASK was distributed last fall to all of the primary care clinics; its impact will be evaluated this fall.

A large trial that illustrates a different adherence challenge, a once-weekly drug dose, is the Azithromycin in Coronary Events Study (ACES). ACES is a trial of a once-a-week dose of antibiotic or placebo for one year in 4000 people with documented prevalent coronary artery disease.[20] To improve adherence in this situation, a telephone reminder system will be used. At the baseline visit, the patient is asked if he or

---

Table 1

Adherence Ideas

- Provide appointment schedule
- Contact before appointment
- Coordinate appointments
- Use automated computer system for reminders
- Arrange socials
- Offer "freebies"
- Personalize visit
- Help arrange travel to clinic with friends
- Check contact information
- Review medication routine each visit
- Invite contributions to newsletter
- Mail greeting cards

Reference: ALLHAT ASK Notebook

she would like a reminder call, and if yes, when and where. At follow-up the same question will be asked.

In addition to adherence-enhancing strategies incorporated into clinical trials sponsored or supported by the National Heart, Lung, and Blood Institute (NHLBI), research has also addressed the issue of how to design interventions to improve adherence in clinical trials. An example of this type of research is the Adherence in Clinical Trials program,[21] which consists of four studies of adherence-enhancing interventions, each conducted within the context of an ongoing clinical trial. Two of these studies were funded by the NHLBI: one examined the effects of adherence interventions in the Childhood Asthma Management—or CAMP—trial,[22] and the other focused on adherence interventions in a study of the effects of lipid-lowering medications on neuropsychological outcomes.[23] The other two studies were supported by the National Institute of Nursing Research (NINR), and consisted of a study of adherence interventions within a trial of potassium supplementation for hypertensive patients,[24] and a Veterans Administration (VA) funded study of warfarin treatment for myocardial infarction (MI) patients.[25] Of the four studies, recruitment for the study ancillary to the VA trial of MI patients was halted early due to problems with recruitment in the parent trial, and data from the study of CAMP patients are not available until closeout of that trial in 2000.

Preliminary findings were reported for two of the Adherence in Clinical Trials projects—those dealing with adherence to antihypertensive (potassium supplementation) and cholesterol-lowering (lovastatin) medications—at the Society for Clinical Trials meeting in May, 1998.[23,24] The data show no effect for the interventions used to promote adherence compared to usual care. The interventions used were behavioral interventions, using strategies such as habit-building and anticipatory problem-solving, and the outcomes included both self-reported and electronically-monitored medication adherence rates. A third paper presented in this symposium showed that for children with asthma, adherence was significantly greater for patients assigned to a twice daily bronchodilator than those assigned to a 4 × a day bronchodilator regimen, confirming other research concerning the value of simpler regimens in promoting adherence.[26]

Reasons for lack of an effect on self-reported adherence in the two projects reporting no effect include the possibility of a "ceiling effect," ie, self-reported adherence rates were extremely high in these trials (eg, 90% to 95%), leaving little room for improvement. However, effects were not found using other, more objective adherence measures (eg, electronic medication monitors) for which lower rates of adherence were found (60% to 80%). Another explanation for lack of effect might be the use of relatively low-intensity interventions, rather than comprehensive or multiple strategy approaches. Lower-intensity interventions were required for these projects because of concern about patient and staff burden in the trials in which the interventions were used. Finally, perhaps the behavioral strategies used did not "match" these patients' reasons for nonadherence. For patients on antihypertensive and cholesterol-lowering medications, the asymptomatic nature of the condition may be one of the most powerful determinants of non-compliance—that is, patients may simply not see therapy as being useful or important to them in the absence of salient symptoms, pain, etc.[27] In that case, interventions that enhance patients' assessments of the benefits of therapy and motivation to adhere to therapy may be needed.

Lessons from Clinical Trials

Experiences using adherence-enhancing strategies in clinical trials can provide insights that may, to some extent, generalize to the clinical practice setting. Identification of those less likely to adhere and use of tools such as the "Red Flags" may allow practitioners to focus resources and educational efforts early in the treatment period on those most likely to be at risk for poor adherence. Selection of the simplest formulation of an agent, such as a once or twice daily dosage schedule rather than four times each day, should also be adopted, where feasible, as a way to promote optimal adherence in clinical care settings.

Another feature of clinical trials—the use of multidisciplinary teams of health care professionals—may be an approach that can be adopted in clinical care to increase patient satisfaction and reinforce instructions regarding the medical regimen. Similarly, materials used routinely in clinical trial settings that explain and describe the exact protocol to be followed by patients may be useful in non-research settings to educate and inform patients. The AHA and the NHLBI have extensive publications and informational items that can be used in patient care and research.[28,29]

Finally, practitioners should use reminders, letters, and telephone calls, and openly discuss their patients' adherence (or lack of it) and potential barriers to adherence. A direct and open approach to addressing these issues with patients along with the maintenance of frequent contact can increase patients' engagement in the treatment process, and thus their willingness to adhere to treatment. It is important to not only engage the patient, but also target multiple levels of the health care system—the patient, the providers, and healthcare organization—in efforts to increase adherence.

References

1. Haynes RB, Taylor DW, Sackett DL, (eds): *Compliance In Health Care*. Baltimore: Johns Hopkins University Press; 1979:1–2.
2. Davis CE. Prerandomization compliance screening: A statistician's view. In Shumaker SA, Schron EB, Ockene JK, (eds): *The Handbook of Health Behavior Change*. New York: Springer; 1990:342–347.
3. Friedman B. Equipoise and the ethics of clinical research. *N Engl J Med* 1987;317:141–145.
4. Piantadosi S: *Clinical Trials A Methodologic Perspective*. New York: John Wiley & Sons, Inc.; 1997:276–277.
5. Friedman LM, Furberg CD, DeMets DL. Issues in data analysis. In *Fundamentals of Clinical Trials*. St. Louis:Mosby Year-Book, Inc.; 1996:289–293B.
6. Bowen D. Determinants/Predictors of Compliance/Noncompliance. In Burke LE, Ockene IS (eds): *Compliance in Healthcare and Research*. Armonk, NY: Futura Publishing, 2001.
7. Davis CE. Analysis Issues in Clinical Trials. In Burke LE, Ockene IS (eds): *Compliance in Healthcare and Research*. Armonk, NY: Futura Publishing, 2001.
8. Friedman LM, Furberg CD, DeMets D. Study population. In *Fundamentals of Clinical Trials*. St. Louis:Mosby Year-Book, Inc.; 1996:36–39.
9. Schron EB, Davey JA, Jensen JM, et al. The Systolic Hypertension in the Elderly Program: Implications for nursing practice and research. *Prog Cardiovasc Nurs* 1989;4:138–145.
10. Cowley SM, Somelofski C, Hill MN, et al. Nursing and cardiovascular clinical trial research: Collaborating for successful outcomes. *Cardiovasc Nurs* 1988;24:25–30.
11. Friedman LM, Furberg CD, DeMets D. Participant adherence. In *Fundamentals of Clinical Trials*. St. Louis: Mosby Year-Book, Inc.; 1996:204–222.
12. Steering Committee of the Physicians' Health Study Research Group. Final report of the aspirin component of the ongoing Physicians' Health Study. *N Engl J Med* 1989;321:129–35.
13. Buring JE, Hennekens CH. The Women's Health Study: Summary of the study design. *J Myocardial Ischemia* 1992;4:27–29.
14. Glynn RJ, Buring JE, Manson JE, et al. Adherence to aspirin in the prevention of myocardial infarction. *Arch Intern Med* 1994;154:2649–2657.
15. SHEP Cooperative Research Group. Prevention of stroke by antihypertensive drug treatment in older persons with isolated systolic hypertension. Final results of the Systolic Hypertension in the Elderly Program (SHEP). *JAMA* 1991;265:3255–3264.
16. Davis BR, Cutler JA, Gordon DJ, et al. Rationale and design for the Antihypertensive and Lipid Lowering Treatment to Prevent Heart Attack Trial (ALLHAT). ALLHAT Research Group. *Am J Hypertens* 1996;9:342–360.
17. Lusk C, Egan D, Carroll L, et al. ALLHAT Adherence Survival Kit. *Controlled Clinical Trials* 1999;20:38S.
18. Probstfield JL, Russell ML, Insull W Jr, et al. Dropouts from a clinical trial, their recovery and characterization. A basis for dropout management and prevention. In: Shumaker SA, Schron EB, Ockene JK (eds): *The Handbook of Health Behavior Change*. New York: Springer; 1990:376–400.
19. Burke LE. Electronic Measures. In Burke LE, Ockene IS (eds): *Compliance in Healthcare and Research*. Armonk, NY: Futura Publishing, 2001.
20. Azthromycin and Coronary Events Study. ACES Manual of Operations, NHLBI, Bethesda, MD 1999.

21. Evaluation of Adherence Interventions in Clinical Trials. NIH Guide, Volume 20, Number 33, September 6, 1991, RFA: HL-91–08-P.
22. Rand C, Huss K, Weeks K. Adherence in the Childhood Asthma Management Program, (UO1 HL48999).
23. Dunbar-Jacobs J, Sereika S. Adherence in clinical trials: Induction strategies. *Controlled Clinical Trials* 1998;19:19S.
24. Hamilton G. Improving adherence in a hypertension clinical trial. *Controlled Clinical Trials* 1998;19:19S.
25. Friedman R, Farzansar R. Computer based adherence interventions in clinical trials. (Cooperative Agreement—Grant Number: U01 NR03318).
26. Rand C, Weeks K, Santopietro V, et al. Patient adherence with bronchodilator therapy is superior with salmeterol. *Am J Respiratory & Critical Care Med* 1998;157(3):A274.
27. Dunbar JM, Stunkard AJ. Adherence to diet and drug regimen. In Levy R, Rifkind B, Dennis B, Ernst N (eds): *Nutrition, Lipids, and Coronary Heart Disease.* New York: Raven Press:79:391–423.
28. National Heart, Lung, and Blood Institute Web site. http://www.nhlbi.nih.gov
29. American Heart Association Web site. http://www.americanheart.org

Chapter 15

Treatment Targets

Harlan M. Krumholz, MD, Mohsen Davoudi, MD, Joan M. Amatruda, RN, and Sarah A. Roumanis, RN

Introduction

The last quarter century has seen a remarkable decrease in the incidence of cardiovascular disease. This reduction in the risk of the population has been paralleled by the emergence of an increasingly sophisticated knowledge of the factors that are responsible for the development of atherosclerotic disease. Public health efforts have successfully targeted modifiable risk factors, reducing risk for many individuals.

Though the success in preventing cardiovascular disease is remarkable, there is substantial evidence that the translation of the science to the individual at risk remains incomplete. For example, despite the successes against high blood pressure, there remain large numbers of patients with undetected hypertension and many more who are undertreated. Despite the successes against elevated lipid levels, there remain many more persons who could benefit from treatment. The potential of the knowledge is incompletely harvested.

The inefficiency in translating knowledge into action has led to a credibility gap. Organizations such as the National Committee for Quality Assurance are developing quality indicators to measure success in risk factor modification. These measures provide a summary of success by focusing on the percentage of patients who reach target levels established by national guidelines. Measuring the percentage of patients who reach target levels incorporates success in screening, treatment and patient adherence to medical advice.

From: Burke LE, Ockene IS (eds). *Compliance in Healthcare and Research.* Armonk, NY: Futura Publishing Company, Inc.; © 2001.

In this chapter we seek to examine the emerging standards for evaluating the success of risk factor modification. For convenience, the chapter will focus on issues relevant to hypertension and hyperlipidemia, but the general principles are broadly applicable. We will begin with a review of the pertinent medical literature regarding deficiencies in screening, treatment and compliance. We will follow the review with several vignettes that illuminate the problems. Then we will describe recent efforts to increase accountability by developing composite measures of success. Finally, we will look to future directions of these efforts.

Review of the Literature

Coronary heart disease (CHD) is the leading cause of mortality in the US. Each year, 1.5 million new patients are diagnosed and one-half million die of it. This costs the country more than $100 billion per year.[1,2] More than half of first myocardial infarctions occur in patients without any prior signs or symptoms of heart disease, and one-third of these are fatal.[1-3] An aggressive risk factor management program geared toward primary and secondary prevention can have a positive impact on the natural history of atherosclerotic cardiovascular disease. The screening and treatment of persons with these modifiable risk factors (hypertension and hyperlipidemia) cannot only improve outcomes, but also is considered to be economically attractive.[4-11]

The relationship between elevated systolic and diastolic blood pressure and cardiovascular risk is considered "strong, continuous, graded, consistent, independent, predictive, and etiologically significant for those with and without coronary heart disease."[2,12, 13] This includes stroke as well as CHD.[14-16] Many studies have observed this direct relationship and how it can be reversed by effective blood pressure control.[12-14,16-23]

Regarding cholesterol, there is compelling evidence that cardiovascular events can be prevented and total mortality and morbidity lowered in patients with hyperlipidemia with known CHD by the implementation of an aggressive lipid-lowering strategy.[24-29] Also, studies have shown this benefit for individuals with hypercholesterolemia without prior cardiac disease and those with CHD but only mild elevations in total cholesterol or LDL levels.[30-33]

The value of controlling hypertension and hyperlipidemia is described in national guidelines that have addressed these conditions. The Sixth Report of the Joint National Committee on Prevention, Detection, Evaluation, and Treatment of High Blood Pressure (JNC VI) was published by the National Institute of Health in 1997.[2,3] By the use of "evidence-based medicine and consensus," the report updates contemporary approaches to hypertension control. Among the issues covered are the important need for prevention of high blood pressure by improving lifestyles, the cost of healthcare, the use of self-measurement of blood pressure, the role of managed care in the treatment of high blood pressure, the introduction of new combination antihypertensive medications and angiotensin II receptor blockers, and strategies for improving adherence to treatment. This document defines hypertension as "systolic blood pressure [SBP] of 140 mmHg or greater, diastolic blood pressure [DBP] of 90 mmHg or greater or taking antihypertensive medication." The guidelines set a goal of "achieving and maintaining SBP below 140 mmHg and DBP below 90 mmHg and lower if tolerated, while controlling other modifiable risk factors for cardiovascular disease." It adds that "lower levels may be useful, particularly to prevent stroke, to preserve renal function, and to prevent or slow heart failure progression." The specific and detailed guidelines in the publication cover such diverse issues as lifestyle modifications (weight reduction, physical activity, dietary control, tobacco avoidance, etc.) pharmacological treatment and biofeedback.

The established effectiveness of aggressive cholesterol assessment and control in positively altering cardiovascular mortality and morbidity caused the National Cholesterol Education Program's Adult Treatment Panel (NCEP) to release its initial guidelines for the screening, diagnosis and treatment of hyperlipidemia in 1988 (NCEP-ATP I).[34] These guidelines were reviewed and revised in 1993 (NCEP-ATP II).[35] NCEP-ATP II recognizes the significant risks of cardiovascular morbidity and mortality posed by elevated lipid levels in both men and women with CHD and postmenopausal women. NCEP combines the overall view of the patient's risk factor status with current lipid levels to create straightforward algorithms to assist physicians in selecting and initiating appropriate treatment. For patients with established CHD, NCEP-ATP II sets a target LDL-cholesterol goal of less than 100 mg/dL.

The promulgation of these guidelines has been accompanied by national efforts to educate the public about the value of risk factor modification. National programs, such as the "Know Your Number" program by the NCEP have been implemented to disseminate information about the value of screening and treatment.

Despite these national efforts, several studies convincingly demonstrate the inadequacy of the current system. National surveys show that approximately 50 million Americans have high blood pressure,[36,37] including 30% of the adult population.[38,39] The National Health and Nutrition Examination Survey published the results of the first phase of its third survey (NHANES III-1, 1988–1991)[36,37] showing that the levels of awareness, treatment and control of hypertension had increased from 51%, 31%, and 10% in the second survey (NHANES II, 1976–1980) to 73%, 55%, and 29% respectively. These improvements have contributed substantially to a decline in the morbidity and mortality attributable to hypertension. As an example, the age-adjusted death rates from stroke have declined by 60%, and those from CHD by 53% in the same period. Unfortunately, the hypertension control rates have not continued to improve (second phase of third survey, NHANES III-2, 1991–1994)[37]. Based on the JNC VI document, "[if] awareness, treatment and control rates had continued the trend established between 1976–80 and 1988–91, there would have been an increase in 1991–94 in awareness to 76.2%, in treatment to 59.6% and in control to 31.2%" instead of a decline to 68.4%, 53.6% and 27.4% respectively[2, 37]. Also, since 1993, stroke rates have risen and the down-sloping curve for age-adjusted incidence of CHD seems to be leveling.[2]

Additionally, reports have demonstrated an increase in the incidence of end-stage renal disease,[40] and the prevalence of congestive heart failure,[41] both of which are primarily predisposed by systemic hypertension. The Minnesota Heart Survey managed to show a decline in the awareness, treatment, and control of hypertension and its consequences.[2,42] Glynn and colleagues found a similar trend in a cohort in Iowa.[43]

Some studies have specifically demonstrated that even patients who are identified as hypertensive are often undertreated. Berlowitz and colleagues[44] examined the care of 800 hypertensive patients in five Veterans Administration (VA) sites in New England over a 2-year period and found that 40% of the patients had a blood pressure greater than or equal to 160/90 mmHg, despite an average of more than six hypertension-related visits per year. In the same period only 6.7% of visits led to an increase in therapy. The study managed to show that patients who received more intensive therapy had significantly better control of their hypertension (blood pressure decline of 6.3 mmHg among those with most intensive treatment, compared to blood pressure increase of 4.8 mmHg among those with least treatment).

Other studies have revealed nonadherence to therapy as a very common reason for not achieving blood pressure control.[45–48] As a result of all of these issues, many persons are not at the target levels suggested by the guidelines.

Many studies show even worse problems with the detection and successful treatment of elevated cholesterol levels. Despite the widespread dissemination of NCEP-ATP II guidelines, there remain many individuals with elevated cholesterol levels. Many studies published between the two NCEP guidelines (1988 and 1993) and afterwards have gathered substantial evidence for the underscreening and undertreatment of all modifiable cardiovascular risk factors, most significantly for cholesterol.[1,28,49–59]

To assess the level of screening for patients with elevated LDL levels, Frolkis and colleagues[1] studied 225 patients admitted in 1996 to the coronary care unit of a university-affiliated teaching hospital. Screening rates among interns (who had the best performance among the tiers of physicians) were 59% for hyperlipidemia and 68% for hypertension. An LDL-level was obtained in less than half of the patients in whom it was indicated on the basis of NCEP-ATP II algorithms.

Danias and colleagues[60] showed that even in a university-affiliated VA hospital in New England, more than 50% of patients meeting NCEP-ATP II criteria for treatment of hypercholesterolemia did not receive appropriate therapy, "largely as a result of incomplete physician adherence to national guidelines." Nieto and his colleagues of the ARIC (Atherosclerosis Risk in Communities) study[57,61] showed that among 15,739 participants aged 45 to 64 years, 42% of hypercholesterolemic subjects were aware of their condition and only 4% had their condition both treated and controlled. This compared with 84% and 50% respectively for hypertension among the same population.

Other studies have observed nonadherence with treatment. Avorn and colleagues[62] studied two groups of hyperlipidemic patients in the US and Quebec who were being treated with lipid-lowering agents and observed that in both populations, patients were without the appropriate medication(s) for at least one-third of the study year on average. After 5 years, one-half of the surviving original cohort in the US had stopped receiving lipid-lowering therapy altogether.

Andrade and colleagues[63] conducted a cohort study on 2369 new users of antihyperlipidemic therapy at two health maintenance organizations (HMOs). They compared the rates of drug discontinuation in these primary care settings with the rates reported in randomized clinical trials from 1975 to 1993. They observed that the risks of discontinuation for most antihyperlipidemics were substantially higher in the HMO settings than in the trials.

In summary, these studies support a disappointing conclusion that despite the progress in risk factor modification, many individuals remain unnecessarily at risk either due to inadequate screening, treatment or compliance. The knowledge exists to reduce mortality and morbidity from cardiovascular disease and stroke, but it is being inadequately implemented.

Vignettes

The previous section described the evidence that demonstrates that many patients having risk factors are not detected. Among those whose risk factors are detected, many persons are not treated adequately and a substantial number do not reach the targets set by national guidelines. The following cases are composites of typical patients we have seen and illustrate many of these issues and the problems inherent in our current system. They are presented to give a human face to this problem.

Case #1

AI is a 77-year-old black woman with a past medical history of an acute myocardial infarction, hospitalized with a reinfarction. Several years ago she underwent bypass surgery. She has been doing fairly well recently without significant complaint. She takes medications for her blood pressure and her cholesterol. In addition, she is on six other medications for her heart and other medical conditions. Her last blood pressure was 165/95 mmHg and her LDL cholesterol was 140 mg/dL. She was interviewed during her admission on issues related to medication compliance and knowledge of specific cardiac risk factors (blood pressure, cholesterol). The patient stated that she frequently forgets to take medications. She was unable to name her medications and was not sure what she was taking to lower her cholesterol and blood pressure. She stated that her medications are expensive and she cannot always afford them. In response to the question: "What can you tell me about the relationship between blood pressure and heart disease?," she stated: "I don't know anything." Although she feels it is very important to take care of her blood pressure, she could not tell the interviewer her blood pressure now or previously. In addition, she did not know her target blood pressure, nor did she know the difference between systolic and diastolic blood pressure. With regard to cholesterol, she felt that taking care of her cholesterol was "important." However, she did not know her cholesterol level, or her target level, or the difference between total cholesterol and LDL. She says that her doctor has told her that her levels are "OK."

Case #2

JM is a 57-year-old white man with past medical history of an acute myocardial infarction and angioplasty who was hospitalized with unstable angina. He had been limited in recent weeks by chest pain and is currently unemployed. He is prescribed medications for his blood pressure and cholesterol, but has not seen a doctor recently nor filled a prescription. He has no health insurance and has not seen a physician in the last year. When he did visit a physician, his blood pressure and cholesterol levels were elevated. During an interview the patient admitted that when he had his medications he would frequently forget to take them and was careless about the timing. He stopped the medications because of cost and his uncertainty about the benefit they were providing. He cannot recall what medications he was taking. He did not know his target blood pressure or cholesterol levels.

What is clear in each of these brief cases is that not only are these patients not 'at target' for cholesterol and/or blood pressure, but they are not educated as to what the targets are, and how to reach their target, despite the fact that both of the patients outlined here have been through the system, having had more than one previous admission for treatment of cardiovascular disease. Moreover, there are multiple barriers to their successful compliance with recommended strategies. These cases exemplify the fact that we are not doing as good a job as we need to in communicating with our patients.

Quality Indicators and Risk Factor Modification

The emergence of evidence about the variability in the screening and treatment of individuals at risk led to interest in measures that would quantify success and allow for comparisons between different clinicians and health care institutions. Moreover, there was interest in developing a fair and feasible measure that would indicate if all of the right processes had taken place and yet not restrict clinicians to practice medicine in a uniform way.

The National Committee for Quality Assurance (NCQA) has led the effort to introduce preventive quality measures on a national scale. NCQA[64] is a not-for-profit corporation governed by a broadly representative board, including payers and policy makers. It is "committed to assessing, reporting on and improving the quality of care provided by organized delivery systems."[38] Its missions are to enable managed care accountability, to provide valid and reliable information on quality of care to purchasers and consumers, and to induce a drive for quality improvement in the healthcare environment.

This organization has developed a set of quality measures called the Health Employer Data Information Set (HEDIS). These measures are used as "an integrated system of comprehensive tools to measure the quality of care and establish accountability in managed care."[38] Presently, HEDIS is becoming a national standard for performance reporting. It is being used by more than 60% of large employers, including the Health Care Financing Administration (HCFA). Currently, 34 states use the HEDIS Report Cards or plan to use them. Hence, HEDIS is emerging as a basis for meaningful judgments about the state of managed care.

In the most recent iterations of HEDIS, indicators for hypertension and hyperlipidemia have been added. The HEDIS hypertension measure is defined as the percentage of hypertensive patients with either SBP greater than or equal to 140 mmHg or DBP greater than or equal to 90 mmHg. The HEDIS hyperlipidemia measure is patients with a serum LDL level of 130 mg/dL or higher drawn at 2 to 12 months after discharge, from a denominator of patients who have been hospitalized for acute myocardial infarction, bypass surgery or percutaneous coronary intervention in the previous year.[38,39]

These measures were added to encourage health plans to focus on risk factor modification in these areas. Moreover, their success would be dependent on not merely the identification and treatment of appropriate persons, but on the success of the treatment. Successful treatment will require the successful engagement of patients to follow the regimen and participate with the clinician in their management.

These measures are superior to chart reviews that are designed to identify documentation of patient counseling or programs to enhance compliance. They indicate whether the patient actually reached the target, and incorporate the consideration of the treatment (including the dosage) and the work with the patient to ensure compliance.

These measures, however, have received criticism. Some clinicians are concerned that a flat blood pressure standard is understandable, but does not give credit for major reductions from high levels that did not reach the target level. Consequently, some clinicians believe that this indicator discriminates against those who treat patients with the most resistant hypertension. Similar concerns have been voiced regarding cholesterol reduction. In addition, some clinicians believe that the NCEP target level is overly restrictive.

While these issues continue to be discussed, the major importance of the measures is their focus on the important outcome. These measures should provide an incentive for health care plans to allocate resources to the successful management of patients with elevated blood pressure and cholesterol.

Future Directions

Paradigms in health care are changing. Clinicians and health care systems are increasingly being asked to be accountable for the care they deliver. These efforts are fueled by studies indicating opportunities to improve detection, treatment and compliance. Many studies are being conducted to discover the reasons behind nonadherence to clinical practice guidelines and testing different methods to improve adherence.[65–82]

The composite measures of our success with patients are likely to proliferate and should challenge the profession to find innovative and inexpensive approaches to risk factor modification. Using measures that incorporate target values, it will not be enough to do part of the job well. Success will require attention to all phases of detection and management. The collection of this information across a continuum of care will provide an opportunity to benchmark best practices and disseminate information about the best approaches.

References

1. Frolkis JP, Zyzanski SJ, Schwartz JM, et al. Physician noncompliance with the 1993 National Cholesterol Education Program (NCEP-ATPII) guidelines. *Circulation* 1998;98:851–855.
2. The sixth report of the Joint National Committee on Prevention, Detection, Evaluation, and Treatment of High Blood Pressure. *Arch Intern Med* 1997; 157:2413–2446.
3. Frohlich ED. The sixth report of the Joint National Committee: An appropriate celebration of the 25th anniversary of the National High Blood Pressure Education Program. *Hypertension* 1997;30:1305–1306.
4. Dustan HP, Roccella EJ, Garrison HH. Controlling hypertension. A research success story. *Arch Intern Med* 1996;156:1926–1935.
5. Ramsey SD, Neil N, Sullivan SD, et al. An economic evaluation of the JNC hypertension guidelines using data from a randomized controlled trial. Joint National Committee. *J Am Board Fam Pract* 1999;12:105–114.
6. Johannesson M, Dahlof B, Lindholm LH, et al. The cost-effectiveness of treating hypertension in elderly people—an analysis of the Swedish Trial in Old Patients with Hypertension (STOP Hypertension). *J Intern Med* 1993; 234:317–323.
7. Edelson JT, Weinstein MC, Tosteson AN, et al. Long-term cost-effectiveness of various initial monotherapies for mild to moderate hypertension. *JAMA* 1990;263:407–413.
8. Littenberg B, Garber AM, Sox HC, Jr. Screening for hypertension. *Ann Intern Med* 1990;112:192–202.
9. Russell LB, Gold MR, Siegel JE, et al. The role of cost-effectiveness analysis in health and medicine. Panel on Cost-effectiveness in Health and Medicine. *JAMA* 1996;276:1172–1177.
10. Weinstein MC, Siegel JE, Gold MR, et al. Recommendations of the Panel on Cost-effectiveness in Health and Medicine. *JAMA* 1996;276:1253–1258.
11. Siegel JE, Weinstein MC, Russell LB, et al. Recommendations for reporting cost-effectiveness analyses. Panel on Cost-effectiveness in Health and Medicine. *JAMA* 1996;276:1339–1341.
12. Stamler J. Blood pressure and high blood pressure. Aspects of risk. *Hypertension* 1991;18(3 Suppl):I95–I107.
13. Flack JM, Neaton J, Grimm R, Jr., et al. Blood pressure and mortality among men with prior myocardial infarction. Multiple Risk Factor Intervention Trial Research Group. *Circulation* 1995;92:2437–2445.

14. Kannel WB. Blood pressure as a cardiovascular risk factor: Prevention and treatment. *JAMA* 1996;275:1571–1576.
15. Kannel WB, Wolf PA, Verter J, et al. Epidemiologic assessment of the role of blood pressure in stroke: The Framingham Study. 1970. *JAMA* 1996;276: 1269–1278.
16. Du X, Cruickshank K, McNamee R, et al. Case-control study of stroke and the quality of hypertension control in north west England. *BMJ* 1997;314: 272–276.
17. Kotchen JM, McKean HE, Jackson-Thayer S, et al. Impact of a rural high blood pressure control program on hypertension control and cardiovascular disease mortality. *JAMA* 1986;255:2177–2182.
18. Morisky DE, Levine DM, Green LW, et al. Five-year blood pressure control and mortality following health education for hypertensive patients. *Am J Public Health* 1983;73:153–162.
19. Anderson KM, Wilson PW, Odell PM, et al. An updated coronary risk profile. A statement for health professionals. *Circulation* 1991;83:356–362.
20. Levy D. A multifactorial approach to coronary disease risk assessment. *Clin Exp Hypertens* 1993;15:1077–1086.
21. Thurmer HL, Lund-Larsen PG, Tverdal A. Is blood pressure treatment as effective in a population setting as in controlled trials? Results from a prospective study. *J Hypertens* 1994;12:481–490.
22. Neaton JD, Grimm RH, Jr., Prineas RJ, et al. Treatment of Mild Hypertension Study. Final results. Treatment of Mild Hypertension Study Research Group. *JAMA* 1993;270:713–724.
23. Lazarus JM, Bourgoignie JJ, Buckalew VM, et al. Achievement and safety of a low blood pressure goal in chronic renal disease. The Modification of Diet in Renal Disease Study Group. *Hypertension* 1997;29:641–650.
24. Randomised trial of cholesterol lowering in 4444 patients with coronary heart disease: The Scandinavian Simvastatin Survival Study (4S). *Lancet* 1994;344:1383–1389.
25. Lipid Research Clinics Program. *JAMA* 1984;252:2545–2548.
26. The Lipid Research Clinics Coronary Primary Prevention Trial results. II. The relationship of reduction in incidence of coronary heart disease to cholesterol lowering. *JAMA* 1984;251:365–374.
27. The Lipid Research Clinics Coronary Primary Prevention Trial results. I. Reduction in incidence of coronary heart disease. *JAMA* 1984;251:351–364.
28. Gotto AM, Jr. Cholesterol management in theory and practice. *Circulation* 1997;96:4424–4430.
29. Pitt B, Mancini GB, Ellis SG, et al. Pravastatin limitation of atherosclerosis in the coronary arteries (PLAC I): Reduction in atherosclerosis progression and clinical events. PLAC I investigation. *J Am Coll Cardiol* 1995;26: 1133–1139.
30. Frick MH, Elo O, Haapa K, et al. Helsinki Heart Study: Primary-prevention trial with gemfibrozil in middle-aged men with dyslipidemia. Safety of treatment, changes in risk factors, and incidence of coronary heart disease. *N Engl J Med* 1987;317:1237–1245.
31. Furberg CD, Adams HP, Jr., Applegate WB, et al. Effect of lovastatin on early carotid atherosclerosis and cardiovascular events. Asymptomatic Carotid Artery Progression Study (ACAPS) Research Group. *Circulation* 1994; 90:1679–1687.
32. Sacks FM, Pfeffer MA, Moye LA, et al. The effect of pravastatin on coronary events after myocardial infarction in patients with average cholesterol lev-

els. Cholesterol and Recurrent Events Trial investigators. *N Engl J Med* 1996; 335:1001–1009.

33. Shepherd J, Cobbe SM, Ford I, et al. Prevention of coronary heart disease with pravastatin in men with hypercholesterolemia. West of Scotland Coronary Prevention Study Group. *N Engl J Med* 1995;333:1301–1307.

34. Report of the National Cholesterol Education Program Expert Panel on Detection, Evaluation, and Treatment of High Blood Cholesterol in Adults. The Expert Panel. *Arch Intern Med* 1988;148:36–69.

35. Summary of the second report of the National Cholesterol Education Program (NCEP) Expert Panel on Detection, Evaluation, and Treatment of High Blood Cholesterol in Adults (Adult Treatment Panel II). *JAMA* 1993; 269:3015–3023.

36. Burt VL, Culter JA, Higgins M, et al. Trends in the prevalence, awareness, treatment, and control of hypertension in the adult US population. Data from the health examination surveys, 1960 to 1991. *Hypertension* 1995;26: 60–69.

37. Burt VL, Whelton P, Roccella EJ, et al. Prevalence of hypertension in the US adult population. Results from the Third National Health and Nutrition Examination Survey, 1988–1991. *Hypertension* 1995;25:305–313.

38. NCQA (National Committee for Quality Assurance). HEDIS 2000, Volume 1: Narrative—What's in it and why it matters, 1999.

39. NCQA (National Committee for Quality Assurance). HEDIS 2000, Volume 2: Technical Specifications, 1999.

40. Incidence and prevalence of ESRD. USRDS. United States Renal Data System. *Am J Kidney Dis* 1997;30(2 Suppl 1):S40–53.

41. Levy D, Larson MG, Vasan RS, et al. The progression from hypertension to congestive heart failure. *JAMA* 1996;275:1557–1562.

42. Brown RD, Whisnant JP, Sicks JD, et al. Stroke incidence, prevalence, and survival: Secular trends in Rochester, Minnesota, through 1989. *Stroke* 1996; 27:373–380.

43. Glynn RJ, Brock DB, Harris T, et al. Use of antihypertensive drugs and trends in blood pressure in the elderly. *Arch Intern Med* 1995;155:1855–1860.

44. Berlowitz DR, Ash AS, Hickey EC, et al. Inadequate management of blood pressure in a hypertensive population. *N Engl J Med* 1998;339:1957–1963.

45. Miller NH, Hill M, Kottke T, et al. The multilevel compliance challenge: Recommendations for a call to action. A statement for healthcare professionals. *Circulation* 1997;95:1085–1090.

46. Setaro JF, Black HR. Refractory hypertension. *N Engl J Med* 1992;327: 543–547.

47. Schultz JF, Sheps SG. Management of patients with hypertension: A hypertension clinic model. *Mayo Clin Proc* 1994;69:997–999.

48. Hill MN, Bone LR, Butz AM. Enhancing the role of community-health workers in research. *Image J Nurs Sch* 1996;28:221–226.

49. Low incidence of assessment and modification of risk factors in acute care patients at high risk for cardiovascular events, particularly among females and the elderly. The Clinical Quality Improvement Network (CQIN) Investigators. *Am J Cardiol* 1995;76:570–573.

50. Aspry KE, Holcroft JW, Amsterdam EA. Physician recognition of hypercholesterolemia in patients undergoing peripheral and carotid artery revascularization. *Am J Prev Med* 1995;11:336–341.

51. Barrett-Connor E. Lowering cholesterol in patients with coronary heart disease: Are we ready yet? *Circulation* 1997;96:4124–4125.

52. Cohen MV, Byrne MJ, Levine B, et al. Low rate of treatment of hypercholes-terolemia by cardiologists in patients with suspected and proven coronary artery disease. *Circulation* 1991;83:1294–1304.
53. Giles WH, Anda RF, Jones DH, et al. Recent trends in the identification and treatment of high blood cholesterol by physicians. Progress and missed opportunities. *JAMA* 1993;269:1133–1138.
54. Hyman DJ, Maibach EW, Flora JA, et al. Cholesterol treatment practices of primary care physicians. *Public Health Rep* 1992;107:441–448.
55. Leaf DA, Neighbor WE, Schaad D, et al. A comparison of self-report and chart audit in studying resident physician assessment of cardiac risk fac-tors. *J Gen Intern Med* 1995;10:194–198.
56. Miller M, Konkel K, Fitzpatrick D, et al. Divergent reporting of coronary risk factors before coronary artery bypass surgery. *Am J Cardiol* 1995;75: 736–737.
57. Nieto FJ, Alonso J, Chambless LE, et al. Population awareness and control of hypertension and hypercholesterolemia. The Atherosclerosis Risk in Communities study. *Arch Intern Med* 1995;155:677–684.
58. Northridge DB, Shandall A, Rees A, et al. Inadequate management of hyp-erlipidaemia after coronary bypass surgery shown by medical audit. *Br Heart J* 1994;72:466–467.
59. Schrott HG, Bittner V, Vittinghoff E, et al. Adherence to National Choles-terol Education Program Treatment goals in postmenopausal women with heart disease. The Heart and Estrogen/Progestin Replacement Study (HERS). The HERS Research Group. *JAMA* 1997;277:1281–1286.
60. Danias PG, O'Mahony S, Radford MJ, et al. Serum cholesterol levels are underevaluated and undertreated. *Am J Cardiol* 1998;81:1353–1356.
61. The ARIC investigators. The Atherosclerosis Risk in Communities (ARIC) Study: design and objectives. *Am J Epidemiol* 1989;129:687–702.
62. Avorn J, Monette J, Lacour A, et al. Persistence of use of lipid-lowering medications: A cross-national study. *JAMA* 1998;279:1458–1462.
63. Andrade SE, Walker AM, Gottlieb LK, et al. Discontinuation of antihyper-lipidemic drugs—do rates reported in clinical trials reflect rates in primary care settings? *N Engl J Med* 1995;332:1125–1131.
64. Iglehart JK. The National Committee for Quality Assurance. *N Engl J Med* 1996;335:995–999.
65. Cabana MD, Rand CS, Powe NR, et al. Why don't physicians follow clinical practice guidelines? A framework for improvement. *JAMA* 1999;282: 1458–1465.
66. Goldman L. Changing physicians' behavior. The pot and the kettle. *N Engl J Med* 1990;322:1524–1525.
67. Lomas J, Anderson GM, Domnick-Pierre K, et al. Do practice guidelines guide practice? The effect of a consensus statement on the practice of physi-cians. *N Engl J Med* 1989;321:1306–1311.
68. Woolf SH. Practice guidelines: A new reality in medicine. III. Impact on patient care. *Arch Intern Med* 1993;153:2646–2655.
69. Hayward RS. Clinical practice guidelines on trial. *CMAJ* 1997;156: 1725–1727.
70. Greco PJ, Eisenberg JM. Changing physicians' practices. *N Engl J Med* 1993; 329:1271–1273.
71. Mansfield CD. Attitudes and behaviors towards clinical guidelines: The clinicians' perspective. *Qual Health Care* 1995;4:250–255.
72. Conroy M, Shannon W. Clinical guidelines: Their implementation in gen-eral practice. *Br J Gen Pract* 1995;45:371–375.

73. Shortell SM, Bennett CL, Byck GR. Assessing the impact of continuous quality improvement on clinical practice: What it will take to accelerate progress. *Milbank Q* 1998;76:593–624.

74. Austin SM, Balas EA, Mitchell JA, et al. Effect of physician reminders on preventive care: Meta-analysis of randomized clinical trials. *Proc Annu Symp Comput Appl Med Care* 1994:121–124.

75. Balas EA, Li ZR, Mitchell JA, et al. A decision-support system for the analysis of clinical practice patterns. *Proc Annu Symp Comput Appl Med Care* 1994: 366–370.

76. Balas EA, Austin SM, Mitchell JA, et al. The clinical value of computerized information services. A review of 98 randomized clinical trials. *Arch Fam Med* 1996;5:271–278.

77. Hunt DL, Haynes RB, Hanna SE, et al. Effects of computer-based clinical decision support systems on physician performance and patient outcomes: A systematic review. *JAMA* 1998;280:1339–1346.

78. Shea S, DuMouchel W, Bahamonde L. A meta-analysis of 16 randomized controlled trials to evaluate computer—based clinical reminder systems for preventive care in the ambulatory setting. *J Am Med Inform Assoc* 1996; 3:399–409.

79. Lomas J. Words without action? The production, dissemination, and impact of consensus recommendations. *Annu Rev Public Health* 1991;12:41–65.

80. Steffensen FH, Sorensen HT, Olesen F. Impact of local evidence-based clinical guidelines—a Danish intervention study. *Fam Pract* 1997;14:209–215.

81. Studnicki J, Schapira DV, Bradham DD, et al. Response to the National Cancer Institute Alert. The effect of practice guidelines on two hospitals in the same medical community. *Cancer* 1993;72:2986–2992.

82. Murrey KO, Gottlieb LK, Schoenbaum SC. Implementing clinical guidelines: A quality management approach to reminder systems. *QRB Qual Rev Bull* 1992;18:423–433.

Section VII

Special Topics

Chapter 16

Analysis of Clinical Trials and Treatment Nonadherence

Susan M. Sereika, PhD and C. E. Davis, PhD

Introduction

The randomized clinical trial has been heralded as the principle method of evaluating the efficacy and effectiveness of therapies in clinical research. An implicit assumption when using a randomized clinical trial design is that the participants adhere, or comply, to their assigned intervention regimen as instructed; however, this assumption is often unwarranted as subjects frequently fail to complete their assigned prescribed treatments. Analysis strategies have been proposed to evaluate efficacy, effectiveness, and safety of treatment in randomized clinical trials in light of treatment nonadherence. One such method is "intention to treat" analysis, which endeavors to maintain the benefits attained through the random assignment of subjects to treatments by including and evaluating in data analysis all subjects in their treatment groups as originally assigned. Although endorsed internationally by regulatory agencies and industry through the International Conference on Harmonization[1] as the primary approach for the analysis of data from clinical trials, intention-to-treat comparisons have been extensively debated in the clinical trials community by statisticians and clinicians alike regarding their universal use as the primary and/or sole method of analysis. This is due to possible losses in statistical power when hypothesis testing and, possible biased estimation of the true treatment effect.[2–7] In response, considerable research reported in the

The authors wish to thank Hilary Lewis for her editorial assistance, Donna Caruthers for her helpful comments, and Sherri Ciocoi for her transcription of the original presentation. This paper was supported in part by the National Heart, Lung, and Blood Institute (U01-HL48992) and the National Institute of Nursing Research (P30-NR03924).

From: Burke LE, Ockene IS (eds). *Compliance in Healthcare and Research.* Armonk, NY: Futura Publishing Company, Inc.; © 2001.

clinical trials literature has centered around various methodologic and analytic strategies to 1) compensate for possible nonadherence through sample size estimation in the design stage,[8-12] 2) improve patient adherence during the conduct of a clinical trial prior to randomization through placebo run-ins[13-15] and postrandomization using adherence-enhancing strategies,[7,16] 3) measure and monitor treatment adherence during the conduct of a clinical trial,[17,18] and 4) take into consideration treatment nonadherence when estimating treatment efficacy.[6,19-25] In what follows, the basic framework of a randomized clinical trial is described to motivate the methodological and statistical issues that may emerge as a result of protocol deviations due to patient's nonadherence to assigned treatment. Methodological and analytic strategies proposed in the clinical trial literature are outlined, and statistical concerns arising from the use of these approaches are discussed.

Treatment Nonadherence in a Randomized Clinical Trial

In concept, a randomized clinical trial is basically a very simple experiment, designed for the evaluation of either the efficacy or effectiveness of a treatment. A sample of participants is assembled and is randomly allocated to a treatment condition. Figure 1 outlines a simple clinical trial of subjects randomly assigned to two treatment arms, placebo control (C) and intervention (I), of sizes n_C and n_I, respectively. The intervention is applied, subjects are monitored, and their responses to the intervention are measured, yielding as responses $\mathbf{y}_C = y_{C,i}(i = 1, \dots, n_C)$ for control subjects and $\mathbf{y}_C = y_{I,j}(i = 1, \dots, n_I)$ for intervention subjects. The effect of the treatment may then be estimated as the difference of the average group responses, $\bar{y}_I - \bar{y}_C$.

Compared with more complex experiments conducted in laboratories and in other settings, these procedures seem quite simple. Indeed, the allocation of subjects to an intervention is typically straightforward, relying on well-described methodologies using approaches that are deterministic, random or a combination[26] in an effort to eliminate potential bias in treatment assignment and to statistically balance groups on known and unknown/unrecorded characteristics.[27] However, while appearing deceptively simple, it is these last steps of a clinical trial—the application of a treatment and the measurement and monitoring of the response—which in fact can be quite difficult to properly implement and, outside of the recruitment of participants into a trial which in itself can be daunting, pose some of the greatest challenges to the clinical trials investigator. In most experiments that take place in laboratories or involve animals as subjects, nonadherence to intervention is usually

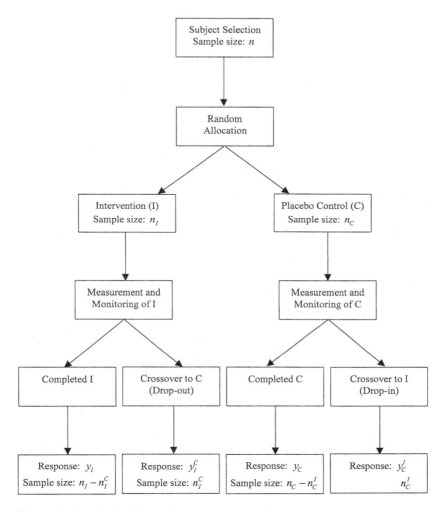

Figure 1. Randomization and treatment nonadherence in simple two-arm, placebo controlled clinical trial.

not an extensive problem and hence has little or no impact on data analysis and interpretation of research findings. In marked contrast, trials involving humans are typified, sometimes dominated by, data imperfections due to deviations from the protocol. An implicit assumption in the conduct of a randomized clinical trial is that participants adhere to their assigned intervention regimen as instructed; however, in human trials this assumption is often not warranted due to the capabilities and autonomy of patients, as well as, the preferences of their personal physicians (eg, patients may not understand the instructions given to them, decide not to fully participate in an assigned intervention through some form of nonadherence, experience side effects inducing their nondaherence with the study treatment, or withdrawal from the study).

Subjects can fail to adhere to almost any aspect of an intervention, such as missing or canceling clinic appointments; failing to administer the study medication as prescribed; participating in other research studies, which may confound the effects of the interventions of either study; and contamination of control subjects by intervention subjects. Specifically, subjects can be *partially adherent* by means of altering the prescribed medication dosing sequence (ie, reducing or increasing the amount taken at an administration, taking additional doses or missing doses all together, and/or adjusting the scheduling or timing of doses).[27] As illustrated in Figure 1, subjects randomized to one arm of a study may, in an unplanned manner, *crossover* to another treatment arm, becoming a "drop-in" or "drop-out" of the intervention. Friedmen et al.[7] defined *drop-ins* as subjects randomly assigned to the control group, who crossover to the intervention arm, while *drop-outs* are subjects randomized to intervention regimen who stop taking the intervention and crossover to the control arm, if either placebo or no standard therapy is used. In this sense, treatment drop-outs and drop-ins are withdrawn, either voluntarily or by the investigator, from their assigned regimen, but not from the observation of study endpoints. As a result, the nonadherent n_C^I placebo control and n_I^C intervention subjects that drop-in and drop-out of their assigned treatment group produce correspondingly the responses $y_{C,i}^I(i = 1,...,n_C^I)$ and $y_I^C(i = 1,...,n_I^C)$, instead of the "true" control and treatment responses under perfect treatment adherence. In effect, the true treatment responses can be viewed as missing data for the nonadherent control and intervention subjects. If a standard, or alternative, active therapy is used as the control regimen as in superiority and equivalence trials, an intervention drop-out assumes the characteristics of patients outside the context of the clinical trial; a control subject, however, can become a drop-out from the standard control therapy.

Such cases of treatment nonadherence have been observed and extensively discussed in the cardiovascular clinical trials literature both for surgical and medical therapies.[28–32] For example, consider a male patient participating in a randomized clinical trial designed to assess the treatment efficacy of new medical therapy compared to a standard surgical procedure on mortality related to myocardial infarction. The subject is randomly allocated to the treatment arm receiving medical therapy and followed for his 10-year survival. During the course of the first year of treatment, this particular subject's adherence with the treatment declines to 50% due to side effects associated with the medication. After 3 years of follow-up, the subject becomes increasingly symptomatic (angina becomes unstable). Always keeping in mind the subject's welfare, the principal investigator crosses the subject over to the surgical control arm and instructs him to continue with his study medication, which the subject adheres to about 40% of the time. On the advice of his personal physician, the subject begins taking a newly approved medical therapy believed to reduce the risk of myocardial infarction and stops taking the original study medication at 5 years of follow-up into the clinical trial. At sixth year of follow-up, the subject dies as a result of a myocardial infarction. Although an extreme example of treatment nonadherence, involving partial adherence, crossover from the treatment to the control condition and contamination by another contending medical regimen, this case is not unlikely, especially in clinical trials involving long periods of follow-up with competing treatments being evaluated (eg, medical therapies vs. surgical therapies, medical therapies vs. behavioral therapies). A case in point from the clinical trials literature is the European Coronary Surgery study,[33] where coronary artery bypass surgery was compared to standard medical therapy. Crossover rates at the end of 5 years of follow-up were 24% (n = 90) from medical therapy to surgery, due to disabling angina pectoris although medically treated, and 7% for subjects randomized to surgery who did not receive the operation. In such instances, the question then becomes how best to analyze the data from subjects who are nonadherent to the assigned treatment regimen in an effort to evaluate treatment efficacy or effectiveness.

Intention to Treat Analysis as the Primary Analysis Strategy

Analogous to the opposing explanatory and pragmatic objectives dictating the design of a clinical trial,[34] Sackett and Gent[35] noted that conflicts also arise with regard to data analysis in light of protocol deviations such as nonadherence to treatment and termed these as "explanatory" and "management" approaches. When an explanatory perspective is adopted, the data analyst's intent is to estimate "biological" efficacy, or the true underlying effect of treatment being evaluated. Assumptions may be made in an effort to answer the biological question. From this standpoint, a clinical trial may be regarded as a test of the treatment received or the "method" effectiveness of the treatment.[6,26] On the other hand, the goal when conducting a management or pragmatic analysis is to compare treatment policies, closely following the design of the clinical trial. In this sense, a clinical trial may be viewed as an assessment of the practical difference between treatment policies or "programmatic," or "use," effectiveness.[6,19,26,36] When perfect adherence exists, the two analytic approaches yield the same results. In the event of treatment nonadherence, conflicting results may emerge when applying both analyses. Careful thought must be given to both the design and analysis of a clinical trial in an effort to yield correct inferences.

The most widely adopted approach, deemed by many in the clinical trials community as the primary method for the analysis of clinical trials data, is *intention to treat* analysis. Based on the deliberations of a working group of the Biopharmaceutical Section of American Statistical Association convened in 1990 to investigate on the qualification and disqualification of subjects in clinical trials, an intention to treat analysis has been defined as an approach that "includes all randomized patients in the groups to which they were randomly assigned, regardless of their compliance with entry criteria, regardless of the treatment they actually received, and regardless of subsequent withdrawal from treatment or deviation from protocol."[27] In terms of treatment adherence, all information concerning the patient's level of adherence following randomization to treatment is essentially ignored when intention to treat is the governing principle for the management of subjects during data analysis. Recalling Figure 1, when analyzing the outcome data using the intention to treat method, the observed average responses (ie, proportion for a binary outcome or mean for a continuous response) for the intervention and placebo control groups become respectively $\bar{y}_I^{ITT} = 1/n_I \left(\sum_{i=1}^{n_I - n_I^C} y_{I,i} + \sum_{i=1}^{n_I^C} y_{I,i}^C \right)$ and $\bar{y}_I^{ITT} = 1/n_C \left(\sum_{i=1}^{n_C - n_C^L} y_{C,i} + \sum_{i=1}^{n_C^L} y_{C,i}^L \right)$ instead of the true mean responses of $\bar{y}_I = 1/n_I \left(\sum_{i=1}^{n_I} y_{I,i} \right)$ and $1/n_C \left(\sum_{i=1}^{n_C} y_{C,i} \right)$ for the treatment and control groups under perfect adherence.

For an extreme illustration of the intention to treat principle, suppose a female patient enters a trial designed to compare the efficacy of a surgical procedure versus medication, and the patient was randomly assigned the surgical procedure. Shortly after enrollment, the subject decides not to have the surgery, but then later has an event and dies. By the intention to treat rule, the death of this patient would be counted in the surgical group, although she did not actually receive the surgery, as exemplified in the primary analysis of the previously mentioned European Coronary Surgery study.[33] Although fairly high rates of crossover were observed in this medical surgical trial monitoring survival in patients with stable angina pectoris, all subjects were analyzed as randomized, including 26 subjects who deviated from surgery (6 died 29 to 82 days following randomization, 19 refused the surgery, and 1 did not receive the surgery due to liver disease).

The same is true for medication regimens or behavioral interventions (eg, diets, exercise, education) for cardiovascular disease when an intention to treat approach is used, as in a randomized clinical trial of beta-blocking drugs[29] and the Hypertension Prevention Trial.[37] In the former study, a double-blind, randomized clinical trial design was used to compare two beta-blocking agents, propranolol and atenolol, with placebo on 1-year mortality in patients hospitalized with suspected myocardial infarction.[29] Mortality data were analyzed retaining the original treatment assignments, although the withdrawals from treatment, due to variety of diagnoses as well as nonadherence with the treatment protocols, ranged from 31% to 40% across the treatment groups. In the Hypertension Prevention Trial,[29] subjects were randomized to either a control condition of no dietary counseling or to one of four dietary counseling treatment groups (calorie restriction, sodium restriction, sodium and calorie restriction, or sodium restriction with increased potassium intake) to assess the effect of dietary changes on blood pressure. Data were analyzed based on randomized assignment, even though attendance at the 12 counseling sessions across the treatment groups decreased over time with the mean percentage attendance across the counseling sessions ranging from 59.4% to 69.3%. Hence, in following the intention to treat principle, a randomized participant who chooses not to follow the directions will still have their response data analyzed in the group to which they were assigned at random regardless of the degree to which they deviate from the course of treatment.

Limitations of the Intention to Treat Analytic Strategy

While most statisticians advocate the use of the intention to treat rule, there has been considerable debate about the comparisons of treatment groups as randomized as the sole method for the analysis of clinical trial data when treatment nonadherence is present. Although the prevailing method of analysis (randomized assignment) is retained and selection bias is not introduced, intention to treat comparisons do not adequately answer the biological question, since subjects may not have received their intended regimen. Instead, intention to treat comparisons address the effectiveness of the treatment, which depends on both the biological action and the subject's adherence to the treatment.[19] In the presence of poor adherence, the intention to treat rule gives a biased estimate of the true treatment effect. For the placebo-controlled trial with a single active treatment, this bias, however, is always toward the null hypothesis of no treatment effect, ie, the bias is always toward finding no difference between the groups. For example, if subjects, who are randomly assigned to take a lipid-lowering drug, refuse to take the medication, their cholesterol values are used in the data analysis as though they received the treatment according to the intention to treat principle. As a result, the true effect of the medication, both therapeutic and adverse, between the groups will be underestimated, since these nonadherent subjects are retained in the intervention group, even though their cholesterol levels likely stayed the same since no medication was taken. In the context of superiority trials, where contending active regimens are being compared with one hypothesized to be more efficacious, an underestimation of the treatment effect would also be observed, dependent on the extent of crossovers and treatment dropouts. Conversely, in equivalency trials, where the underlying hypothesis is that the active interventions being compared have similar therapeutic responses, yet one may have less adverse effects, "an intention to treat analysis generally increases the chance of erroneously concluding that no difference exists," producing "bias in anti-conservative direction."[5]

Along with this biased estimation of the treatment effect is a loss of statistical power in detecting this effect, that is, the probability of the treatment effect being found, when the intervention is truly efficacious, is diminished. Weinstein and Levin[38] discussed the impact of unplanned crossovers on the statistical power of randomized studies of surgical therapies and developed a binomial model to generate power curves under various mortality rates, crossover rates from the medical control group to the surgical treatment group, and sample sizes. Statistical power to detect differences in mortality rates diminished substantially as the rate of crossover increased for a given sample size. For example, with a sample size of 400 per group and death rates for the surgical and medical control groups of 0.05 and 0.10, respectively, the statistical power would be 0.77 with no crossovers and 0.57 with 25% crossover.

Rather than treating nonadherence as a simple binary variable, Freedman[39] studied patterns of nonadherence over time and their impact on the incidence of disease and ultimately the statistical power in prevention trials focusing on dietary fat intake in women with an above-average fat intake. Four patterns of adherence over time were considered for both the treatment (low fat diet) and control (high fat diet) groups: perfect adherence, almost immediate nonadherence, gradual nonadherence, and linear nonadherence. As anticipated, the largest treatment difference in terms of the incidence of disease was observed between groups demonstrating perfect adherence, since no treatment crossovers were observed over time and the true treatment effect was observed. Considerably smaller differences were noted between the groups having variable adherence profiles over time. The smallest differences were observed when assuming immediate nonadherence, where the estimation of the true response rates in both groups is most compromised and the statistical power is reduced to as low as 0.48.

This reduction in statistical power implies that some truly beneficial interventions may not be identified as efficacious when using the intention to treat rule, thus missing true treatment effects. On the other hand, an intervention will not be deemed beneficial when in fact it is not. Under this argument, if a statistically significant intervention effect is found, under the intention to treat rule, then a real intervention effect exists with high probability. This is true because an effect, known to be biased toward no effect in the presence of nonadherence, is still found to be statistically significant. It is for this reason that the Food and Drug Administration (FDA) requires that an intention to treat analysis be included for all new drug applications.[40] By taking this conservative viewpoint, the FDA limits the approval of new treatment regimens to only those found to be effective even in the presence of nonadherence when using the intention to treat principle.

Strategies to Limit Bias and Maintain Power When Employing the Intention to Treat Rule

These empirical studies point to a need for the consideration of the level and time course of nonadherence in the planning, conduct and analysis of research studies, in particular clinical trials. Advocates of the intention to treat rule start from the position that measuring adherence is not so vital, because subjects are counted in the group to which they were assigned regardless of their treatment adherence. Rather than investing in methods to measure adherence, resources are allocated in maintaining adherence, since treatment effects are reduced and statistical power is lessened in the presence of heavy treatment nonadherence. Various strategies have been proposed in an effort to maintain treatment adherence during a clinical trial including sample selection based on prerandomization screen for adherence[3,10,13,14,41,42] and the use of adherence enhancing strategies and removing barriers to poor adherence once enrolled.[7,16] With the placebo run-in, the potential for poor adherence from promising subjects is identified before randomization to a treatment group.[13] For the prerandomization screen for adherence or placebo run-in, all potentially eligible subjects for the clinical trial are given placebo in a single masked manor (ie, where only subjects are masked with regard to the regimen) prior to random assignment. Subjects are then monitored for their adherence to the placebo during a relatively short period of time (eg, 2 weeks to 1 month period). Adherence to the placebo is determined for each potential subject, and, if adherence is poor, based on some pre-established definition of poor adherence (eg, ≤ 75% of the prescribed pills taken), he/she is not entered into the randomized clinical trial. The rationale for this exclusion of eligible subjects based on poor adherence to the placebo is that if adherence is poor during this short placebo run-in, then the adherence during a long trial, which may last 1 or more years, is also likely to be poor. This idea is empirically supported by research studies suggesting that the initial treatment adherence may be predictive of future adherence in a clinical trial.[43] Dunbar and Knoke[44] observed that in the Lipid Research Clinics Coronary Primary Prevention Trial (LRC-CPPT) about 35% of the variance in adherence to study medication in the first year could be accounted by medication adherence during the first month immediately following randomization. Furthermore, this initial adherence continued to predict long-term adherence in the LRC-CPPT at the end of 7 years.

Davis et al.[15] tested this assumption using data from the Cholesterol Reduction in Seniors Program (CRISP) study. The purpose of this pilot study was to assess the lipid-lowering response and safety of two daily dosage levels (20mg and 40mg) of lovastatin compared to placebo in adults over 64 years of age with elevated cholesterol levels. To evaluate the effects of a placebo run-in at enhancing adherence during a clinical trial, 431 subjects satisfying general entry criteria were screened for their adherence to placebo administered in a single-blinded fashion over a 3-week period, at the end of which they were classified according to their adherence based on pill count. Rather than using these results as an entry criterion as in a true placebo run-in, all subjects were then randomized to one of three treatment arms and followed to at most 12 months.

Based on the results of this run-in, 15% (n = 66) were classified as poor run-in adherers (ie, having less than 80% adherence or failed to return unused medication) and would have been excluded from further participation had this been an actual prerandomization adherence screen. Examination of regimen adherence and low-density lipoprotein (LDL) cholesterol at follow-up revealed that the use of the adherence information from the placebo run-in to exclude poor adherers would have had little effect on the outcome results. The mean adherence at 3 and 6 months follow-up of 89.3% and 83.4%, respectively, for all participants would have increased slightly to 90.9% at 3 months and 85.5% at 6 months once poor run-in adherers were excluded. All subjects randomized to lovastatin had lower LDL cholesterol values at follow-up, including those who would have been excluded by the placebo run-in. Exclusion of poor run-in adherers would have increased the treatment effect (ie, differences in mean changes from baseline to follow-up between lovastatin and placebo groups) in terms of lowering

LDL cholesterol at 3 months follow-up on the order of 1.6 when comparing 20mg/day lovastatin with placebo, and 2.9 when comparing 40mg/day lovastatin with placebo. Even more modest increases in the treatment effect for LDL cholesterol were observed at 6 months with the omission of poor run-in adherers.

In general, prerandomization adherence screening is used to improve the efficiency of a clinical trial by excluding participants using prerandomization adherence estimates as a proxy for postrandomization adherence in an effort to increase the treatment effect and decrease costs associated with nonadherence. In their test of a placebo run-in, Davis et al.[15] found that the presumed efficiency gains with respect to increased study power were not realized, since only small increases in the treatment effect were found with the exclusion of poor adherers, yet the sample size reduced by 15%. Placebo run-ins also increase the costs and difficulties associated with recruitment in a clinical trial by delaying the start of the actual trial.[14] In the CRISP pilot study, Davis et al.[15] noted that recruitment difficulties would increase, especially for individuals with lower educational attainment, and concluded that the placebo run-in would most likely not improve efficiency in the larger scale study of lipid-lowering in older adults. Additionally, by limiting subject selection to only run-in adherers, the generalizability of the results may be affected.[13,15,42] For example, Davis et al.[15] reported that educational attainment appeared to be related to adherence during run-in. Although not generally an issue in efficacy studies since adherence may be thought of as a nuisance variable and the sample is usually restricted to subjects demonstrating good adherence, limiting the generalizability of results is particularly problematic in effectiveness trials, where the goal is to determine whether the targeted patient population in practice will use biologically efficacious regimens.[13] Based on empirical evaluation through simulation and using actual trial data, Brittain and Wittes[45] questioned the use of the run-in period when the proportion of exclusions based on prerandomization adherence is low and misclassification of postrandomization adherence based on prerandomization adherence status is high. Friedman and colleagues[7] asserted that run-ins should be considered as a viable option in the design of a clinical trial so long as exclusion rates are at least 8% to 10% and impart no substantial delays in the start of the actual trial. Given the additional costs and possible limitations of run-ins, careful consideration should be given before implementation of a prerandomization adherence screen in a clinical trial.

The maintenance of adherence during the clinical trial following randomization may also be achieved through the use of various strategies to enhance adherence to study regimens and improve the appointment keeping of study visits. Clark and Becker[16] presented theoretical models that have been put forth to explicate regimen nonadherence and identify long-established practice-based strategies used to improve adherence. Although presented in the context of clinical practice, the approaches have utility in the clinical research setting. These methods target such areas as the provision of information to the patient, the modification of characteristics of the regimen and evaluation of the patient's skill at administering the regimen, modification of the patient's health attitudes and beliefs, reinforcement of aspects of the treatment, enlistment of support of family and friends, and enhancement of the healthcare provider-patient relationship. These methods are typically used in combination in a trial and often provide a cost-effective means of enhancing treatment adherence.

Additionally, adjustments to sample size in the planning stage of a clinical trial have been proposed to help recompense for potential treatment nonadherence due to drop-ins and drop-outs.[8–12,36,46,47] Lachin[9] presented a simple, conservative adjustment for the sample size to allow for nonadherence relating to drop-out in a simple clinical trial comparing treatment and placebo control groups. Using the terminology developed for Figure 1, to account for the proportion of drop-outs in the treatment group, $p_I^C = n_I^C/n_I$, the sample size under perfect adherence, n, would be inflated to $n/(1 - p_I^C)^2$. Davis[42] illustrated the profound impact of nonadherence on power and sample size when following the intention to treat rule. For example, if the projected proportion of nonadherent subjects in the treatment group is 0.50, the sample size of the clinical trial would need to be inflated to $n/(1 - .50)^2 = 4n$ to have the same power as a clinical trial with perfect adherence. Lachin and Foulkes[11] later generalized this inflation factor to also take into consideration the proportion of drop-ins into the treatment group, $p_C^I = n_C^I/n_C$, as $n/(1 - p_I^C - p_C^I)^2$.

More elaborate models have also been advanced for planning the size of a clinical trial when treatment nonadherence is anticipated.[8,10–12,36,46,47] Schork and Remington[8] developed procedures that adjust event rates assuming constant rates of treatment nonadherence. Halperin et al.[46] furthered these efforts by developing a general model that incorporates nonadherence to treatment in addition to taking into account the time to reach maximum treatment effectiveness. These models have been extended to include losses to follow-up[47] and time-dependent drop-out and event rates.[10,12] Newcombe[36] formulated sample size estimation considering not only protocol deviations but also whether a pragmatic or explanatory approach is to be adopted. Although viewed as a less efficient approach to increase study power compared to the prerandomization adherence screen,[14] the adjustment of the study sample size may be warranted when contraindications exist for the use of run-ins (eg, abbreviated prerandomization period due to the underlying disease process or clinical trial constraints; possible unblinding during or following randomization) and nonadherence is likely to be a concern.

Analytic Strategies to Recover the Treatment Effect

Some clinical trials researchers, however, have argued that analysis following the intention to treat principle fails to evaluate the "actual" effect of the treatment when treatment nonadherence is a concern, especially when crossovers and drop-outs from the assigned treatment are heavy.[48] In an attempt to account for nonadherence and recover the "true" treatment effect, various methods for the analysis of clinical trials data have been proposed, including *per-protocol* analysis and *as-treated* analysis. With the per-protocol method, only those subjects who adhere to the assigned treatment are considered in the analysis stage.[6,49–51] Also referred to as *efficacy subset* analysis, this *adherers-only* approach requires that a subject's adherence with the assigned treatment be quantified and a cutoff for treatment adherence be specified *a priori* to identify the efficacy analyzable sub-sample. Reflecting on the simple trial outlined in Figure 1, limiting the analysis of outcome data to only the adherent subjects would yield as the observed average group responses $\bar{y}_I^{PP} = 1/n_I - n_I^C \ (\sum_{i=1}^{n_I - n_I^C} y_{I,i})$ for the intervention subjects and $\bar{y}_C^{PP} = 1/n_C - n_C^I \ (\sum_{i=1}^{n_C - n_C^I} y_{C,i})$ for placebo control subjects. A classic clinical trials illustration of this approach was the re-analysis of the results from the Coronary Drug Project,[28] where subjects demonstrating good cumulative adherence based on pill counts of capsules prescribed during the first 5 years of follow-up (at least 80% adherence) were retained for the analysis of the efficacy of an active cholesterol-lowering medication, clofibrate, compared to a lactose placebo on total mortality.

When using an as-treated, or treatment-received, approach one analyzes responses based on the treatment the subject *ultimately received*, thus ignoring the subject's random assignment as well as his/her treatment history.[49,50] Using the treatment-received approach, the resulting estimator of the average response for the intervention group becomes $\bar{y}_I^{TR} = 1/n_I - n_I^C + n_C^I \ (\sum_{i=1}^{n_I - n_I^C} y_{I,i} + \sum_{i=1}^{n_C^I} y_{C,i}^I)$, incorporating both the responses of adherent intervention subjects and nonadherent placebo control subjects who dropped into intervention into the estimate of the response for treated subjects. Likewise, to estimate the average response for the placebo control group, the response data from both adherent placebo control subjects and nonadherent intervention subjects would be combined, producing $\bar{y}_C^{TR} = 1/n_I - n_C^l + n_I^C$ ($\sum_{i=1}^{n_I - n_C^l} y_{C,i} + \sum_{i=1}^{n_C^C} y_{I,i}^C$). For example, if subjects who are assigned to the active therapy in a placebo controlled trial elect not to take that regimen, their outcome data would be analyzed as though they were in the control group when using a treatment-received approach. In the Boston Area Anticoagulation Trial for Atrial Fibrillation, subjects were randomized to either warfarin or control and followed for the occurrence of stroke.[52] Following an intention to treat analysis of warfarin with control, a treatment-received analysis was conducted to evaluate the effects of warfarin relative to aspirin, since control subjects could elect to take aspirin during follow-up.[53]

Two additional methods—*censored* analysis and *transition* analysis—have also been considered in the analysis of time to event type data such as time to death in surgical/medical clinical trials. Rather than omit a subject entirely from the analysis, the censored method retains a subject in the analysis up to the point of their treatment nonadherence at which point the subject is treated as being censored and no longer contributes to the analysis of the response.[38,49,54] In the Coronary Artery Surgery Study clinical trial, secondary descriptive comparisons were conducted between medical and surgical groups on selected descriptors of quality of life (chest pain status, use of β-receptor blocking drugs), using a censored analysis, that is, where only information prior to coronary revascularization surgery were used for subjects randomized to medical therapy and only data following surgery were retained for analysis for the subjects randomized to surgery.[30] Some subjects who were randomized to surgery (n = 31; 8%) never received coronary revascularization and were completely censored from the descriptive re-analysis.

As a variation to the as-treated idea, the transition approach handles the treatment actually received by the subject as a time-dependent quantity, which may vary over the course of study, such as in the survival analysis of mortality in the Stanford Heart Transplant program,[55,56] where subjects were transferred to the transplant group following a heart transplantation. Peduzzi and colleagues[49,50] utilized this method in a re-analysis of mortality data collected in the Veterans Administration Coronary Artery Surgery Cooperative Trial,[31] in which subjects with stable angina pectoris and coronary artery disease were randomly assigned to either surgical or medical treatments. In this re-analysis, crossovers were counted as members of their originally assigned treatment groups until the point of crossover whereupon they became members of their new treatment group. In this way, deaths among crossovers are attributed to the treatment received following the transition.

Among statisticians, there is a strong consensus that these alternate approaches—treatment-received, per-protocol, censored, and transition—in lieu of intent to treat analysis should be avoided, due to the potential for bias when excluding or transferring subjects based on their treatment adherence following randomization.[7,26,32,49,50] The selection bias that may be introduced when subjects self-select to adhere or not adhere, or when trial investigators or personal health care providers withdraw or modify a subject's treatment causes these analyses to be highly unreliable. Not only may adherence be related to treatment assignment with varying reasons for nonadherence, but it may also be related to the characteristics of the subject. For instance, in the Coronary Drug Project[28] researchers found that adherence to the assigned treatment was related to a number of baseline factors, which varied by treatment group. Adjustment of the excess prevalence of baseline risk-factors found in poor adherers to placebo failed to eliminate the difference observed in 5-year mortality observed between poor and good adherers (25.8% vs. 16.4%). This suggests that other risk factors, not measured in the Coronary Drug Project, must discriminate between poor and good adherers and account for the differences in mortality. Collins and Dorus[57] reported that subject characteristics varied by adherence status (adherent, nonadherent, and dropouts) in the Department of Veterans Affairs Cooperative Study on Lithium Treatment in Alcohol Dependence, a double-blind, placebo-controlled clinical trial to assess the efficacy of lithium as a maintenance therapy for patients with alcohol dependence who may or may not have a history of depression. Differences in subject characteristics were noted across adherence-based groups within and between treatment groups suggesting that use of a per-protocol analysis has a lack of comparability between treatment groups based on only adherent subjects in addition to impacting the generalizability of findings back to the clinical population. Assuming that the efficacy analysis is not biased by subset selection, Lachin[51] reported that intention to treat analysis may be more powerful than efficacy subset analysis when the subjects excluded from the efficacy analysis in fact demonstrate positive therapeutic effects. Moreover, when using an adherers-only analysis, a large loss of information may occur with high rates of crossovers and drop-outs, clearly making this approach ill-advised.

Such is also the case when using a more practical definition of intention-to-treat as proposed by Gillings and Koch.[58] Combining some aspects of the per-protocol and as-treated approaches, a refinement of the traditional intention to treat analysis is suggested by limiting the analysis to "all patients randomized who were known to take at least one dose of treatment and who provided any follow-up data for one of more key efficacy variables; in turn intention to treat patients are allocated to treatments actually received."[58] Gillings and Koch[58] qualified the use of this definition to when "this population does not differ from the population of all patients randomized to their intended treatments by more than five percent." Lewis and Machin[5] cautioned the use of this guide as it is based on the selection of subjects using postrandomization responses (adherence and key efficacy endpoints) and may lead to selection bias.

In the cases of censored and transition analyses, each method attempts "to minimize bias by assigning survival time to the treatment being received" and thus corrects for length-sampling bias inherent treatment-received and per-protocol methods.[50] Some have argued that there may be instances where adjusting for baseline factors related to nonadherence may limit selection bias and permit the use of an alternate strategy such as a censored analysis.[54] Unfortunately, there may be other unmeasured variables that may be related to adherence, which limits the usefulness of such methods as shown in the Coronary Drug Project.[28] Peduzzi and colleagues[49,50] later stated that when empirically testing the four above approaches and intention to treat analysis using time-to-death data from the Veterans Administration Coronary Artery Surgery Cooperative Trial, each method based on adherence is subject to biases and that intention to treat analysis is preferred as the primary analysis when treatment nonadherence exists. Since much is unknown about the selection bias process, it is highly unwise, in general, to trust these as the only analyses to be conducted.

Use of Model-Based Analyses to Estimate Treatment Efficacy

Unlike the previous approaches described, model-based analysts seek to incorporate information on both the *intended* and *received treatment* when estimating treatment responses.[6,19–21,23,25,59–61] When using a model-based approach, the objective is not to test the hypothesis that an intervention is efficacious or not. Instead, the goal is to estimate the treatment effect under perfect adherence, that is, what would be the treatment effect if all subjects in the study administered their intervention as prescribed.

In contrast to intention to treat comparisons, the precise measurement of treatment adherence throughout the clinical trial is vital when conducting model-based analyses. Recent advances in measurement of adherence using electronic event monitoring[18,62] now allow for the longitudinal assessment of medication taking behavior and have greatly improved the accuracy of adherence measurement. Using the adherence information that has been accumulated, the model-based analyst can estimate what the treatment effect would be under perfect adherence.

For each subject, there are four possible responses that can be measured: y_I, the endpoint response if receiving the intervention; y_C, the endpoint response if receiving the control regimen; a_I, adherence if using the treatment; and a_C, adherence when using the control regimen. However, due to the constraints of study design and randomization, for subjects in the intervention group, only their response on the intervention and their adherence on intervention are observed. Outcome responses and adherence to the control regimen are missing for intervention subjects. Likewise for subjects in the control group, the outcome responses and adherence to the control regimen are observable, while the response and adherence to intervention are missing. Since randomization was used for the assignment of subjects to treatment groups, the data that are unobserved are missing completely at random, that is, the missingness of the information is unrelated to the endpoint response and adherence.

Using this mathematical property, models relating adherence to endpoint response may then be constructed. To accomplish this requires that some assumptions be made. For instance, one might assume that adherence to the intervention is the same as adherence to the control regimen and that the relationship between the endpoint response and adherence is similar, ie, $A_I = A_C : Y = F(A)$. This might be a reasonable assumption if the administered treatment had very few, or no, side effects so that adherence to the regimen would largely be behavioral. This would be a very bad assumption with a medication that has side effects, because one would expect adherence to be related to those side effects. In that case, one might assume different adherence levels between the groups and even different relationships between the endpoint response and adherence, ie, $Y_I = F_I(A_I) : Y_C = F_C(A_C)$. The assumptions that the model-based analyst makes concerning the nature of these functional relationships within and between groups may be quite simple (linear) or extremely complex (nonlinear). Some of these assumptions are testable; however, other assumptions are not.

In general, the growing body of work in model-based methods supports the use of supplementary comparative analyses for estimating treatment efficacy by incorporating information on adherence to treatment assignment, with a few caveats.[63] First, model-based methods require estimates of treatment adherence that are comprehensively, consistently, and reliably measured. Although more precise methods of adherence measurement now are available (eg, electronic event monitoring), the costs of implementing such adherence measurements may be prohibitive in large-scale studies and difficulties may arise in the incorporation of complex adherence information when modeling treatment efficacy. Secondly, empirical work has shown that model-based methods may be extremely sensitive to departures from the underlying assumptions.[22] Pocock and Abdulla[63] pointed to a need "to provide a balanced account of the model assumptions, selection biases and data limitations which affect the ability to make causal inference from observational compliance data."[63]

Summary

The impact of partial adherence, crossovers, drop-ins, and drop-outs on estimation and hypothesis testing when evaluating the effects of intervention has been well-described in the clinical trials literature.[36,39,48] Nonadherence with an intervention can lead to the underreporting of both therapeutic and adverse effects, thus comprising the validity of results based on estimation and hypothesis testing and seriously devaluing even the most well designed trial.[7] Approaches to the analysis of clinical trials have been proposed when nonadherence to treatment exists. Regardless of the method, tradeoffs are made regarding bias and the underlying assumptions one makes when conducting data analysis in the presence of treatment nonadherence. As demonstrated, the intention to treat analysis can be a fairly conservative approach when treatment nonadherence exists, in that it is biased toward the null hypothesis of no treatment effect. As it makes few assumptions, intention to treat analysis is simple to implement. Since subjects are analyzed based on their original treatment assignments, emphasis is placed on maintaining adherence throughout the duration of follow-up. In contrast, model based analysis requires that strong assumptions be made and stresses the measurement of adherence. By incorporating information about the adherence to treatment, it may yield a more logical and more interesting estimate of the actual effect, in many regards, compared to an intention to treat approach. Although empirical work still supports the use of intention to treat analysis as the primary approach for the analysis of clinical trials data,[7,26,51] supplemental analyses using model-based approaches may be used in conjunction with intention to treat comparisons.

References

1. ICH E9 Expert Working Group. ICH Harmonized Tripartite Guideline—Statistical Principles for Clinical Trials. *Stat Med* 1999;18:1905–1942.
2. Gail MH. Eligibility exclusions, losses to follow-up, removal of randomized

patients and uncounted events in cancer clinical trials. *Cancer Treat Rep* 1985;69:1107–1113.

3. Feinstein AR. Intent-to-treat policy for analyzing randomized trials: Statistical distortions and neglected clinical challenges. In Cramer JA, Spilker B (eds): *Patient Compliance in Medical Practice and Clinical Trials.* New York, NY: Raven Press, 1991;359–370.

4. Newell DJ. Intention-to-treat analysis: Implications for quantitative and qualitative research. *Int J Epidemiol* 1992;21:837–841.

5. Lewis JA, Machin D. Intention to treat – Who should use ITT? *Br J Cancer* 1993;68:647–650.

6. Sheiner LB, Rubin DB. Intention-to-treat analysis and the goals of clinical trials. *Clin Pharmacol Ther* 1995;57:6–10.

7. Friedman LM, Furberg CD, Demets DL. *Fundamentals of Clinical Trials* (3rd ed.). St. Louis: Mosby-Year Book Inc; 1996.

8. Schork MA, Remington RD. The determination of sample size in treatment-control comparisons for chronic disease studies in which drop-out or non-adherence is a problem. *J Chronic Dis* 1967;20:233–239.

9. Lachin JM. Introduction to sample size determination and power analysis for clinical trials. *Control Clin Trials* 1981;2:93–113.

10. Wu M, Fisher M, DeMets D. Sample sizes for long-term medical trials with time-dependent drop-out and event rates. *Control Clin Trials* 1980;1: 111–121.

11. Lachin JM, Foulkes MA. Evaluation of sample size and power for analyses of survival with allowance for nonuniform patient entry, losses to follow-up, noncompliance, and stratification. *Biometrics* 1986;42:507–519.

12. Lakatos E. Sample size determination in clinical trials with time-dependent rates of losses and non-compliance. *Control Clin Trials* 1986;7:189–199.

13. Lang JM. The use of a run-in to enhance compliance. *Stat Med* 1990;9:87–95.

14. Probstfield J. Clinical Trial Prerandomization Compliance (Adherence) Screen. In Cramer JA, Spilker B (eds). *Patient Compliance in Medical Practice and Clinical Trials.* New York: Raven Press; 1991:332–333.

15. Davis CE, Applegate WB, Gordon DJ, et al. An empirical evaluation of the placebo run-in. *Control Clin Trials* 1995;16:41–50.

16. Clark NM, Becker MH. Theoretical models and strategies for improving adherence and disease management. In Shumaker SA, Schron EB, Ockene JK, McBee WL (eds): *The Handbook of Health Behavior Change* (2nd ed.). New York: Springer Publishing Co, Inc, 1998; 5–32.

17. Dunbar J. Adherence measures and their utility. *Control Clin Trials* 1984;5: 515–521.

18. Rand CS, Weeks K. Measuring adherence with medication regimens in clinical care and research. In Shumaker SA, Schron EB, Ockene JK, McBee WL (eds). *The Handbook of Health Behavior Change* (2nd ed.). New York: Springer Publishing Co, Inc, 1998;114–132.

19. Sommer A, Zeger SL. On estimating efficacy from clinical trials. *Stat Med* 1991:10:45–52.

20. Efron B, Feldman D. Compliance as an explanatory variable in clinical trials (with discussion). *J Am Stat Assoc* 1991;86:9–26.

21. Mark SD, Robins JM. A method for the analysis of randomized trials with compliance information: An application to the multiple risk factor intervention trial. *Control Clin Trials* 1993;14:79–97.

22. Albert JM, DeMets DL. On a model-based approach to estimating efficacy in clinical trials. *Stat Med* 1994;13:2323–2335.

23. Rochon J. Supplementing the intent-to-treat analysis: Accounting for covariates observed postrandomization in clinical trials. *J Am Stat Assoc* 1995; 90:292–300.
24. Angrist JD, Imbens GW, Rubin DB. Identification of causal effect using instrumental variables. *J Am Stat Assoc* 1996;91:444–472.
25. Goetghebeur E, Molenberghs G, Katz J. Estimating the causal effect of compliance on binary outcome in randomized controlled trials. *Stat Med* 1998; 17:341–355.
26. Piantadosi S. *Clinical Trials: A Methodologic Perspective.* New York: John Wiley and Sons, Inc, 1997.
27. Fisher LD, Dixon DO, Herson J, et al. Intention to treat in clinical trials. In Peace KE (ed): *Statistical Issues in Drug Research and Development.* New York: Marcel Dekker; 1990:331–350.
28. The Coronary Drug Project Research Group. Influence of adherence to treatment and response of cholesterol on mortality in the Coronary Drug project. *N Engl J Med* 1980;303:1038–1041.
29. Wilcox RG, Roland JM, Banks DC, et al. Randomised trial comparing propranolol with atenolol in immediate treatment of suspected myocardial infarction. *Br Med J* 1980;1:885–888.
30. CASS principal investigators and their associates. Coronary Artery Surgery Study (CASS), a randomized trial of coronary artery bypass surgery. Survival data. *Circulation* 1983;68:939–950.
31. The Veterans Administration Coronary Artery Bypass Surgery Cooperative Study Group. Eleven-year survival in the Veterans Administration randomized trial of coronary bypass surgery for stable angina. *N Engl J Med* 1984;311:1333–1339.
32. Oakes D, Moss AJ, Fleiss JL, et al. Use of compliance measures in an analysis of the effect of diltiazem on mortality and reinfarction after myocardial infarction. *J Am Stat Assoc* 1993; 88:44–49.
33. European Coronary Surgery Study Group. Long-term results of prospective randomised study of coronary artery bypass surgery in stable angina pectoris. *Lancet* 1982;2:1173–1180.
34. Schwarz D, Lellouch J. Explanatory and pragmatic attitudes in therapeutic trials. *J Chronic Dis* 1967;20:637–648.
35. Sackett DL, Gent M. Controversy in counting and attributing events in clinical trials. *N Engl J Med* 1979;301:1410–1412.
36. Newcombe RG. Explanatory and pragmatic estimates of the treatment effect when deviations from allocated treatment occur. *Stat Med* 1988;7: 1179–1186.
37. Hypertension Prevention Trial Research Group. The Hypertension Prevention Trial: Three-Year Effects of Dietary Changes on Blood Pressure. *Arch Intern Med* 1990;150:153–162.
38. Weinstein GS, Levin B. Effect of crossover on the statistical power of randomized studies. *Ann Thorac Surg* 1989;48:490–495.
39. Freedman LS. The effect of partial noncompliance on the power of a clinical trial. *Control Clin Trials* 1990;11:157–168.
40. Food and Drug Administration. International Conference on Harmonisation; Guidance on statistical principles for clinical trials; Availability. *Federal Register* 1998;63:49583–49598.
41. Knipschild P, Leffers P, Feinstein AR. The qualification period. *J Clin Epidemiol* 1991;44(6):461–464.
42. Davis CE. Prerandomization compliance screening: A statistician's view.

In Shumaker SA, Schron EB, Ockene JK, McBee WL (eds): *The Handbook of Health Behavior Change* (2nd ed.). New York: Springer Publishing Co, Inc; 1998:485–490.

43. Dunbar-Jacob JM, Schlenk EA, Burke LE, et al. Predictors of patient adherence: Patient characteristics. In Shumaker SA, Schron EB, Ockene JK, McBee WL (eds): *The Handbook of Health Behavior Change* (2nd ed.). New York: Springer Publishing Co, Inc; 1998:491–511.

44. Dunbar J, Knoke J. Prediction of medication adherence at one year and seven years: Behavioral and psychological factors. *Control Clin Trials* 1986; 7:223.

45. Brittain E, Wittes J. The run-in period in clinical trials. The effect of misclassification on efficiency. *Control Clin Trials* 1990;11:327–338.

46. Halperin M, Rogot E, Gurian J, et al. Sample sizes for medical trials with special reference to long-term therapy. *J Chronic Dis* 1968; 21:13–24.

47. Palta M, McHugh R. Planning the size of a cohort study in the presence of both losses to follow-up and non-compliance. *J Chronic Dis* 1980;33: 501–512.

48. Feinstein A. Clinical Biostatistics. XXX. Biostatistical problems in "compliance bias." *Clin Pharmacol Ther* 1974;16:846–857.

49. Peduzzi P, Detre K, Wittes J, et al. Intent-to-treat analysis and the problem of crossovers. *J Thorac Cardiovasc Surg* 1991;101:481–487.

50. Peduzzi P, Wittes J, Detre K, et al. Analysis as-randomized and the problem of non-adherence: An example from the Veterans Affairs Randomized Trial of Coronary Artery Bypass Surgery. *Stat Med* 1993;12:1185–1195.

51. Lachin JM. Statistical considerations in the intent-to-treat principle. *Control Clin Trials* 2000;21:167–189.

52. The Boston Area Anticoagulation Trial for Atrial Fibrillation Investigators. The effect of low-dose warfarin on the risk of stroke in patients with nonrheumatic atrial fibrillation. *N Engl J Med* 1990;323:1505–1511.

53. Singer DE, Hughes RA, Gress DR, et al. The effect of aspirin on the risk of stroke in patients with nonrheumatic atrial fibrilliation: The BAATAF Study. *Am Heart J* 1992;124:1567–1573.

54. Detre K, Peduzzi P. The problem of attributing deaths of nonadherers: The VA coronary bypass experience. *Control Clin Trials* 1982;3:355–364.

55. Mantel N, Byar DP. Evaluation of response-time data involving transient states: An illustration using heart-transplant data. *J Am Stat Assoc* 1974;69: 81–86.

56. Crowley J, Hu M. Covariance analysis of heart transplant survival data. *J Am Stat Assoc* 1977;72:27–36.

57. Collins JF, Dorus W. Patient selection bias in analyses using only compliant patients. In Cramer JA, Spilker B (eds): *Patient Compliance in Medical Practice and Clinical Trials*. New York: Raven Press; 1991:335–338.

58. Gillings D, Koch G. The application of the principle of intention-to-treat to the analysis of clinical trials. *Drug Inf J* 1991;25:411–424.

59. Robins JM, Tsiatis AA. Correcting for non-compliance in randomized trials using rank preserving structural failure time models. *Commun Stat-Theory Methods* 1991;20:2609–2631.

60. Rubin DB. Comment on "Compliance as an explanatory variable in clinical trials" by Efron B, Feldman D. *J Am Stat Assoc* 1991;86:9–26.

61. Rubin DB. More powerful randomization-based p-values in double-blind trials with non-compliance. *Stat Med* 1998;17:371–385.

62. Dunbar-Jacob J, Sereika S, Rohay JM, et al. Electronic methods in assessing adherence to medical regimens. In Krantz DS, Baum A (eds): *Technology and Methods in Behavioral Medicine*. Mahwah, NJ: Lawrence Erlbaum Associates Inc; 1998:95–113.
63. Pocock S, Abdalla M. The hope and the hazards of using compliance data in clinical trials. *Stat Med* 1998;17:303–317.

Chapter 17

Compliance of Providers to Guidelines

Thomas A. Pearson, MD, PhD and
Laurie A. Kopin, MS, ANP

Introduction

The terms "noncompliance" or "nonadherence" are used most frequently when referring to the behavior of patients who ignore the medical advice provided by their healthcare providers. Oftentimes, there is a tendency to "blame the patient" when a therapeutic intervention is not implemented in the way intended. Conversely, there is another dimension to the problem of failure to implement well-established and effective therapeutic guidelines, namely, the lack of compliance of the healthcare provider themselves to provide the necessary recommendations. In this instance, it may be easy to merely "blame the doctor," and simply assume clinical incompetence on the part of the health care provider. After all, this is, in essence, the same type of superficial reasoning used to explain the complex problem of patient noncompliance.

The purpose of this chapter is to explore some of the issues related to healthcare providers' noncompliance with implementing well-accepted, standardized guidelines for screening and treatment. Specifically, potential barriers for healthcare providers to comply with guidelines for screening and treatment will be identified. Evidence supporting the importance of identifying these barriers as causes of noncompliance with well accepted guidelines related to the prevention of coronary heart disease (CHD) will then be reviewed. Finally, strate-

From: Burke LE, Ockene IS (eds). *Compliance in Healthcare and Research.* Armonk, NY: Futura Publishing Company, Inc.; © 2001.

Table 1

Databases Used to Illustrate Issues in Healthcare Provider Compliance

Database	Years	Number of patients	Number of providers	Guidelines examined
ACCEPT*	1996–7	5620	–	AHA Secondary Prevention
RLRC**	1991–2	1400	36	NCEP ATP-1
LTAP***	1996–7	4888	619	NCEP ATP-2

* American College of Cardiology Evaluation of Preventive Therapeutics
** Rural Lipid Resource Center
*** Lipid Treatment Assessment Program

gies to remove these barriers will be suggested, as a means to better implement CHD prevention guidelines.

To illustrate these issues, three large data sets will be used to draw examples of the barriers present (Table 1). First, the American College of Cardiology Evaluation of Preventive Therapeutics (ACCEPT) Study[1] randomly selected 53 US hospitals and recruited 5620 patients admitted in 1996 with CHD. The patients, with diagnoses including coronary artery bypass surgery, coronary angioplasty, myocardial infarction, and unstable angina, had their medical records reviewed at the time of admission and were then followed for 6 months after discharge. During this time, they were interviewed and examined for levels of CHD risk factors in an effort to determine the extent to which the American Heart Association guidelines for secondary prevention of CHD were followed.[2] Second, The Rural Lipid Resource Center performed audits of 1400 randomly selected medical records from 16 rural practices and 34 primary care providers in upstate New York,[3] to assess the extent to which the National Cholesterol Education Program Adult Treatment Panel – I (NCEP ATP-I) guidelines were being followed. These guidelines were initially released in 1988,[4] and then updated in 1991. In 1994, another 1720 records were reviewed in these same rural practices. Third, the Lipid Treatment Assessment Program (L-TAP) assessed 4888 patients from 619 primary care practices in the US in 1996,[5] to determine the extent to which patients under treatment for dyslipidemia have met risk-specific goals set by the National Cholesterol Education Program Treatment Panel II (NCEP ATP-II).[6] These three data sets will be discussed to illustrate issues in healthcare providers' compliance with guidelines.

Compliance of Healthcare Providers in Inpatient Settings

When looking for opportunities for intervention on CHD risk factors in clinical settings, multiple levels can be identified, including health systems/programs/governmental agencies, the inpatient setting, ambulatory care sites, and the patient and his/her family (Figure 1). This discussion will focus on the healthcare provider, as they have opportunities within both the inpatient and ambulatory care settings to positively impact secondary prevention efforts.

There is an unfortunate tendency for healthcare providers positioned in clinical settings to neglect the initiation of a vital aspect of patient care, namely, coronary risk factor modification. However, there are a number of reasons to integrate this much-needed care into the acute care setting.[7] First, the patient, their family members, and the primary care provider need to understand that treatment of the primary disease process, atherosclerosis, is as important (if not more important over the long-term) as the treatment of acute manifestations of CHD. The impression that coronary risk factor modification can wait until months later sends the incorrect message that this is not an important part of overall care. Second, clinical trials have repeatedly identified both short-term and long-term benefits of such interventions, and patients should not be denied these proven benefits of care in the months soon after CHD onset. Third, coronary risk factor reduction can yield added benefits to the disease process in other vascular beds outside the cardiovascular system. Fourth, the benefits of risk factor modification are certainly additive to other cardiologic therapies, such as the use of pharmaceutical agents. However, they need integration into the entire plan of care to avoid deleterious interactions between interventions (eg, bile acid-binding resins interacting with cardioprotective drug absorption). Finally, in the acute care setting soon after the cardiac

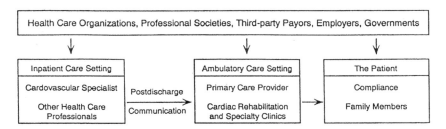

Figure 1. The chain of opportunities for integration of comprehensive risk reduction strategies into the overall care of the patient.[7]

event, there is a window of opportunity known as the "teachable moment." It is during this time when the patient and family members may be highly motivated for behavior change, whereas days or weeks later, the receptivity tends to be markedly diminished.

Nonetheless, there remain barriers to the implementation of guidelines for secondary prevention through risk factor modification at the patient, physician, healthcare organization, and community levels (Table 2).[8] In the inpatient setting, these include a priority for acute care of the CHD syndrome or procedure prompting the admission. Despite the advantages described previously, the main focus of care is on the acute symptoms or short-term interventions. Often, hospitals are simply not organized or staffed to provide preventive services. Nursing and other allied health-care personnel are continually faced with the dilemma of increasing patient/staff ratios. At the same time,

---

Table 2

Barriers to Implementation of Preventive Services

Patient
Lack of knowledge and motivation
Lack of access to care
Cultural factors
Social factors
Physician
Problem-based focus
Feedback on prevention is negative or neutral
Time constraints
Lack of incentives, including reimbursement
Lack of training
  Poor knowledge of benefits
  Perceived ineffectiveness
  Lack of skills
Lack of specialist-generalist communication
Lack of perceived legitimacy
Health-care setting (hospitals, practices, etc.)
Acute care priority
Lack of resources for preventive services
Lack of systems for preventive services
Time and economic constraints
Poor communication between specialty and primary care providers
Lack of policies and standards
Community/Society
Lack of policies and standards
Lack of reimbursement

From Pearson TA, McBride PE, Houston-Miller N, Smith SC. Organization of preventive cardiology service, *J Am Coll Cardiol* 1996;27:1039–1047.

criteria for hospital admission are becoming more stringent, patients are requiring more acute care services as they are sicker, and the length of stay is decreasing. This lack of designated personnel assigned the responsibility of providing preventive services and necessary tools for them to be effective makes difficult the provision of even minimal inpatient preventive services. Finally, many hospitals continue to lack policies, procedures, and standards, despite the adoption of secondary prevention guidelines by most professional and quality assurance groups.[2]

There is ample evidence that these barriers do affect care. For example, in the ACCEPT Study, of the 5620 medical records of patients admitted with various CHD diagnoses and procedures, there was a wide range of documentation of risk factors. On the positive side, 92.2% of medical records documented the history of cigarette smoking as affirmative or negative. Moderate proportions of records made note of obesity (69.3%), hypertension (70.3%), or a family history of CHD (71.6%). Disappointing proportions of records noted the presence or absence of hyperlipidemia (48.1%) or diabetes (54.7%). There was also a dearth of action taken as part of the hospital admission. For example, in the ACCEPT Study, 40% of patients admitted were current smokers. Only half of them had any evidence that smoking cessation advice was given and only 3.5% of patients were referred to a formal smoking cessation program. Regarding hyperlipidemia detection and management, a total cholesterol level or lipid profile was available in the medical record in only 57.4% of patients. In about half (44.7%), no action was taken with regard to counseling about hyperlipidemia. In 11.5%, general lifestyle counseling was provided, and one-third received advice from a nutritionist. As for lipid-lowering pharmacotherapy, 12.8% continued their medication and 8% had these agents started. Only 21% of patients were discharged on these effective agents.

A variety of opportunities exist to correct this lack of detection and management of risk factors in the inpatient setting. Since acute coronary syndromes often appropriately occupy the attention of hospital staff, a variety of "automatic" procedures should be incorporated into the patient's plan of care so that, after the acute interventions are initiated, the stage is set for implementation of prevention guidelines. Examples include protocols for the measurement of serum lipids within the first 24 hours of admission for coronary patients, and the identification of abnormal laboratory values by hospital staff, including reminders of NCEP-LDL cholesterol goals. One means to assure the assessment and documentation of the inpatient's coronary risk factor profile is through the completion of a risk factor inventory checklist (Figure 2). The checklist is completed by specially trained staff, usually deployed by the Phase I cardiac rehabilitation program. The team generally consists of nurses, exercise physiologists/physical therapists,

Risk Intervention	Recommendations				Initial Status	Follow-Up
Smoking: **Goal** Complete Cessation	Strongly encourage patients and family to stop smoking. Provide counseling, nicotine replacement, and formal cessation programs as appropriate.					
Lipid Management: **Primary Goal** LDL <100 mg/dL **Secondary Goals** HDL >35 mg/dL; TG <200 mg/dL	Start AHA Step II Diet in all patients: ≤30% fat, <7% saturated fat, <200 mg/d cholesterol. Assess fasting lipid profile. In post-MI patients, lipid profile may take 4 to 6 weeks to stabilize. Add drug therapy according to the following guide:					
	LDL <100 mg/dL	LDL 100 to 130 mg/dL	LDL >130 mg/dL	HDL <35 mg/dL		
	No Drug Therapy	Consider adding drug therapy to diet, as follows:	Add drug therapy to diet, as follows:	Emphasize weight management and physical activity.		
		Suggested Drug Therapy		Advise smoking cessation.		
	TG <200 mg/dL	TG 200 to 400 mg/dL	TG >400 mg/dL	If needed to achieve LDL goals, consider niacin, statin, fibrate.		
	Statin Resin Niacin	Statin Niacin	Consider combined drug therapy (niacin, fibrate, statin)			
	If LDL goal not achieved, consider combination therapy.					
Blood Pressure Control: **Goal** ≤140/90 mm Hg	Initiate lifestyle modification—weight control, physical activity, alcohol moderation, and moderate sodium restriction—in all patients with blood pressure >140 mm Hg systolic or 90 mm Hg diastolic. Add blood pressure medication, individualized to other patient requirements and characteristics (i.e. age, race, need for drugs with specific benefits) if blood pressure is not less than 140 mm Hg systolic or 90 mm Hg diastolic in 3 months or if *initial* blood pressure is >160 mm Hg systolic or 100 mm Hg diastolic.					
Physical Activity: **Minimum Goal** **30 minutes 3 to 4 times per week**	Assess risk, preferably with exercise test, to guide prescription. Encourage minimum of 30 to 60 minutes of moderate-intensity activity 3 or 4 times weekly (walking, jogging, cycling, or other aerobic activity) supplemented by an increase in daily lifestyle activities (e.g. walking breaks at work, using stairs, gardening, household work). Maximum benefit 5 to 6 hours a week. Advise medically supervised programs for moderate to high risk patients.					
Weight Management:	Start intensive diet and appropriate physical activity intervention, as outlined above, in patients >120% of ideal weight for height. Particularly emphasize need for weight loss in patients with hypertension, elevated triglycerides, or elevated glucose levels.					
Antiplatelet Agents/ Anticoagulants:	Start aspirin 80 to 325 mg/d if not contraindicated. Manage warfarin to international normalized ratio = 2 to 3.5 for post-MI patients not able to take aspirin.					
ACE Inhibitors Post MI:	Start early post-MI in stable high-risk patients (anterior MI, previous MI, Killip Class II, [S₃, gallop, rales, radiographic CHF]). Continue indefinitely for all with LV dysfunction (ejection fraction ≤40%) or symptoms of failure. Use as needed to manage blood pressure or symptoms in all other patients.					
Beta-blockers:	Start in high-risk post-MI patients (arrhythmia, LV dysfunction, inducible ischemia) at 5 to 28 days. Continue 6 months minimum. Observe usual contraindications. Use as needed to manage angina, rhythm, or blood pressure in all other patients.					
Estrogens:	Consider estrogen replacement in all postmenopausal women. Individualize recommendation consistent with other health risks.					

Figure 2. Checklist for hospitalized patients with coronary disease incorporating the American Heart Association guidelines for secondary prevention[2] with a plan for assessment and follow-up.[7]

and other designated health care personnel. This valuable assessment tool serves to identify the level of coronary risk factors present, list the goals for intervention, and recommendations for ambulatory follow-up care.

Another opportunity for inpatient risk factor management is the development of protocols or care maps that incorporate risk factor assessment and modification. The advantage of integrating coronary risk factor management into the overall patient care map is that preventive care can then be initiated without specific written orders, thereby expediting secondary prevention. Utilization of a multidisciplinary team approach is the optimal strategy, incorporating nursing, physical therapy, nutrition, and psychology/social work staff. Ideally, the protocols should include the initiation of either nurse case management programs or referral to Phase II cardiac rehabilitation programs.

Poor Communication Between Inpatient and Ambulatory Care Providers: A Major Cause of Noncompliance?

A special problem arises when the patient is discharged from the increasingly shortened length of hospital stay, which is very common today. The need for communication between the inpatient cardiac rehabilitation specialist and the primary care provider is vital regardless of whether or not there was an opportunity to assess and modify coronary risk factors. Very often, the written and verbal communication between providers deals solely with highly technical information regarding the findings of invasive diagnostic procedures, and monitoring of various cardiologic and revascularization procedures. All too often, the discharge summaries fail to communicate the coronary risk factor assessments, steps taken to modify those risk factors, and a comprehensive intervention plan to address the identified risk factors. The unfortunate result is the primary care provider then receives the wrong message that either risk factor assessment and intervention is not important, or that no further risk factor modification needs to be performed. The specialist, on the other hand, often assumes that the primary care provider will take responsibility for risk factor assessment and modification. Some specialists even fear loss of referral of patients from primary care providers if they initiate this type of care. To clarify this issue, the 27th Bethesda Conference of the American College of Cardiology states clearly: "The management of cardiovascular risk factors is an integral part of the optimal care of the patient with established cardiovascular disease or at high risk for development of the disease."[9] Therefore, risk factor management is an appropriate and necessary aspect of care to be delivered by all health care providers, including specialists, primary care physicians, and nurses.

There is considerable evidence to suggest that post discharge communication (or lack of it) is a major cause of noncompliance by healthcare providers. In the ACCEPT Study, review of 31% of 5620 medical records could not identify a discharge plan. While over 90% of patients with a plan were prescribed cardiac drugs and scheduled for a follow-up visit with the cardiologist, less than half were provided with an exercise prescription and only one in four were referred to a cardiac rehabilitation program. Only about half of the patients with medical histories significant for hypertension and smoking, had discharge plans for blood pressure control or smoking cessation, respectively. The medical record review also made mention of the need for further assessment and treatment of lipid disorders in 41% of patients.

Sadly, in less than 1% of patients was there a plan to screen first degree relatives for risk factors. Clearly, this must negatively affect both the patients' opportunity to modify their risk factors, as well as the primary care provider's abilities to incorporate these steps into a long-term plan of care.

The opportunity to rectify this dilemma might be as simple as the consistent utilization of a well-designed and comprehensive risk factor checklist as previously discussed (Figure 2). In any case, the risk factors identified and the goals for their modification should be an integral part of the post discharge communication to the primary care provider. Moreover, any interventions initiated during the inpatient setting should be adequately relayed, therefore, avoiding both costly and unnecessary duplication of efforts. Another benefit of the checklist, especially if time during hospitalization did not allow initiation of risk factor intervention, is to provide the necessary recommendations to guide the primary care provider in their follow-up and long-term care.

Compliance of Healthcare Providers in Ambulatory Care Settings

Ambulatory care settings, by virtue of their long-term relationship and frequency of interactions with the high-risk patient, present another ideal opportunity to implement guidelines for risk factor management. Unfortunately, care providers find additional barriers to implementation of preventive services in this setting as well (Table 2). Once again, the care has a problem-based focus, often related to an underlying sign or symptom, rather than CHD risk. For many providers, the value of preventive care services is not realized because if prevention succeeds, the provider hears less from the patient as the need for acute office visits diminish. Paradoxically, if the preventive intervention causes an adverse reaction or deleterious effect in the patient's perceived quality of life, the feedback relayed to the provider is negative. Also, similar to inpatient length of stay, the duration of ambulatory care visits is growing increasingly shorter. Visits are typically scheduled at 10–15 minute intervals, not allowing adequate time to initiate profound discussions about lifestyle modification and cardiovascular risk reduction. Another limiting factor rests with the providers themselves often not believing they possess the necessary skills to be effective counselors in areas such as behavioral modification, nutrition, etc. Tragically, the tendency is to then neglect this important aspect of patient care. Several surveys of physicians have identified them as experiencing considerable discomfort in the provision of dietary counseling, while at the same time, physicians have been identified as the most credible source of nutrition information.[10,11] In addition to perceived ineffectiveness, providers often are not aware of the benefits of risk factor modification relative to those of more traditional cardiologic care. Finally, as previously discussed, there remains confusion as to whom has responsibility for risk factor modification.

There is ample evidence that a number of opportunities are missed for risk factor modification in ambulatory care settings. For example, in the Rural Lipid Resource Center, a 1991 survey of 1400 medical records from 34 care providers in 16 rural practices showed only 56.9% of patients had a total cholesterol measured since 1988, and in only 58.8% of these patients was the cholesterol measurement noted in the record.[3] Thus, only about one-third of patients had a cholesterol level actively taken into account. Tests for secondary causes, dietary therapy, and pharmacologic intervention were infrequently performed. Interestingly, the 34 care providers were assessed for their knowledge and attitudes about the NCEP-ATP-1 guidelines. Most were rather knowledgeable and accepting of these guidelines. However, there was absolutely no correlation between these knowledge and attitude measures and the successful implementation of the guidelines. This suggests that barriers other than providers' knowledge and attitudes are responsible for noncompliance with established guidelines. Nonetheless, among these practices, those practitioners with the best adherence to the guidelines, in fact, showed the best abilities to reduce LDL-cholesterol levels in hyperlipidemic individuals.

Another type of noncompliance with guidelines is the quantitative rather than qualitative type. In the Lipid Treatment Assessment Program, 4888 patients receiving care for hyperlipidemia were recruited by 619 primary care providers.[5] While all of them were under care, the proportions of patients who reached NCEP-ATP II goals were disappointing. Overall, only 39% of patients on drug therapy and only 34% of patients on dietary therapy reached their NCEP goal (Table 3). For CHD patients, only 18% and 7% of patients on drug and diet therapies, respectively, reached their LDL-C goal. Furthermore, the patients were not nearly at goal; as many CHD patients had LDL-C levels above 160 mg/dL as below 100 mg/dL. A search for the reasons for these poor levels of compliance revealed a number of likely causes. These included the lack of dietary therapy, or in postmenopausal women, estrogen therapy, concomitant with lack of drug therapy or inadequate drug therapy (especially the lack of use of statins). The most common problem was the initiation of drugs without further titration of dose to reach the LDL-C goal. Finally, combinations in drug therapy were infrequently used. This provides evidence that ambulatory care providers may be initiating appropriate therapies, but perhaps not using the correct type and/or dosages of medication to achieve desired goals,

Table 3

Number and Percent of 4888 Patients Achieving LDL Cholesterol Goals by Risk Group and Diet vs. Drug Therapies: The Lipid Treatment Assessment Project*

Risk Group**	LDL-C Goal (mg/dL)	Nondrug therapy		Drug therapy	
		Number	Percent Success	Number	Percent Success
No CHD, <2 Risk Factors	<160	282	59	861	70
No CHD, ≥2 Risk Factors	<130	361	22	1924	40
CHD	<100	108	7	1352	18
Total		751	34	4137	39

* Reference 5.
** As defined by the National Cholesterol Education Program (6).

thereby, representing another form of noncompliance. Unfortunately, this is becoming an increasingly common problem.

A number of opportunities exist for improvements in compliance with risk factor management guidelines in ambulatory care settings. First the ambulatory care clinic or office needs to be organized to allow preventive services to be rendered. A key element to success is the clear delineation of roles and responsibilities of the staff toward this effort. Certainly, roles can be identified and assignments made accordingly to efficiently utilize the time and talents of the physicians, nurses, technicians, and office support staff.

If the ambulatory care site is unable to provide adequate levels of preventive services, several alternative models exist. First, nurse case manager programs have been shown to be an effective means to organize and implement secondary prevention guidelines.[12,13] For example, Debusk and Houston-Miller demonstrated striking improvements in levels of lipid management, smoking cessation, and exercise capacity in those patients referred to a nurse case managed program as compared to usual care (Table 4).[12] Nurse Managers who possess excellent organizational skills and are given the responsibility and provided with the necessary tools, are clearly an important and cost-effective means to comply with secondary prevention guidelines. Similarly, cardiac rehabilitation programs, with up to 12 weeks of regular contact with

Table 4

Risk Factor Modification Rates in Patients after Myocardial Infarction: Comparison of Nurse Case Manager-Based Program with Usual Care*

Risk factor modification	Nurse case-manager	Usual care
N	293	292
Smoking cessation at 12 months (%)	70	53
LDL Cholesterol <100 mg/dL at 12 months (%)	42.4	15.2
Functional capacity at 6 months (METS)	9.3	8.4

* Reference 12

the high-risk patient, can provide an effective platform for risk factor control. Finally, preventive cardiology clinics and other specialty programs often provide a multidisciplinary staff (physicians, nurses, nutritionists, exercise physiologists, behavioral scientists), as well as, tools such as computerized risk assessment, specialized laboratory testing, and noninvasive cardiac function testing that might be useful in risk factor management.

Interventions in Healthcare Providers to Improve Compliance

Both physicians and nurses alike might benefit from additional steps to improve their compliance with established guidelines for the assessment and management of cardiovascular disease. Many curricula in medical and nursing schools have minimal content discussing noncompliance as a health issue and contain few opportunities to build skills in enhancement of patient compliance. Continuing education programs are often bereft of such discussions and use formats that are not conducive to adult learning.[14] Another means of improving compliance is performance feedback. Among interventions in clinical settings, performance feedback is among the most consistently shown to influence provider behavior.[14–17] The development of tools to assist providers with patient compliance would also be useful, particularly if incorporated into educational programs with instruction on how to best use the tools. Finally, the reorganization of practices, such as with nurse case management, allows the clear designation of a team approach to implement the guidelines. Responsibilities are assigned to those with the most appropriate level of skill, and provided with the necessary tools and time to complete the task of secondary prevention.

Conclusion

While there is a tendency to first "blame the patient" for lack of compliance with guidelines, a second major contributor to noncompliance lies with the ownership of healthcare providers at both the inpatient and ambulatory care settings. Considerable barriers continue to persist at both of these sites, yet there are numerous occasions to seize the opportunity for prevention in both settings. The inpatient providers must better communicate findings and improve plans for the transition of the patient from the inpatient to the ambulatory care setting. Various strategies to improve and reorganize the ambulatory care setting to foster preventive efforts can also be cited. Attention needs to be given to barriers other than knowledge and attitudes of providers. Numerous alternative strategies, such as nurse case managed programs, provide viable alternatives to current practices, and likely have their greatest impact by improving compliance with guidelines from both the providers and patient perspectives. When a patient is not compliant with a treatment of proven effectiveness, the reason for noncompliance likely resides both with the patient and his/her healthcare provider.

References

1. Pearson TA, Peters TD. The treatment gap in coronary artery disease and heart failure: Community standards and the post-discharge patient. *Am J Cardiol* 1997;80:45H–52H.
2. Smith SL, Blair SN, Criqui MH, et al. Preventing heart attack and death in patients with coronary disease. *Circulation* 1995;92:2–4.
3. Ammerman A, Caggiula A, Elmer P, et al. Putting medical practice guidelines into practice: The cholesterol model. *Am J Prev Med* 1994;10:209–216.
4. Report of the National Cholesterol Education Program Expert Panel on Detection, Evaluation, and Treatment of High Blood Cholesterol in Adults. *Arch Intern Med* 1988;148:36–69.
5. Pearson TA, Laurora I, Chu H, Kafonek S. The Lipid Treatment Assessment Project (L-TAP): A multicenter survey to evaluate the percentages of dyslipidemic patients receiving lipid-lowering therapy and achieving NCEP target LDL-C goals. *Arch Int Med* (in press).
6. Expert Panel on Detection, Evaluation and Treatment of High Cholesterol in Adults. Summary of the Second Report of the National Cholesterol Education Program (NCEP) on Detection, Evaluation, and Treatment of High Blood Cholesterol in Adults (Adult Treatment Panel II). *JAMA* 1993;269:3015–3023.

7. Pearson TA. An integrated approach to risk factor modification. In Topol EJ (ed): *Comprehensive Cardiovascular Medicine*. Philadelphia: Lippincott-Raven☐98:297–311.

8. Pearson TA, McBride PE, Houston-Miller N, et al. Organization of preventive cardiology service. *JACC* 1996;27:1039–1047.

9. Pearson TA, Fuster V. 27th Bethesda Conference: Matching the intensity of risk factor management with the hazard for coronary disease events. *JACC* 1996;27:958–963.

10. Shea S, Gemson DH, Mossel P. Management of high blood cholesterol by primary care physicians: Diffusion of the National Cholesterol Education Adult Treatment Panel guidelines. *J Gen Intern Med* 1990;5:327–334.

11. Roberts WC. Getting cardiologists interested in lipids. *Am J Cardiol* 1993; 72:744–745.

12. DeBusk RF, Houston-Miller N, Superko HR, et al. A case-management system for coronary risk factor modification after acute myocardial infarction. *Ann Intern Med* 1994;120:721–729.

13. Taylor CB, Houston-Miller N, Killen JD, et al. Smoking cessation after acute myocardial infarction: Effects of a nurse-managed intervention. *Ann Intern Med* 1990;113:118–123.

14. Orlandi MA. Promoting health and preventing disease in health care settings: An analysis of barriers. *Prev Med* 1987;16:119–130.

15. Siscovick DS, Strogatz DS, Wagner EH, et al. Provider-oriented interventions and management of hypertension. *Med Care* 1987;28:254–258.

16. Tierney WM, Hui SL, McDonald CJ. Delayed feedback of physician performance versus immediate reminders to perform preventive care. Effects on physician compliance. *Med Care* 1986;24:659–666.

17. Boekeloo BO. Evaluation of Strategies for Increasing Intern Cholesterol Management in Inpatients. (dissertation). Baltimore (MD): Johns Hopkins University, 1988.

Chapter 18

Impact on Clinical Outcomes

Michel Burnier, MD, and
Hans R. Brunner, MD

Introduction

Many large clinical trials have demonstrated the benefits of normalizing blood pressure in hypertensive patients.[1,2] Thus, physicians are well aware that an adequate control of blood pressure enables patients to reduce the incidence of strokes, myocardial infarction, congestive heart failure, or chronic renal failure. Yet, there is still a major gap between the official recommendations and the actual rate of blood pressure normalization in the community. Despite the fact that the control of hypertension has improved considerably in some countries, only a small fraction of hypertensive patients have blood pressure values below the recommended target in industrialized countries. For example, the results of the Third National Health and Nutrition Examination Survey (NHANES III) have shown that approximately 70% of hypertensive patients are aware of their disease and half are being treated with antihypertensive medication.[3] However, the proportion of hypertensives with a blood pressure below 140/90 mmHg is only 27%. The situation is much worse in the UK, the corresponding figure being only 6% in that country.[4]

Why is Blood Pressure Control So Poor?

There may be several reasons that explain the poor blood pressure control achieved in general practice. Many physicians do not adhere

This concept has been developed based on clinical studies made possible with the financial help of Pfizer, Bristol Myers Squibbs and the Drug Information Association.

From: Burke LE, Ockene IS (eds). *Compliance in Healthcare and Research.* Armonk, NY: Futura Publishing Company, Inc.; © 2001.

to the official recommendations and set the therapeutic goal at higher levels.[5] In this respect, it is also important to realize that major differences exist between various national guidelines and these variations influence considerably the assessment of hypertension control. Thus, in a recent study, Fahey et al. have demonstrated using the blood pressure data of a sample of 876 treated hypertensive patients, that the proportion of patients with normalization of blood pressure would vary from 17.5% to 84.6% depending on whether the guidelines established in New Zealand, Canada, the United States, Great Britain, or by the World Health Organization were used.[6] The physician's willingness to change patients' medications or to intensify treatment plays an important role in the control of blood pressure. A recent study performed in a selected population of older men has indeed shown that patients who received more intensive medical therapy had better blood pressure values, suggesting thereby that many physicians are not aggressive enough in their approach to hypertension.[7] The high blood pressure values commonly found in treated hypertensive patients can also not be accounted for only by a white-coat effect. Indeed, the number of patients with inadequate blood pressure control is high not only when measured in the physician's office, but also when assessed at home or by ambulatory blood pressure monitoring.[8] On the other hand, the results of the Hypertension Optimal Treatment (HOT) study have demonstrated that it is possible to achieve a good control of blood pressure using combinations of the four classes of antihypertensive agents commonly recommended for first line therapy in hypertension.[9]

Patient compliance (which refers to the willingness and ability of an individual to follow health-related advice, to take and persist in taking medication as prescribed, to attend scheduled clinic appointments and to complete recommended investigations) is a major health issue with outcomes related to levels of morbidity, mortality, and cost utilization. Studies of patient compliance with medical treatment have consistently demonstrated a high level of noncompliance in hypertension.[10] Interestingly, poor adherence to treatment is the first cause of failure to normalize blood pressure evoked by physicians, whereas patients claim that they always take their medication and attribute the failure to reach the therapeutic goal to the poor efficacy of antihypertensive drugs.[11] This discrepancy clearly illustrates that the patient's and the doctor's perceptions of the role of compliance in reaching the therapeutic goals differ markedly. This gap in perception may be due to a poor communication on the topic of compliance. Indeed, physicians often feel uncomfortable talking about compliance because they are concerned with the possibility that some patients might consider their questions on compliance as an invasion of their privacy or as a lack of confidence.

The Need for an Objective Monitoring of Compliance

A clinical problem cannot be solved unless it can be detected and quantitated adequately using reliable and objective methods. Today, the detection of noncompliance remains a major issue. Indeed, assessing patient's compliance in everyday practice is a difficult task. Several methods are available to examine drug adherence but most of them are used almost exclusively in clinical trials and not in the day to day management of hypertensive patients.

Many physicians claim that they have no problem recognizing poorly compliant patients because they have known their patients for many years. There is increasing evidence that this assumption is incorrect. Indeed, studies have demonstrated that the physician's estimate is as precise as flipping a coin with a positive predictive value of about 30% when compared to the pill count.[12] In clinical practice, the physician's estimate of compliance is based on several aspects such as the respect of appointments, a direct questioning, the occurrence of side-effects or the outcome of therapy. These approaches are limited in various ways. Direct questioning of the patients is highly subjective and depends on the patient's memory. Thus, only short-term information can be obtained. The only situation in which questioning may be helpful is when the patient admits spontaneously to a noncompliant behavior. In clinical studies, the reported compliance correlates poorly with the rate of blood pressure normalization.[13] The occurence of drug-specific untowards effects indicates that the prescribed drug has been taken recently. However, it does not provide any information on the dynamic of compliance and does not ascertain a good compliance to concomitant treatments. Finally, the fact that a patient does not achieve the therapeutic goal cannot be taken as an evidence of poor compliance. Indeed, in hypertension, any medication given in monotherapy is ineffective in approximately 50% of the patients even if the drug is taken regularly.

The pill count and the prescription refills can hardly be used in the office if the doctor is not at the same time the prescriber and the dispenser of the medications. Otherwise, the physician must be in close contact with the pharmacist to obtain the information. However, several studies have even demonstrated that the pill count overestimates the actual compliance because patients may intentionally discard tablets before returning the container to the physician or the pharmacist.[14,15] Prescription refills may be of interest for epidemiological studies or investigations in a community of hypertensive patients, but can hardly be used in taking care of an individual subject.

Detection of Non-Compliance: The Place of Electronic Monitoring

In recent years, new approaches to measure drug compliance have been developed using microelectronic monitoring systems.[16-19] The newest devices such as the Medication Event Monitoring System (MEMS, Aprex Corporation, Fremont, California, USA) consists of a container which can contain pill and capsule medication formulations, fitted with a special cap containing a microprocessor which records each opening of the cap as a presumptive dose.[18] These devices have now been used extensively in large phase II and phase III clinical trials where it is essential to assess the efficacy of new therapeutic agents by taking compliance into consideration and by drawing the relation curve between the medication really taken and the clinical outcome. These systems, which offer the unique opportunity to collect dynamic data on compliance, have also been used in smaller groups of patients to characterize the patterns and the frequency of noncompliance in various diseases.[18,20-28]

Yet, these electronic monitors can be very useful to detect compliance problems in ambulatory medicine and to help patients to follow the prescriptions for medications. Indeed, the MEMS system, which is the most widely used system in Europe and the US, is simple, easy to handle and relatively cheap if one takes into account the price of drugs and the savings that could potentially be generated by improved treatment efficacy and outcome.[27] The reading of the data takes only a few minutes. In contrast to blood and urine samples which are sometimes considered as the gold standard, the MEMS is the only system to provide dynamic data regarding time and date of container opening over the whole period between physicians visits. This aspect is crucial because compliance is by definition a dynamic parameter which varies in time depending on the patient's life. The printed compliance report which is based on the collected data is a rather important element of the monitoring (Figure 1). The dose frequency is displayed as a calender plot indicating the number of openings occuring each day. This calender plot is very simple for the patient to understand, and represents an interesting support enabling the physician to start a discussion with the patient based on real data and not on suspicion. It is of course mandatory to inform the patient and to obtain his consent before starting monitoring, and one has to be clear that the goal of the procedure is to support and not to police drug compliance. This condition contributes to enhancing the patient's responsibility. The patient will feel very much concerned by the data since he/she will have collected the information. With the compliance report in hand, it will be possible to in-

COMPLIANCE REPORT   5 Jul 1999

Patient ID **8341**	Start date	**13 Feb 1999 03:00**	Dose regimen	**1X**
Device # **87132**	Stop date	**01 Jun 1999 02:59**		
Drug **Reniten 20 mg**	# of days **108**		# of doses taken **105**	

% days correct number of doses taken **93.52%**	% prescribed doses taken on schedule **82.41%**

CALENDAR PLOT

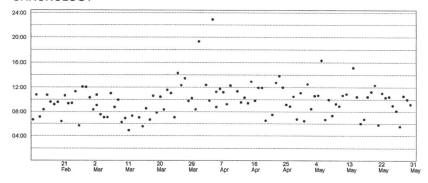

February 1999

Mon	Tue	Wed	Thr	Fri	Sat	Sun
1	2	3	4	5	6	7
8	9	10	11	12	13 1	14 1
15 1	16 1	17 1	18 1	19 1	20 1	21 1
22 1	23 1	24 1	25 1	26 1	27 1	28 1

March 1999

Mon	Tue	Wed	Thr	Fri	Sat	Sun
1 1	2 1	3 2	4 1	5 1	6 1	7 1
8 1	9 1	10 1	11 1	12 1	13 1	14 0
15 1	16 1	17 1	18 1	19 1	20 1	21 1
22 1	23 1	24 1	25 1	26 1	27 1	28 1
29 1	30 1	31 1				

April 1999

Mon	Tue	Wed	Thr	Fri	Sat	Sun
			1 1	2 0	3 1	4 1
5 1	6 2	7 1	8 1	9 1	10 1	11 0
12 1	13 1	14 1	15 1	16 1	17 1	18 1
19 1	20 1	21 0	22 1	23 1	24 1	25 1
26 1	27 1	28 1	29 1	30 1		

May 1999

Mon	Tue	Wed	Thr	Fri	Sat	Sun
					1 1	2 1
3 1	4 1	5 1	6 1	7 1	8 1	9 1
10 1	11 1	12 1	13 1	14 0	15 1	16 1
17 1	18 1	19 1	20 1	21 1	22 1	23 1
24 1	25 1	26 1	27 1	28 1	29 1	30 1
31 1						

CHRONOLOGY

Figure 1. Example of a compliance report obtained with the MEMS system. Enalapril 20 mg once daily was prescribed. As can be seen on the calender plot, the patient sometimes takes two tablets a day rather than one, and the timing of his taking habit is very variable. There are some omissions on Sundays.

volve the patient during an interactive feedback discussion in reviewing and choosing among possible solutions to avoid the omissions.

Can Adequate Compliance Be Defined More Precisely?

In clinical studies, the patients' compliance is often analyzed using arbitrary cut-offs chosen to discriminate "good" from "partial" compliers. The limit, which is frequently set at 80%, has hardly been validated and may not correspond to anything practically relevant for most of the prescribed drugs. Today, a more precise definition of compliance is needed which should not consider the number of doses taken but rather the number of days with a correct dosing. Because they record the date and hour each time the pillbox is opened, electronic monitors can provide such information. The monitors also enable calculation of the dosing intervals and, by knowing the duration of action of a given drug, allow assessment of the therapeutic coverage. This important clinical information might help to define more accurately what a good compliance rate is. Thus, although a 100% adherence to treatment is the ideal goal, it is conceivable that perfect compliance is not always necessary to obtain the full benefit of all drugs, depending on their mechanism and duration of action. With some drugs, a prolonged duration of action could potentially compensate for imperfect medication-taking behavior. Today, many drugs are approved for once-daily use, but actually do not provide a consistent effect over the 24-hour period. Considering the limitations in human behavior, it may be of interest to evaluate drugs not only for their efficacy when properly used but also for the persistence of their effects during partial compliance. In this respect, Leenen et al. have recently demonstrated that although amlodipine and diltiazem are fairly similar in lowering blood pressure from an efficacy point of view, during short periods of noncompliance, blood pressure control persists markedly better with the agent with a long elimination half-life.[28]

When Should Electronic Monitors Be Used?

Today, there is only limited experience of the use of electronic monitors of compliance in everyday practice. Conceivably, the clinical appplication of these devices will depend on the disease as well as on the treatment. Thus, the place of electronic monitoring will be different in diseases with measurable outcomes such as hypertension, dyslipidemia or diabetes from those with less well measurable endpoints such as preventive chemotherapy of tuberculosis. In hypertension, there is apparently no need to investigate compliance when blood pressure is well controlled. On the other hand, whether drug adherence should be investigated in patients whose blood pressure is not normalized with a monotherapy is highly debatable because there is only roughly a 50% chance to control blood pressure with a single antihypertensive agent. In this case, the probability of an ineffective treatment is probably greater than the probability of noncompliance. The situation differs when blood pressure is not normalized by a combination of two or more antihypetrensive agents. In that case, more than 80% of patients should respond to treatment and have a well-controlled blood pressure. There is some evidence that in this case, monitoring of compliance can improve the outcome.[29] "Refractory hypertension" raises questions regarding the effectiveness of the prescribed therapeutic regimen, the need for investigating secondary hypertension, and of course compliance.[30] As physicians we are faced by these questions daily, and because of the lack of a rational assessment of compliance, we usually choose to change the doses and mix of the therapeutic agents. It is a fact that the assumption on which these decisions are based, ie appropriate compliance, is not often wrong. Yet, for a rational management of refractory hypertension, decisions should be made based on objective measurements of compliance in order to avoid unecessary, costly investigations and prescriptions of excessive doses and combinations of antihypertensive drugs.

The patient's history presented in Figure 2 illustrates these potential benefits of using electronic monitoring of compliance in refractory hypertension. This young male hypertensive patient was very hypertensive despite the prescription of a quadruple therapy of losartan 50mg/day, torasemide 10mg/day and a fixed combination of felodipine 10mg/metoprolol 100mg/day. With the consent of the patient, the treatment was reconditioned into three electronic monitors without any change in prescription. After 2 months of such monitoring without any other action taken by the physician, office blood pressure fell from 160/120 mmHg to 140/98 mmHg and compliance was excellent (> 95% for all drugs). The improvement was confirmed by ambulatory blood pressure monitoring which revealed an even slightly lower daytime average blood pressure of 135/85 mmHg. Thus, just the electronic monitoring per se had already a very marked positive effect on the treatment results. Immediately after interrupting the monitoring, blood pressure rose again to 180/140 mmHg. The compliance issue was discussed at the next visit based on the previous monitoring data and possible solutions to improve pill taking habits were generated. This resulted in a sustained improvement in blood pressure control without any modification of therapy.

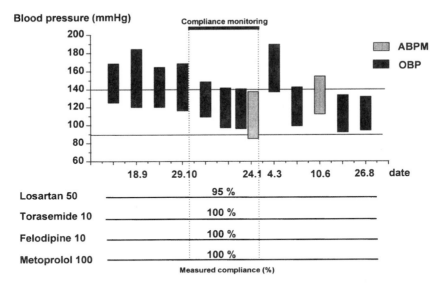

Figure 2. Office and ambulatory blood pressures in a patient with refractory hypertension treated with losartan, torasemide, felodipine and metoprolol. Note that during electronic monitoring of compliance, blood pressure falls dramatically without any other intervention of the physician. OBP = office blood pressure; ABPM = ambulatory blood pressure monitoring.

This case history reflects several aspects of compliance monitoring which have been observed repeatedly in our experience. First, compliance was excellent when the patient was monitored, suggesting that monitoring drug adherence per se improves the medication-taking behavior. Second, this improvement in compliance was reflected by a drastic fall in blood pressure, demonstrating that the treatment was effective when taken adequately. This provided the knowledge to the physician that blood pressure could be perfectly normalized with the prescribed therapy. Thirdly, once the problem of noncompliance is recognized, patients may be helped by additional encouragements or by specific modifications of either the regimen itself or their habits in trying to maintain it. A major improvement in clinical outcome can be expected from this approach. Today, forty patients with refractory hypertension (triple association) have been investigated using the same protocol and one-third of them normalized their blood pressure during monitoring without any other physician interaction. Another 20% of patients had a low compliance with an uncontrolled blood pressure.[31,32] Together these preliminary results indicate that electronic monitors are indeed useful tools to detect noncompliance and improve the management of patients with hypertension "resistant" to therapy.

Can Electronic Monitors Contribute to Support Compliance?

As mentioned above, the adherence to treatment tends to improve when patients receive a monitor. Several studies have reported this phenomenon which could be attributed to the so-called "study bias" whereby a parameter improves as soon as it is measured. Still, this clinical observation suggests that the device per se may help partially compliant patients to take their drugs. Because of their unusal shape and size, which might represent a form of mnemonic stimulation, electronic monitors of compliance are not only useful to detect but even more so to support compliance. So far, these devices have not been promoted for this purpose and hence, there is not much experience on the potential benefits of electronic monitoring to improve long-term drug adherence in "treatment resistant" patients. In our experience, many patients have chosen to continue monitoring for a year and more. These patients experienced the monitor as a useful helper to take their drugs. In addition, they appreciate the opportunity to discuss the print-out of the compliance pattern with their physician. Clearly, more studies are needed to investigate this new way of using electronic monitors.

Conclusions

Noncompliance is recognized as a major clinical problem in many guidelines or recommendations for clinical practice. Yet, there exists an enormous discrepancy between the increasingly frequent emphasis of poor compliance as an important cause of less than optimal blood pressure control and the complete lack of action taken to objectively measure and enhance compliance in everyday practice. The frequently encountered resistance of a given hypertensive patient to an association of two or more antihypertensive agents always raises the unanswerable question of inadequate pharmacological regimen versus inadequate compliance. Without any objective measurement of drug compliance, we have become used to almost always opting for inadequate pharmacologic regimen, and consequently for enhancing doses or prescribing new drug combinations without even realizing anymore the completely irrational basis to these decisions. The recent development of electronic monitors offers a unique opportunity to improve the detection and quantitation of noncompliance. In the near future, additional information should be gathered to define more precisely the recommendations for the use of these devices in clinical practice and the long-term benefits that can be expected from a more frequent use by physicians.

References

1. MacMahon S, Peto R, Cutler J, et al. Blood pressure, stroke, and coronary heart disease. Part 1, prolonged differences in blood pressure : Prospective observational studies corrected for the regression dilution bias. *Lancet* 1990; 335:765–774.
2. Kannel WB, Castelli WP, McNamara PM, et al. Role of blood pressure in the development of congestive heart failure. The Framingham Study. *N Engl J Med* 1972;287:781–787.
3. Burt VL, Whelton P, Roccella EJ, et al. Prevalence of hypertension in the US adult population: Results from the Third National Health and Nutrition Examination Survey, 1988–1991. *Hypertension* 1995;25:305–313.
4. Colhoun HM, Dong W, Poulter NR. Blood pressure screening, management and control in England: Results from the health survey for England 1994. *J Hypertens* 1998;16:747–752.
5. Dickerson REC, Brown MJ. Influence of age on general practitioners definition and treatment of hypertension. *BMJ* 1995;30:574.
6. Fahey TP, Peters TJ. What constitutes controlled hypertension? Patient based comparison of hypertension guidelines. *BMJ* 1996;313:93–96.
7. Berlowitz DR, Ash AS, Hickey EC, et al. Inadequate management of blood pressure in a hypertensive population. *N Eng J Med* 1998;339:1957–1963.
8. Mancia G, Sega R, Milesi C, et al. Blood pressure control in the hypertensive population. *Lancet* 1997;349:454–457.
9. Hansson L, Zanchetti A, Carruthers SG, et al. Effects of intensive blood-pressure lowering and low-dose aspirin in patients with hypertension: Principal results of the Hypertension Optimal Treatment (HOT) randomised trial. HOT study group. *Lancet* 1998;351:1755–1762.
10. Cramer JA. Consequences of intermittent treatment for hypertension: The case for medication compliance and persistence. *Am J Managed Care* 1998; 4:1563–1568.
11. Ménard J, Chatellier G. Limiting factors in the control of blood pressure: Why is there a gap between theory and practice? *J Hum Hypertens* 1995; 9(suppl. 2):19–23.
12. Gilbert JR, Evans CE, Haynes RB, et al. Predicting compliance with a regimen of digoxin therapy in family practice. *Can Med Assoc J* 1980;123:119.
13. Hershey JC, Morton BG, Davies JB, et al. Patient compliance with antihypertensive medication. *Am J Public Health* 1980;70:1081–1089.
14. Lee JY, Kusek JW, Green PG, et al. Assessing medication adherence by pill count and electronic monitoring in the African American Study of Kidney Disease and Hypertension (AASK) pilot study. *Am J Hypertens* 1996;9: 719–725.
15. Fallab-Stubi CL, Zellweger JP, Sauty A, et al. Electronic monitoring of adherence to treatment in the preventive chemotherapy of tuberculosis. *Int J Tuberc Lung Dis* 1998;(7):525–530 .
16. Cramer JA. Microelectronic systems for monitoring and enhancing patient compliance with medication regimens. *Drugs* 1995;49(3):321–327.
17. Urquhart J. The electronic medication event monitoring. Lessons for pharmacotherapy. *Clin Pharmacokinet* 1997;32(5):345–356.
18. Cramer JA, Mattson RH, Prevey ML, et al. How often is medication taken as prescribed? A novel assessment technique. *JAMA* 1989;261(22):3273–3277.
19. Elliott WJ. Compliance strategies. *Curr Opin Nephrol Hypertens* 1994;3: 271–278.

20. Kruse W, Rampmaier J, Ullrich G, et al. Patterns of drug compliance with medications to be taken once and twice daily assessed by continuous electronic monitoring in primary care. *Int J Clin Pharmacol Ther* 1994;32(9): 452–457.
21. Waterhouse DM, Calzone KA, Mele C, et al. Adherence to oral tamoxifen: A comparison of patient self-report, pill counts, and microelectronic monitoring. *J Clin Oncol* 1993;11:1189–1197.
22. Guerrero D, Rudd P, Bryant-Kosling C, et al. Antihypertensive medication-taking. Investigation of a simple regimen. *Am J Hypertens* 1993;6:586–592.
23. Kruse W, Eggert-Kruse W, Rampmaier J, et al. Compliance and adverse drug reactions: A prospective study with ethinylestradiol using continuous compliance monitoring. *Clin Invest* 1993;71:483–487.
24. Matsuyama JR, Mason BJ, Jue SG. Pharmacists' intervention using an electronic medication event monitoring device's adherence data versus pill counts. *Ann Pharmacother* 1993;7:851–855.
25. Kruse W, Koch GP, Nikolaus T, et al. Measurement of drug compliance by continuous electronic monitoring: A pilot study in elderly patients discharged from hospital. *J Am Geriatr Soc* 1992;40:1151–1155.
26. Kruse W, Nikolaus T, Rampmaier J, et al. Actual versus prescribed timing of lovastatin doses assessed by electronic compliance monitoring. *Eur J Clin Pharmacol* 1993;45:211–215.
27. Matsui D, Hermann C, Klein J, et al. Critical comparison of novel and existing methods of compliance assessment during a clinical trial of an oral iron chelator. *J Clin Pharmacol* 1994;34:944–949.
28. Leenen FHH, Fourney A, Notman G, et al. Persistence of antihypertensive effect after "missed doses" of calcium antagonists with long (amlodipine) vs short (diltiazem) elimination half life. *Br J Clin Pharmacol* 1996;41:83–88.
29. Waeber B, Vetter W, Darioli R, et al. Improved blood pressure control by monitoring compliance with antihypertensive therapy. *J Clin Pract* 1999; (in press).
30. Setaro JF, Blocak HR. Refractory hypertension. *N Engl J Med* 1992;327: 543–547.
31. Burnier M, Schneider MP, Chioléro A, et al. Objective monitoring of drug compliance : An important step in the management of hypertension resistant to drug therapy. *Am J Hypertens* 1999;12(4, part 2):129A.
32. Bertholet N, Favrat B, Fallab-Stubi C, et al. Why objective monitoring of compliance is important for the mangement of hypertension. *J Clin Hypertens* 2000;2:258–262.

Chapter 19

Managed Care

Thomas H. Lee, MD, MSc

Introduction

Managed care organizations are unlikely to win many popularity contests in the US today, and are often assumed to place economic priorities ahead of quality of care. Health maintenance organizations (HMOs)—as well as indemnity insurers—are indeed under tremendous financial pressure, as several factors conspire to raise health care costs. These factors include the aging of the population, advances in medical technologies, new pharmaceutical agents, and consumer demand that is often cultivated by direct-to-consumer advertising.

For insurers, the factors driving increased costs are complicated by other considerations, including the relatively short time that members are likely to stay with any single insurance plan. In addition, for-profit insurers must be aware of the importance of quarterly balance statements. Therefore, many insurers do not have a strong financial incentive to adopt the "long-term" view of what is in their patients' interests.

These perspectives would logically lead to the conclusion that managed care organizations and other insurers are not likely to be interested in improving physician compliance with guidelines or patient compliance with pharmaceutical therapy. Indeed, short-term financial interests might be better served by a strategy in which the insurer hopes that compliance with recommended interventions is poor.

However, some recent developments suggest that the opposite may be true. Some managed care organizations are investing resources in improving compliance with guidelines by physicians, and in detecting patients who are not using their medications as prescribed. The

From: Burke LE, Ockene IS (eds). *Compliance in Healthcare and Research*. Armonk, NY: Futura Publishing Company, Inc.; © 2001.

reasons make sound business sense. An optimistic assessment is that some managed care organizations may far outperform indemnity medicine in improving compliance in cardiovascular care over the next several years.

NCQA and HEDIS

The two most important areas in which HMOs are now developing programs to improve compliance in cardiovascular medicine are:

- LDL cholesterol control after acute myocardial infarction, coronary artery bypass graft surgery, or percutaneous transluminal angioplasty; and
- control of high blood pressure.

A major reason why HMOs are giving these two issues such attention is the implementation in the year 2000 of two new Health Employer Data Information Set (HEDIS) measures. The first will require HMOs to follow patients after these coronary events, and report the percentage of patients who achieve an LDL cholesterol level below 130 mg/dL.[1] The second will involve chart review of a random sample of patients with hypertension; the HMOs will report the percentage with blood pressure below 140/90 mmHg.

The potential impact of these two new HEDIS measures is considerable, and has great implications for public health. One of the ironies of modern medicine is that the effectiveness of interventions demonstrated in randomized trials is usually only partially realized in the general population, in part because patient compliance with the intervention strategy is not reinforced by clinical personnel as in a clinical trial. In theory, managed care organizations have the potential to improve quality of care through development of supportive systems.

The National Committee for Quality Assurance (NCQA) and its HEDIS performance measures therefore have considerable potential to accelerate translation of insights into what cardiovascular interventions are effective into lower cardiovascular morbidity and mortality. NCQA is a nonprofit organization that evaluates the quality of care delivered by managed care organizations. It provides accreditation to organizations that undergo and pass its periodic reviews. NCQA accreditation in many marketplaces is critical to the competitiveness of HMOs.

A stated goal of NCQA is to promote competition among HMOs on the basis of quality, and much of the framework for this competition is HEDIS. HMO performance on HEDIS measures is often published and compared in lay publications; hence, many HEDIS measures (eg mammography and influenza vaccination rates) have become key focuses for HMO quality improvement initiatives. Recent changes in NCQA accreditation standards will result in a portion of accreditation decisions being driven directly by HEDIS performance levels.

In the past, HEDIS measures focused on "process" variables such as the use of screening tests. Many physicians complained that these measures had little to do with the quality of care for people with acute or chronic illness. However, that situation is changing with more recent measures, which have been developed by multidisciplinary Measurement Advisory Panels (MAPs). These MAPs include physicians and scientists nominated by leading professional societies and managed care organizations, and researchers from the Centers for Disease Control and Prevention, the National Institutes of Health, academic settings and other research organizations.

The clear focus of many of these MAPs has been on outcomes and key process variables for patients with chronic disease. The historical focus of HEDIS on "process measures" was due in part to the difficulty of collecting outcome data and then adjusting for other factors that influence risk for poor outcomes. Process measures, such as whether or not cholesterol was measured, can usually be determined from readily available claims data, and are considered valid across populations.

The NCQA's decision to use a specific LDL-cholesterol level for a performance measure thus represents a major departure from prior versions of HEDIS in two important ways. LDL-cholesterol control is an "intermediate outcome," because LDL levels have been convincingly linked to risk for CHD events. In addition, LDL-cholesterol and other laboratory data are not currently available to most managed care organizations. Therefore, collection of data for this measure will pose new administrative burdens for HMOs.

Similarly, the new performance measure for control of hypertension will require review of a random sample of charts. NCQA commissioned research to determine the cost and reliability of such chart review. The expenses related to such chart review will be borne by the managed care organizations. In truth, these HMOs will bear other costs as well, as they develop systems to improve their performance on these measures. However, the investments are already being made within some HMOs, and some employers are already considering financial incentives to promote HMO initiatives to improve blood pressure and cholesterol control.

Reaching the New HEDIS Goals

The new HEDIS goals will indeed pose considerable challenges for HMOs. Recently published data from the Framingham Heart Study showed that the rate of use of antihypertensive medications has increased from 2% to 28% from 1950 to 1989 in that cohort,[2] but research has demonstrated that only a minority of patients are under active treatment.[3,4]

Compliance with cholesterol guidelines is also poor.[5] Research performed by NCQA in cooperation with the Robert Wood Johnson Foundation in 1996 at two large HMOs showed that only 28% (and 39%) of patients had their LDL levels checked in the year after a hospitalization for acute myocardial infarction (unpublished data). This research also showed that, even when lipids were checked, only 32% (and 58%) achieved an LDL-cholesterol level below 130 mg/dL within 18 months of a hospitalization for an AMI.

The reasons for these disappointing statistics are multifactorial, and covered in greater detail elsewhere in this monograph. The causes include the many factors contributing to poor patient compliance with prescribed regimens, physician reluctance to advance regimens to reach goals,[4] and loss of patients to follow-up care.

These problems are difficult to address systematically in fee-for-service care, but managed care organizations have the capacity to develop and implement programs that identify and correct "errors" in physician and patient compliance. The new HEDIS measures now provide a strong financial incentive for these organizations to use these programs.

These initiatives are often labeled "disease management" programs,[6] and are now increasingly implemented in HMOs either through "carve-out" or "carve-in" models. "Carve-out" models are those in which an outside organization (eg, a pharmacy benefits management company or a for-profit disease management company) implements a system that follows patients with the condition of interest. The care delivered through these systems is essentially independent of that given by the physician. This fragmentation of the delivery system is an important source of discontent about "carve-out" models, many of which have failed to achieve goals because physicians either resist or simply fail to refer patients to the program.

Carve-in models are more difficult to implement, and are best demonstrated in staff model HMOs. In such organizations, specialists and other physicians do not have financial disincentives to resist the programs, which may actually decrease their workload while improving care and follow-up of the patient. However, most of the health care system is not sufficiently integrated to make such carve-in models practical.

Structure Of Disease Management Programs

Although many physicians believe that disease management consists of reaching consensus among physicians about clinical guidelines, and then disseminating the information, this is actually just the first step. The key programmatic steps in most managed care disease management initiatives include:

- Identification of patients. For example, pharmacy and medical claims data are now being used in many systems to identify patients who have had coronary events or have hypertension.
- Obtaining permission of physician for referral of patient to the program. This step is extremely labor intensive, but is believed to improve patient participation and overall program effectiveness.
- Collection of further information. Review of charts and direct surveys or interviews of patients are often used to determine symptomatic status, whether they have had side effects to any medications, and other key clinical information.
- Risk stratification of patients. In general, more costly but more effective interventions should be targeted on the patients with the highest risk for complications, and therefore the greatest chance of benefiting from the interventions.
- Interventions performance.
- Measurement of impact.

The types of interventions that are being used to improve compliance with blood pressure and LDL cholesterol management include:

- Identification of patients who are not under treatment at all through use of medical and pharmacy claims data.
- Identification of patients who are using significantly less than the expected number of pills/month through analysis of pharmacy claims data.
- Identification of patients who have been lost to follow-up through analysis of medical claims data.
- Chart review to detect patients who are not reaching guideline targets for LDL cholesterol or blood pressure.
- Feedback to physicians of patients whose care would not meet HEDIS performance measure goals.
- Assistance for physicians in implementing changes.

Although the analysis of claims data may sound easy, the development of a data warehouse with integrated pharmacy and medical claims data is actually a costly and technically challenging goal. In addition, considerable costs are required to perform chart review, and then seek physician participation in implementing changes to improve patients' care. These costs are not welcomed by the business leadership of many HMOs.

However, the new HEDIS measures are likely to make such programs a business imperative in many marketplaces. The results will be better care and lower cardiovascular event rates for managed care patients.

References

1. Lee TH, Cleeman JI, Grundy SM, et al. Clinical goals and performance measures for cholesterol management for secondary prevention of coronary heart disease. *JAMA* 2000;283:94–98.
2. Mostero A, D'Agostino RB, Silbershatz H, et al. Trends in the prevalence of hypertension, antihypertensive therapy, and left ventricular hypertrophy from 1950 to 1989. *N Engl J Med* 1999;340:1221–1227.
3. The sixth Report of the Joint National Committee on Detection, Evaluation, and Treatment of High Blood Pressure. *Arch Intern Med* 1997;157:2413–2446. [Erratum, *Arch Intern Med* 1998;158:573.]
4. Berlowitz DR, Ash AS, Hickey AC, et al. Inadequate management of blood pressure in a hypertensive population. *N Engl J Med* 1998;339:1957–1963.
5. Expert Panel on Detection, Evaluation, and Treatment of High Blood Cholesterol in Adults. Summary of the second report of the National Cholesterol Education Treatment Program (NCEP) Expert Panel on Detection, Evaluation, and Treatment of High Blood Cholesterol in Adults (Adult Treatment Panel II). *JAMA* 1993;269:3015–3023.
6. Bodenheimer T. Disease management: Promises and pitfalls. *N Engl J Med* 1999;340:1202–1205.

Section VIII

Future Directions

Chapter 20

Innovative Approaches to Compliance

Deborah J. Aaron, PhD, MSIS, Kimberly A. Morris, PhD, Patricia A. Nixon, PhD, Jeffrey P. Martin, MBA, Deborah Echement, BA, Ronald E. LaPorte, PhD

Introduction

Epidemiology is the study of the distribution of a disease or a physiological condition in human populations and of the factors that influence this distribution.[1] There are primarily three focuses of epidemiologic research; 1) to determine the prevalence and incidence of disease, 2) to identify associated causes and risk factors of disease, and 3) to design, implement, and evaluate intervention programs for reducing disease. The underlying concept behind the field of epidemiology is the acquisition and dissemination of information. We are currently in an information revolution and our ability to transmit information is increasing in magnitudes that are unprecedented in the history of communication. It has been estimated that there has been a 100,000–fold increase in information processing, a 1,000,000,000-fold increase in information transmission, and a 1,000,000-fold increase in information storage since 1950.[2] These dramatic increases have been brought about by advancing computer and network technology, and in particular the Internet. However, for the most part, epidemiology is using outdated information technology such as, face-to-face communication, postal system, telephone, and fax. All of which have severe drawbacks in regards to cost, timeliness, and/or accuracy. The integration of an In-

Funded, in part, by a Seed Money Grant from the Children's Hospital of Pittsburgh

From: Burke LE, Ockene IS (eds). *Compliance in Healthcare and Research.* Armonk, NY: Futura Publishing Company, Inc.; © 2001.

ternet backbone, with its high-speed and high-capacity information technology, in epidemiological research could dramatically improve our ability to impact on the identification, causes, and prevention of disease.

Other disciplines have embraced new information technologies. For example, businesses have incorporated information technology to redesign their operations. Business Process Reengineering is the "fundamental rethinking and radical redesign of business processes to achieve dramatic improvements in critical contemporary measures of performance, such as cost, quality, service, and speed."[3] To achieve this goal involves Business Process Automation; the strategic use of information technology to automate all or part of a critical process is incorporated into each process of the business. This automation ultimately leads to more satisfied customers, quicker product introduction, increased revenue, lower costs, reduced cycle time, and increased capacity. Perhaps it is time that epidemiology begins to view itself as a business and reengineers itself. The goals of epidemiology are not unlike those of a business (Table 1) and have the potential to be dramatically enhanced by the incorporation of information technology.

The purpose of this chapter is to provide an example of how information technology can be used to reengineer the process of conducting epidemiological intervention studies. Our example will be related to an intervention study designed to increase physical activity. However, the information technology model could be easily incorporated into any epidemiologic study to enhance communication, particularly in multicenter studies, facilitate subject recruitment and data entry, and increase the speed by which results are summarized and disseminated.

Table 1

Comparison of Goals Related to Business and Goals Related to Epidemiology

Business	Epidemiology
More Satisfied Customers	More Compliant Subjects
Quicker New Product Introduction	Quicker Processing of Data
Increased Revenue	Increased Knowledge to Field
Lower Costs	Lower Costs
Reduced Process Cycle Time	Reduced Time to Disseminating Results
Increased Capacity	Increased Ability to Process Information

Intervention Studies

An intervention study is one in which the investigator *intervenes* on a known risk factor of a disease before the disease has developed in individuals with characteristics that increase their risk of developing the disease.[1] Once the subjects are recruited, they are normally allocated to either the experimental (eg, intervention) or control groups. The experimental group receives the new treatment or preventive agent and the control group receives the "usual" treatment.

The primary goal of an intervention study of physical activity is to motivate and encourage the subjects in the experimental group to appropriately increase their level of physical activity. The intervention protocol can be very costly, in terms of both the researcher and the subject, and in both money and time. The only way to be sure that an intervention is successful is to be confident that the experimental group is actually receiving the treatment. Thus, it is critical in an intervention study to monitor the subject's compliance with the treatment. In order to prevent noncompliance or withdrawal from the study it is necessary for the research staff to provide motivation and feedback to the subjects. Monitoring of physical activity usually involves the subjects keeping track of daily activity with the use of a logbook. Periodically, the logbooks are returned to the study office for review and data entry. Motivation and feedback are provided through a variety of methods, such as reminder post cards, educational material, phone calls from the research staff, supervised exercise groups, and support groups. Monitoring, motivation, and feedback all involve the transfer of information from researcher to subject, subject to researcher, and subject to subject. However, the current communication tools used in intervention studies are expensive, require a large staff, delay feedback to subjects, and impose a high burden on the subjects. Several items suggest that the incorporation of an Internet based information system holds some promise for reengineering intervention studies.

- Internet based programs can be flexible to time and content. Contact between the researchers and a participant does not need to be confined to real-time contact.
- Internet access is relatively inexpensive, about $20 per month, and can be easily accessed over a computer equipped with a modem or with the new Web TV technology. In addition, the Internet is based upon existing network structures.
- A World Wide Web based intervention may also motivate

subjects. Home pages and hypertext links generally spur users to explore for more information.

Work-Centered Analysis Framework

The concept of this paper is derived from the Work-Centered Analysis (WCA) model that has been used to describe the general framework for thinking about work processes and the information systems that support them.[4] The WCA consists of six linked elements (Figure 1), which are described below. The links between elements of the WCA model are two-way and indicate that all must be in balance for an effective and efficient information system.

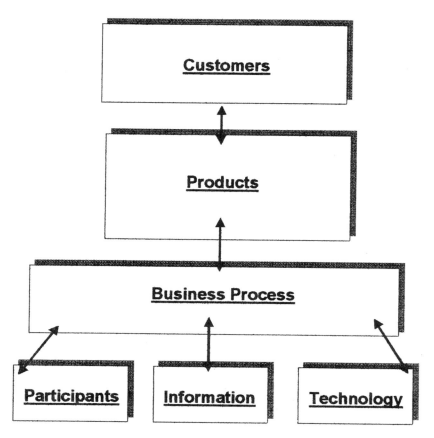

Figure 1. The WCA Framework.

Customers: Customers are the people who use the output of an information system.

Product: The product is the output of the business process.

Business Process: A business process is a series of steps or activities that utilizes people, information, and other resources.

Participants: The participants are the people who enter, process, or use the information within the system.

Information: The information in a system can take a variety of forms, including, data, sounds, pictures, graphics, and video.

Technology: Technology refers to the tools that perform work or help people perform work. The primary focus of technology in this framework is the extent to which it can support and enhance the business processes.

The WCA model will be used to evaluate the application of an information system approach to a physical activity intervention study. This chapter describes an information technology approach to a physical activity intervention study and illustrates how this approach impacts on the components of the WCA to increase the effectiveness and efficiency of the overall information system.

Basic Equipment and Technology

The physical activity intervention would be an Internet-based system. The primary Internet services to be incorporated into this system include electronic mail (email), a list server, and the World Wide Web. In order to use these services, subjects need to have not only access to a computer connected to the Internet, but also a minimal working knowledge of the technology. Current advances in technology allow Internet access at a minimal cost. For participants who already have a computer, access will be obtained by purchasing a modem, if needed, and the monthly access charges. The total cost would be less than $100 for the modem and $240/year for access charges. The cost would be only slightly increased for participants who do not have a computer. Web TV technology has advanced to the level that it is affordable to most Americans with a television set and a telephone. The cost would include the Web TV unit, at a current price of $150 and $240/year for access charges. It is anticipated that in addition to providing access for some subjects, many will also require a period of training and indoctrination to the Internet.

World Wide Web Site for Physical Activity Intervention

A World Wide Web site will be the primary tool used in the IT approach to physical activity intervention. The main component of the web site will be individual password protected pages where the subjects can enter information related to daily physical activity, an "electronic log book." Using current encryption technology, these web pages will be very secure and the confidentiality of submitted information will not be compromised. Each subject will have a calendar form (Figure 2), where if any day is selected, details on the type and amount of physical activity undertaken that day can be entered and immediately posted on the calendar. Once entered, the data will be immediately transmitted to a secure database on a computer located at the study office. This eliminates the burden on subjects to mail/return their logbooks to the study office and allows the data to be immediately available for analysis. In addition, the web calendar can be programmed so that the subject must enter their data for a particular day within a certain time frame, ie, 48 hours. Thus, if the subject attempts to enter data for Monday on Thursday, an error message will be returned indicating that data can no longer be entered for that date. An additional

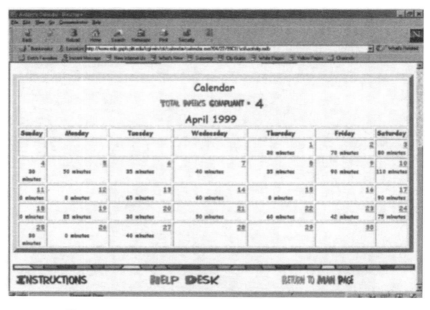

Figure 2. Web calendar for recording physical activity.

feature of this "electronic log book" is that the research staff can monitor each subject's compliance and progress daily, as all of the subject activity calendars will be accessible by the research team. Thus, if a subject shows a pattern of nonadherence to the physical activity program, the researcher can provide immediate feedback and motivation to the subject via an email message. Likewise, a continued pattern of compliance can be acknowledged with encouragement to keep up the good work. Providing subjects the opportunity to send email questions to the research staff will also enhance communication.

Support groups have been used in traditional intervention studies to allow subjects to interact and discuss issues related to their problems and successes in attempting to change behaviors. However, this face-to-face interaction places additional demands on both the subject and researcher with regards to time and scheduling. To overcome these barriers, a list server would be established for subject-to-subject interaction. The list server would function as a "virtual support group" and allow a subject to post a message and engage in an ongoing communication with other subjects without the constraints of time and distance. The web site will also be utilized to provide the subjects with educational material related to the health benefits of physical activity. Links to other activity and health web sites will be available to obtain additional information.

WCA Applied to Intervention Study

The application of the WCA to an Internet-based physical activity intervention study is illustrated in Figure 3. The *primary business processes* of an intervention study are recording daily physical activity by the subjects and monitoring compliance and providing feedback by the researchers. To implement these processes the participants, the information, and the technology must be defined. The *participants* of an intervention study are both the subjects and the researchers as both are involved with the entering, processing and utilization of information. The *information* obtained via the system is the date, time, type, and amount of physical activity. Secondary information includes questions from the subjects and feedback from the researchers. As previously described, the *technology* used in this system is the Internet and in particular, email and the World Wide Web. The integration of these four components of the WCA forms the information system. The end result of an information system is the product and the customer who benefits from that product. The *products* of an intervention study include increased compliance to lifestyle modification by the subject and more efficient monitoring and feedback by research staff. The *customers* in-

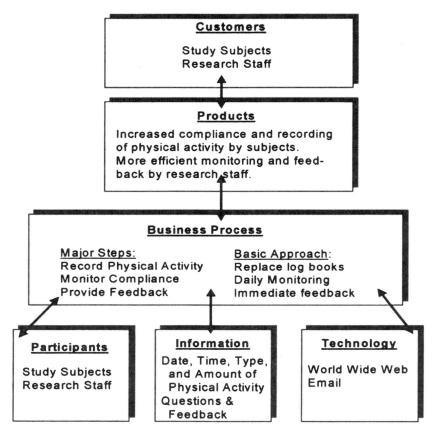

Figure 3. WCA model for epidemiologic physical activity intervention study.

clude both the subjects, who will have adopted a healthier lifestyle, and the researchers, who can disseminate important findings to the public health community. The remainder of this section will focus on evaluating the Internet-based information system for intervention studies compared to a traditional intervention model. The evaluation will focus on system performance variables such as capacity, productivity, consistency, cycle time, flexibility, and security and factors that contribute to improving the product and increasing customer satisfaction such as cost, quality, responsiveness, reliability, and conformance to standards.[4]

Evaluating System Performance

A summary of performance variables as applied to an intervention study is presented in Table 2. The application of an Internet-based infor-

Table 2

Process Performance Variables and Application to Intervention Studies

	Definition	Application to intervention study
Capacity:	Amount of work the system can perform.	Number of subjects in study.
Productivity:	Relationship between output and amount of money, time, and effort it consumes	Number of research staff required. Amount of time between subject recording activity and review by researcher. Number of phone calls to contact one subject.
Consistency:	Application of same techniques in same way.	Subject recording of activity. Manual data entry.
Cycle Time:	Length of time between start of process and completion.	Periodic contact of all subjects. Data entry.
Flexibility:	Ease of adjustment to meet immediate need	Increase motivation/feedback. Provide additional education.
Security:	Likelihood that information is invulnerable to unauthorized use.	Assurance of subject confidentiality.

mation system has the potential to dramatically increase the majority of these performance measures. The ability to draw conclusions from a study is directly related to the number of subjects, more subjects means greater statistical power to detect differences between the experimental group and the control group. An Internet-based system could increase the number of subjects that could be recruited for a study by performing many of the tasks automatically, such as monitoring and data entry. Traditionally, study resources such as personnel and funds have limited the number of subjects. An Internet-based intervention study will not only allow the recruitment of a greater number of subjects, but also allow better utilization of some resources. The traditional approach is to use a number of study personnel to maintain contact with subjects via postal mailings or telephone calls. These methods of communication are extremely costly in both time and funds. However, using email and/or a list server, one researcher can contact ALL subjects within a matter of seconds. The enhanced communication via the Internet will also reduce the cycle time for monitoring and increase the flexibility of the intervention. Rather than reviewing hard copy logbooks of physical activity on a monthly basis, the researcher can monitor physical activity on a daily basis. If a pattern of noncompliance is observed for a subject, the researcher can immediately target the individual for increased motivation and feedback, as well as provide necessary educational material. The only area where the Internet based intervention may not positively impact is security. When agreeing to participate in a research study, subjects are guaranteed that all information will remain confidential. There are many concerns regarding the security of information submitted and transmitted via the Internet. However, with the continued development of security technologies, such as data encryption, the concern over unauthorized access to subject information will be diminished.

Evaluating Product Performance

The end result of any business process is the product and the value it holds for the customers. Application of an Internet based information system for intervention studies will have a significant impact on the product and customers (Table 3). The structure of the Internet intervention will permit feedback, reinforcement, and independent learning among the subjects at a higher level than is possible with the traditional

---

Table 3

Impact of Internet Based Intervention Study on Products and Customers

Cost:	Reduce internal costs of performing study through decreased personnel time, telephone charges, and mailing cost.
	Reduce cost to subject by eliminating need to maintain hardcopy logbooks and reducing time to interact with researchers.
Quality:	Ensure that the data are entered and verified in a more consistent manner.
	Increases the ability of the researchers to process and interpret data.
Responsiveness:	Increase the speed of data availability and thus, reporting results.
	Increase speed of response to subjects and increase ability to manage individual needs.
Reliability:	Eliminate human error by automating monitoring and data entry.

methods of monitoring physical activity. The underlying assumption is that this type of interaction will motivate the subjects to maintain activity regimens to a greater degree. The impact on the researchers is related to decreased cost of conducting the study, increased availability of data, enhanced ability to monitor and provide feedback to subjects, and increase the speed by which information is processed and disseminated.

Acceptance of IT Approach to Intervention Studies

Prior to incorporating an Internet-based approach to intervention studies, the system must be evaluated in terms of subject acceptability and cost effectiveness. The acceptability could be assessed in three ways. First, monitoring each subject's use of her individual calendar web page to record physical activity. Second, monitor the number of times email is used by each participant to communicate with the researchers and the number of messages posted to the list server. Finally, a survey should be completed by the participants to query them on the degree to which they found the Internet-based system to be user friendly and provide relevant information. Detailed records relating to time, effort, equipment, and supplies needed to develop and implement the Internet-based intervention should be maintained. These records will allow a comparison of the "cost" of conducting a physical activity intervention to the traditional methods. The final step in this process of evaluating the IT approach to intervention studies will be to conduct a randomized trial to compare compliance and change in behavior between an Internet-based intervention group and a "traditional approach" intervention group.

Summary

A successful intervention study depends on the efficient and timely collection and transfer of information between researchers and subjects. The Internet has increased our ability to communicate and manage information in a way that is unprecedented with earlier technologies. Other disciplines, such as business, have embraced these new technologies to redesign and reengineer their processes. However, epidemiology is still using outdated and inefficient information technology. The purpose of this chapter was to begin to view epidemiology as a business, with processes, products, and customers. As shown through the WCA model, the application of an Internet-based information system has the potential to dramatically increase the effectiveness and efficiency of conducting epidemiological intervention studies.

References

1. Lilienfeld DE. *Foundations of Epidemiology*. Oxford: Oxford University Press; 1980.
2. Spring MB, Campbell JD. *The Document Processing Revolution*. (unpublished manuscript).
3. Yablonsky D. Reengineering with Knowledge: Getting the Most Value from Your Most Valuable Asset. *Harvard Business Review*; Sept-Oct. 1992, pp. 95–104.
4. Alter S. *Information Systems: A Management Prospective*. New York: Benjamin/ Cummings Publishing Company; 1996.

Chapter 21

Future Directions: What Paths Do Researchers Need to Take?
What Needs to be Done to Improve Mulit-Level Compliance?

Neil B. Oldridge, PhD

"The real challenge of the new millennium may indeed be to strike an appropriate balance between the pursuit of exciting new knowledge and the *full application of strategies known to be extremely effective, but considered underused.*"[1]

Introduction

The American Heart Association (AHA) is to be recognized for organizing this monograph on Compliance in Healthcare and Research. I understand that this is the AHA's first monograph on adherence/compliance and that the AHA recognizes this as a multilevel concern, ie, a patient, provider, and system concern, that is critical to the clinical effectiveness of interventions known to be effective.[2] Approximately 10% of all hospital and 23% of all nursing home admissions are associated with poor patient adherence with effective medication regimens which, together with the associated lost productivity, costs the US an estimated $100 billion annually at a minimum.[3] Recent systematic reviews on the issue of patient adherence/compliance have reinforced the importance of examining various patient-focused adherence-enhancement strategies in order to optimize treatment effectiveness.[4–6] However, it is increasingly important that we acknowledge that more emphasis should be placed on measures that increase adherence by *physicians* with regimens with proven benefits.[7]

From: Burke LE, Ockene IS (eds). *Compliance in Healthcare and Research.* Armonk, NY: Futura Publishing Company, Inc.; © 2001.

The major focus in patient adherence with health care recommendations naturally has been on *patient and characteristics and behaviors* with the assumption that altering these will improve his or her treatment adherence and outcome. This line of research has not been particularly useful or helpful. In fact, Donovan has pointed out that for many patients with chronic conditions, such as heart disease, treatment nonadherence is not an issue, as they make reasoned decisions about their treatment based on their own beliefs, personal circumstances, and the information available to them.[8, 9] The literature increasingly supports the "notion that patients evaluate medication based not only on its clinical effectiveness but also on how it affects their lives."[10] Surely the same holds true for lifestyle behavior changes that are recommended to patients with heart disease?

Another area of adherence-enhancing research has focused on *regimen factors*. Haynes suggests that although strategies for improving adherence with long-term interventions are seldom very effective on their own, there are time-proven, effective, and simple adherence-enhancing approaches which, *if implemented*, can work.[11] These approaches include keeping the regimen straightforward, providing clear instructions and periodic checks, promoting good communication with the patient, and reinforcing their accomplishments.

Based on the evidence for treatment effectiveness, comprehensive risk reduction guidelines for patients with established heart disease have been formulated and promulgated by various scientific and policy agencies.[12-14] Despite this, "evidence from the United Kingdom and Europe, and estimates from the United States, suggest that a large 'treatment gap' exists between recommended therapies for patients with cardiovascular disease and the care that they are actually receiving."[15] If this is the case, can there be any doubt that this 'treatment gap' significantly amplifies the impact on the effectiveness of proven interventions that poor patient adherence plays? Reducing this 'treatment gap' by enhancing *provider adherence* (as well as organization and system adherence) with evidence-based medicine and appropriate standards of care is a critical area of future investigation.

The question of what this poor adherence by providers with guidelines for proven treatment is due to remains unclear. Has it to do with patient characteristics and their behavior and attitude? Or is it rather a disagreement with the manner in which the recommendations are made and treatment regimens designed? Or is it because providers simply do not agree with or like to follow established guidelines? The answer surely is some combination of the above and other factors.[16] However, there can be little doubt that the problem of poor adherence by providers to guidelines for treatments proven to be effective needs considerably more attention in the future than it receives at this time.

Adherence and Outcome

The 1997 report on the prevention, detection, evaluation, and treatment of high blood pressure[17] clearly demonstrates that, despite increased evidence of treatment effectiveness, the awareness, treatment, and control of hypertension in 1994 did not continue to follow the improvements seen between 1976 and 1991. Had the 1976–1991 trends continued, the awareness, treatment, and control of high blood pressure in 1994 would each have increased by about 15%.[17]

The assumption, rightly or wrongly, is that higher adherence with effective treatments automatically is associated with better outcomes. Research to enhance adherence is not of itself a justifiable end, and ethical standards dictate that attempts to increase adherence must be judged on their effects on adherence rates as well as on clinical benefits.[18] If high adherence with effective treatment for heart disease is associated with improved outcome, are effective adherence-enhancing strategies associated with outcome? A recent systematic review of randomized controlled trials (RCT) of interventions to assist patients to improve adherence with their prescriptions for medications[6] extended earlier observations by the same researchers.[4] Nineteen interventions were identified in 17 RCTs, with eight heart disease intervention trials, seven hypertension trials, and one hyperlipidemia trial, met eligibility criteria (documentation of both adherence rates and treatment outcome) for further analysis.[6] In these eight cardiovascular RCTs, neither adherence nor outcome improved in three (37.5%), adherence only improved in two (25%), and both adherence and outcome improved significantly in three (37.5%) which was consistent with the proportion seen in all 19 interventions when both outcomes were positive.[6]

Judgement about adherence and clinical outcome raises interesting questions about adherence with treatment and placebo interventions. If high adherence with effective treatments for cardiovascular disease is associated with improved outcomes, might this also hold true for high adherence with placebo interventions? There are data in at least two cardiovascular medication RCTs which support the suggestion by Epstein and Cluss that "adherence may ignite changes that directly or indirectly influence outcome."[19] The first of these is the Coronary Drug Project (CDP) in which lipid-lowering medications were evaluated for efficacy and safety;[20] the second is the β-Blocker Heart Attack Trial (BHAT) in which the efficacy of propanolol hydrochloride to reduce mortality was evaluated.[21]

In the CDP, the 5-year mortality of 20% in those treated with clofibrate was not significantly different from the 21% seen in the control group.[22] In the BHAT, 1-year mortality was lower ($P < 0.005$) in treated patients (7.2%) as compared to placebo patients (9.8%).[21] When analyzed by adherence level, there were unexpected adherence effects on mortality. Mortality in the CDP treatment group high adherers was 15% compared to 25% in low adherers; surprisingly, in the CDP placebo group mortality in high adherers was also 15% compared to 28% in low adherers.[22] A similar mortality pattern was seen in the BHAT where the odds ratio for mortality among treatment low versus high adherers was 3.1 (95% confidence intervals, 0.9 to 10.3) compared to 2.5 (95% confidence intervals, 0.9 to 7.0) in the placebo group.[23] These observations appear to support the statement by Epstein and Cluss[19] that adherent behavior, in and of itself and regardless of intervention, may influence outcome.

The conclusion in the review of adherence-enhancing strategies and clinical outcome by Haynes and colleagues[6] was that " . . . full benefits of medications cannot be realised at currently achievable levels of adherence. Current methods of improving adherence for chronic health problems are mostly complex and not very effective. More studies of innovative approaches to assist patients to follow medication prescriptions are needed." Based on evidence from two cardiovascular medication trials where high adherence with both intervention and placebo patients was associated with positive outcomes,[22,23] Horwitz and Horwitz[24] concluded that ". . . what is needed are experimental and observational studies that will enable us to understand the impact of adherence on the 'nonspecific' effects of an intervention." And surely these conclusions also apply equally to lifestyle behavior change interventions designed to reduce cardiovascular risk?

Enhancing Adherence

In the opening presentation at this Conference, Haynes stated that, "because the 'state of the art' for improving adherence is relatively static while new treatments abound, the gap is widening between what we could achieve with full application of current best care and what we are achieving."[11] Does this suggest that there is no future for adherence-enhancing research? Absolutely not. And the timeliness of this symposium on Compliance in Healthcare and Research is clear. There is little doubt that adherence-enhancement is a multilevel task, ie, patient, provider, and healthcare organization,[2,25,26] and a number of exciting, new lines of adherence-enhancing research were discussed in this scientific conference. These included the increasing emphasis on standards of care and the role played by the clinician,[27] the potential of healthcare organizations, such as managed care, to promote strategies to enhance adherence,[28] as well as technology advances such as the internet and electronic monitoring,[29,30] and the use of computer-assisted surveys.[31]

A number of recent reviews have focused on adherence and adherence-enhancing strategies in the promotion of risk factor management in populations at risk for the development of cardiovascular disease or in populations with established disease.[2,26,32–34] Unfortunately, effective treatments for heart disease often are limited by poor adherence rates, frequently associated with poor outcomes. In clinical practice, poor 1-year adherence rates with lipid-lowering medication range from 13% to 45% in health maintenance organizations, which is considerably higher than the 4% and 31% rates reported in clinical trials.[35] We have reported that as many as 50% of patients referred to cardiac rehabilitation exercise programs dropout within 6 months of starting to exercise[36] although this does not necessarily mean that the poor program adherers stop exercising.[37] Poor adherence with medication and dietary regimens accounts for more than 30% of preventable hospital admissions in patients with heart failure[38,39] and poor adherence has been suggested as a "risk factor" in heart disease.[40] Observations in studies of β-blockers and cholesterol-lowering medications demonstrate this notion well. In a case-control study, when compared to the event rate in patients with heart disease who were 100% adherent with prescribed β-blockers, patients who adhered 80% to 99% of the time had twice the event rate (confidence interval, 0.62 to 6.25) while those adhering less than 80% of the time had four times the event rate (confidence interval, 1.1 to 18.5).[41] In a primary prevention RCT of simvastatin, the reduction in the risk of definite coronary heart disease death or non-fatal myocardial infarction was 38% in those with $> 75\%$ adherence which is in stark contrast to no reduction in event rate in those with an adherence rate of $< 75\%$.[42] In a secondary prevention RCT, the 1-year post-trial cholesterol level among current statin users was 5.1 compared to 5.7 mmol/L ($P < 0.001$) in those not continuing with the medication.[43] In another RCT, adherence with comprehensive lifestyle changes, but without use of lipid-lowering drugs, over a 5-year period of time in patients with documented heart disease was associated with a 7.9% regression of coronary artery diameter stenosis compared to a 27.7% worsening in the control group.[44]

Approaches To Adherence-Enhancement Research

Much of the available adherence research has focused either on a) identifying factors that contribute to poor adherence or on b) developing patient adherence-enhancing strategies.[11] As stated previously, the available research suggests that the adherence problem is a multilevel one.[2,25,26] Factors considered in adherence-enhancing research traditionally have fallen into three categories: patient-related factors, regimen-related factors, and provider-related factors. While there is some agreement that successful adherence-enhancement strategies need to be individualized and personalized, multifactorial, with regular periodic reinforcement, the focus has tended to be on changing patient rather than provider behaviors by incorporating strategies like reinforcement control, stimulus control, and cognitive, self-control procedures.

The early adherence-enhancing literature, and much of the recent literature, has focused on patient and regimen characteristics. The former are notoriously difficult to alter while the latter have had some success in enhancing adherence with both short-and long-term health care behaviors – whether medication-taking or lifestyle behavior changes. For example, Burke and colleagues listed 13 strategies "deemed to be successful in enhancing compliance" but she pointed out that "the majority of these have not been tested in controlled studies for comparative efficacy."[33] In addition, and as part of the multilevel challenge to improving adherence and clinical outcomes in patients with heart disease,[2,25,26] strategies to reduce the 'treatment gap' by enhancing provider adherence with evidence-based medicine and appropriate standards of care urgently need to be addressed.[15]

Patient-Related Factors

A considerable body of knowledge has been generated on patient-related factors that affect adherence levels in treatments for patients with heart disease. It appears that certain patient characteristics are more likely to be associated with adherence than other characteristics.[32-34] These factors include

- Knowledge and understanding of what needs to be done;
- Previous levels of adherence;
- Perceived confidence in the ability, or self-efficacy, to perform behaviors;
- Perceptions of treatment effectiveness;
- Availability of social support;
- Satisfaction with health care.

Regimen-Related Factors

Haynes has pointed out that many of the strategies designed to help patients follow their treatment regimens don't work well, are expensive to implement, involve reinventing the wheel; are not creative, are impractical, that no one strategy is very effective if applied in isolation; and that little of what is known and practical is in fact applied in routine clinical practice.[11] Regimen-related factors appear to be more useful in improving patient adherence than trying to change deeply rooted patient behaviors. The following regimen-related factors deserve special attention by health care professionals and include:

- Regimen complexity, intensity, duration, side effects, convenience, and costs;
- Social support;
- Process variables, such as waiting time, frequency of appointments;
- Continuity of care including factors such as access to the facility.

Provider-Related Factors

Recognition of the fact that "measures that will increase compliance by both physicians and patients to regimens with proven benefit are necessary"[7] is explicit recognition of the importance of the role played by the provider in patient adherence. For example, improving provider communication skills is important because patient adherence and outcomes depend to a considerable extent on good provider-patient communication.[45] Provider-related factors associated with poor patient adherence typically include:

- Poor provider-patient communication;
- Complex regimens and recommendations;
- Exclusion of patients from decision-making;
- Inadequate follow-up, use of reminders, and reinforcement about patient progress;
- Lack of training, eg, use of behavioral strategies in patient counseling;
- Time constraints;
- Lack of incentive, including reimbursement.

At least one other provider factor must be added to the list of factors associated with poor patient adherence and outcome. This is

- Poor adherence by providers to the results of evidence-based medicine and appropriate clinical practice guidelines or standards of care.

The Treatment Gap

The 'treatment gap' is the differential between recommended effective therapies and the care that they actually receive.[15] Efforts to close the gap between research and clinical practice include continuing education activities to improve performance and optimize health outcomes. Systematic reviews of these continuing education activities suggest that the process of health care, and on occasion, health care outcomes, may be improved by interventions designed to increase the use of what are known to be effective treatments.[46, 47] As part of the continuing education activity spectrum, clinical practice guidelines have been developed as a means to improve the process of health care and health outcomes, to decrease practice variation and costs, to optimize resource utilization, and foster evidence-based decision-making.[48]

Cardiovascular Disease Treatment Gaps

In cardiovascular disease, effective therapies often are underutilized.[1] There is evidence of poor adherence with risk factor guidelines in the children of parents with premature coronary heart disease[49] just as there is evidence of poor adherence with the use of oral coagulation in older people.[50] Surveys in the United Kingdom document that the prevalence of pharmacotherapies with proven efficacy for males following coronary artery bypass surgery was 18% for β-blockers and lipid-lowering therapy, and 17% for ACE inhibitors, and as low as 9% for lipid-lowering therapy in patients with myocardial infarction.[51] In the United States, an estimated 30% of patients surviving a myocardial infarction in 1996 were recommended cholesterol-lowering drugs, 20% cholesterol-lowering dietary or smoking cessation advice, and <10% were referred to cardiac rehabilitation.[52] "... Without better compliance [on the part of both provider and patient], the knowledge we have won in so many expensive and laborious trials is not being put to use preventing atherosclerosis – the most common cause of death in the world".[7]

Cholesterol

In the 2 years following the release of the National Cholesterol Education Program 1993 Adult Treatment Panel II guidelines for patients with heart disease, adherence by primary care physicians to the screening and management recommendations was not consistent.[53] As many as 33% of patients with heart disease were not screened with lipid panels, 45% were not given dietary counseling, and 67% were not prescribed cholesterol medications, with the result that only 14% of the patients had achieved the recommended LDL lipoprotein level of 100 mg/dL.[53] In a similar analysis, Sueta and colleagues report that only 44% of 48,586 patients with heart disease had annual diagnostic testing of low-density lipoprotein cholesterol and only 39% were prescribed lipid-lowering therapy, and as few as 25% of patients reached target LDL levels of 100 mg/dL.[54]

High Blood Pressure

Controlling high blood pressure has long been recommended as effective.[17] Yet there is consistent documentation that, despite improved hypertension awareness, treatment, and control over the last 30 years or more, hypertension control is still a problem. In 1974 only 16% of all people with hypertension were controlled at <160/95 mmHg compared to 64% in 1991; however, also in 1991, only 29% of people with hypertension were controlled at <140/90 mmHg, now recognized as controlled hypertension.[55] Notably, this level of control had decreased to 27% by 1994.[17] Inadequate management of blood pressure in a hypertensive population is still a problem, as documented in a 1998 Department of Veterans Affairs study.[56] In this study, as many as 40% of patients with >6 hypertension-related visits in a year had blood pressures >160/90 mmHg with increased therapy reported in <10% of the visits; importantly, those patients receiving more intensive therapy had better control.[56]

β-Blockers

Despite a recent improvement in utilization of β-blocker therapy after acute myocardial infarction between 1992 and 1995, there is considerable evidence that β-blocker therapy is underutilized. For example, underutilization rates in the GUSTO trial ranged from 19% to 49% despite the fact that β-blocker therapy was mandated in the trial.[57] Among patients of all ages eligible to receive β-therapy after hospitalization for an acute myocardial infarction, 65% are not receiving it[58] and this underutilization rate increases to 79% of patients with no strong contraindications seen during an office visit.[59] The underutilization rate also is high in elderly patients with no contraindications after myocardial infarction[60] with 73% of patients between 67 and 96 years[61] and as many as 92% of nursing home patients with a mean age of 81 years not receiving β-blocker therapy.[62]

This high underutilization rate for β-blockers is an important example of the 'treatment gap' as it occurs despite the approximately 30% to 40% reduction in mortality with β-blockers.[58,63]

ACE Inhibitors

Underutilization of ACE inhibitors, a highly effective medication, in patients with heart failure is high. In 1997, Stafford and colleagues[64] reported that the use of ACE inhibitors in patients with heart failure increased from 24% in 1989 to only 31% in 1994, with fewer than 1 in 2 cardiologists and 1 in 4 of all other physicians prescribing ACE inhibitors. In one study, there was no evidence of the use of ACE inhibitors, digoxin, diuretics, or other vasodilators in 23% of the visits coded as heart failure.[64] A more recent 1999 article points out that as few as 44% of patients defined as meeting "ideal" criteria for ACE inhibitor therapy were prescribed doses recommended on the basis of evidence from large clinical trials.[65] In the same report, only 9% of current smokers had documented advice to quit smoking.

The statement below, from an editorial on the use of ACE inhibitors in heart failure, presumably also holds equally true for interventions to control cholesterol and high blood pressure and for the use of β-blockers and cardiac rehabilitation, as discussed in the next section. " It would therefore be reasonable to assume that many, if not all, of these patients were deprived of an effective therapeutic regimen that could have had significant impact on the progression of their disease and related prognosis."[66]

Cardiac Rehabilitation

With as few as 11% of eligible patients participating in rehabilitation in one review[67] and as many as 38% in one RCT,[68] it is estimated that less than 20% of the 12 million patients in the USA with established coronary heart disease are referred to cardiac rehabilitation programs. This is so despite the fact that cardiac rehabilitation has been shown to be associated with reduced mortality,[69] increased exercise tolerance,[70] physical function,[71] and health-related quality of life,[72] and that the improved exercise tolerance and health-related quality of life reportedly is associated with long-term survival.[73,74] However, information from the United Kingdom suggests that, although cardiac rehabilitation guidelines recommend a menu of services including an individual assessment, adherence to the guidelines is poor and that few physicians play an active role in the programs.[75]

Research Into Provider Adherence with Recommended Guidelines

Clinical practice guidelines are developed to reduce the gap between research and practice by improving clinical decision-making about effective interventions, with the expectation that the process and outcomes of health care will improve. Guidelines are usually developed as an amalgam of clinical experience, expert opinion, and research evidence.[76] For guidelines to be successful and improve the process and outcomes of health, no matter how well they are developed, requires provider adherence with the guidelines and, of course, patient adherence to provider recommendations. What is the evidence for improving provider adherence with guidelines, which are one attempt to close the gap between research and practice, if their utilization is low?

Utilization of, and adherence with, guidelines by providers may be low for various reasons. These include not being aware of them,[77,78] lack of agreement, self-efficacy, and outcome expectation,[79] not believing that they decrease health care costs, defensive practices, or malpractice suits,[80] and that they threaten provider autonomy.[78] Evidence from general practitioners suggests that they have a generally positive attitude to standard-setting but that, even when they know what to do, they often do not practice in accordance with their knowledge or skill[81] and often do not adopt guidelines.[78] Finally, there is some support for the model that suggests that adopting clinical practice guidelines is related to at least four determinants: clinician characteristics, patient characteristics, social factors, and practice characteristics.[16] This all suggests that behavior change on the part of the provider requires more than dissemination of information and standards; specific guideline implementation strategies are necessary as a barrier in one setting may well not be a barrier in another setting.[79]

Data from systematic reviews of interventions to translate guidelines into practice suggest a considerable range in the strength of the evidence on changing clinician performance.[46,47,82–84] The evidence is relatively strong for the effectiveness of reminder systems, academic detailing and multiple interventions; moderately effective for audit and feedback targeted to specific providers and delivered by peers or opinion leaders; and weak for didactic, traditional continuing medical education, and mailings.[84] Systematic reviews of the implementation of, and adherence with, clinical practice guidelines by clinicians suggest an inconsistent impact on patient outcomes.[82,84,85] However, this conclusion could be biased by a lack of methodologically sound studies, the use of out-of-date clinical practice guidelines, and uncertainty whether the outcomes such as "hard" biochemical or physical outcomes are more or less appropriate than "soft" outcomes such as health-related quality of life or patient satisfaction.

While guideline adoption strategies are integral to the ultimate success of clinical practice guidelines for treatments known to be effective and safe, there are serious deficiencies in their adoption. This makes it imperative that developing strategies to enhance guideline adoption be made a high priority for the immediate future in order to close the gap between research and practice. Research into interventions to improve the implementation of guidelines into clinical practice, and so reduce the 'treatment gap' has been identified by the National Health Service in the UK as such a priority area.[86]

Conclusion

Effective therapies in cardiovascular disease often are underutilized and poor adherence by providers with guidelines and by patients with recommendations are major barriers to improving the process of health care and patient outcomes.

Improved patient adherence with proven treatments can improve health outcomes. On one hand, research suggests that patient behaviors and attitudes are not clearly correlated with adherence and may not be particularly useful in enhancing patient adherence with interventions. On the other hand, regimen-related factors are associated with patient adherence. Therefore, future research efforts should focus on regimen characteristics associated with increased adherence and to develop strategies to enhance patient adherence with interventions that have been proven effective.

Improved provider adherence with guidelines for effective treatments has the potential to make a large, positive impact on patient outcomes but, unfortunately, there is considerable evidence of a 'treatment gap' with poor provider adherence with clinical practice guidelines. Adherence by providers to guidelines that are based on sound research evidence appears to improve the process of health care and, by extension, patient outcomes. Therefore, research into provider adherence-enhancing strategies is imperative in the attempt to close the gap between research and practice and to improve the process of health care and patient outcomes.

The existence of 'treatment gaps', despite the proven efficacy of many interventions to improve the health and health-related quality of life of patients with heart disease, is well established. The recommendation by the American Heart Association[2] that ". . . emphasis must be placed on implementing [adherence-enhancing] strategies at the patient, provider, and organizational level . . . [which,] . . . if integrated into a multilevel approach, offers enormous promise for decreasing risk and improving patient outcomes" is an important one that deserves serious attention by researchers and funding agencies.

References

1. Lenfant C. Conquering cardiovascular disease: Progress and promise. *JAMA* 1999;282:2068–2070.
2. Miller NH, Hill M, Kottke T, et al. The multilevel compliance challenge: Recommendations for a call to action. A statement for healthcare professionals. *Circulation* 1997;95:1085–1090.
3. Berg JS, Dischler J, Wagner DJ, et al. Medication compliance: A healthcare problem. *Ann Pharmacother* 1993;27:S1-S24.
4. Haynes RB, McKibbon KA, Kanani R. Systematic review of randomised trials of interventions to assist patients to follow prescriptions for medications. *Lancet* 1996;348:383–386.
5. Roter DL, Hall JA, Merisca R, et al. Effectiveness of interventions to improve patient compliance: A meta-analysis. *Med Care* 1998;36:1138–1161.
6. Haynes RB, Montague P, Oliver T, et al. Interventions for helping patients to follow prescriptions for medications (Cochrane Review). Oxford: The Cochrane Library. Update Software; 2000.
7. LaRosa JC. Future cardiovascular end point studies: Where will the research take us? *Am J Cardiol* 1999;84:454–458.
8. Donovan JL, Blake DR. Patient non-compliance: Deviance or reasoned decision-making. *Soc Sci Med* 1992;34:507–513.
9. Donovan JL. Patient decision making. The missing ingredient in compliance research. *Int J Tech Ass Health Care* 1995;11:443–455.
10. Morris LS, Schulz RM. Medication compliance: The patient's perspective. *Clin Ther* 1993;15:593–606.
11. Haynes RB. Improving patient adherence: State of the art, with a special focus on medication taking for cardiovascular disorders. In Burke LE, Ockene IS (eds.) *Compliance in Healthcare and Research.* Armonk, NY: Futura, pp 3–22.
12. Braunwald E, Mark DB, Jones RH, et al. Unstable angina: Diagnosis and management. Clinical Practice Guideline Number 10. AHCPR Publication No. 94–0602. Rockville, MD: Agency for Health Care Policy and Research and the National Heart, Lung, and Blood Institute, Public Health Service, U.S. Department of Health and Human Services; 1994.
13. Smith SC, Jr., Blair SN, Criqui MH, et al. AHA consensus panel statement. Preventing heart attack and death in patients with coronary disease. The Secondary Prevention Panel. *J Am Coll Cardiol* 1995;26:292–294.
14. Wenger NK, Froelicher ES, Smith LK, et al. Cardiac Rehabilitation. Clinical Practice Guideline #17. AHCPR # 96–0672. Rockville, MD: U.S. Dept of Health & Human Services, Public Health Service, Agency for Health Care Policy & Research and the National Heart, Blood & Lung Institute; 1995.
15. Pearson TA, Peters TD. The treatment gap in coronary artery disease and heart failure: Community standards and the post-discharge patient. *Am J Cardiol* 1997;80:45H-52H.
16. Tudiver F, Herbert C, Goel V. Why don't family physicians follow clinical practice guidelines for cancer screening? Family Physician Study Group, Sociobehavioral Cancer Research Network, National Cancer Institute of Canada. *CMAJ* 1998;159:797–798.

17. The sixth report of the Joint National Committee on prevention, detection, evaluation, and treatment of high blood pressure. *Arch Intern Med* 1997; 157:2413–2446.
18. National Heart, Lung, and Blood Institute Working group on Patient Compliance. Management of patient compliance in the treatment of hypertension. *Hypertension* 1982;4:415–423.
19. Epstein LH, Cluss PA. A behavioral medicine perspective on adherence to long-term medical regimens. *J Consult Clin Psychol* 1982; 50: 950–971.
20. Coronary Drug Project Research Group. Clofibrate and niacin in coronary heart disease. *JAMA* 1975;231:360–381.
21. Beta-blocker Heart Attack Trial. A randomized trial of propranolol in patients with acute myocardial infarction. I. Mortality results. *JAMA* 1982; 247:1707–1714.
22. Coronary Drug Project Research Group. Influence of adherence to treatment and response of cholesterol on mortality in the Coronary Drug Project. *N Engl J Med* 1980;303:1038–1041.
23. Horwitz RI, Viscoli CM, Berkman L, et al. Treatment adherence and risk of death after a myocardial infarction. *Lancet* 1990;336:542–545.
24. Horwitz RI, Horwitz SM. Adherence to treatment and health outcomes. *Arch Intern Med* 1993;153:1863–1868.
25. Hill MN, Miller NH. Compliance enhancement. A call for multidisciplinary team approaches. *Circulation* 1996;93:4–6.
26. Miller NH. Compliance with treatment regimens in chronic asymptomatic diseases. *Am J Med* 1997;102:43–49.
27. Krumholz HM. Treatment targets and the influence of standards of care. In Burke LE, Ockene IS (eds). *Compliance in Healthcare and Research.* Armonk, NY: Futura, pp 247–260.
28. Lee TH. How managed care thinks about compliance. In Burke LE, Ockene IS (eds). *Compliance in Healthcare and Research.* Armonk, NY: Futura, pp 311–316.
29. Aaron DJ, Morris KA, Nixon PA, et al. Reengineering epidemiology: An internet-based model for intervention studies. In Burke LE, Ockene IS (eds). *Compliance in Healthcare and Research.* Armonk, NY: Futura, pp 319–330.
30. Burke LE. Electronic measures. In Burke LE, Ockene IS (eds). *Compliance in Healthcare and Research.* Armonk, NY: Futura, pp 117–138.
31. Turner CF. Self-report measures: Their utility, how to structure. (in press.)
32. Burke LE, Dunbar-Jacob J. Adherence to medication, diet, and activity recommendations: From assessment to maintenance. *J Cardiovasc Nurs* 1995; 9:62–79.
33. Burke LE, Dunbar-Jacob JM, Hill MN. Compliance with cardiovascular disease prevention strategies: A review of the research. *Ann Behav Med* 1997;19:239–263.
34. Oldridge NB, Pashkow FJ. Adherence and motivation in cardiac rehabilitation. In Pashkow FJ, Dafoe WA (eds): *Clinical Cardiac Rehabilitation. A Cardiologist's Guide.* Baltimore: Williams & Wilkins; 1999:487–503.
35. Andrade SE, Walker AM, Gottlieb LK, et al. Discontinuation of antihyperlipidemic drugs—Do rates reported in clinical trials reflect rates in primary care settings? *N Engl J Med* 1995;332:1125–1131.
36. Oldridge NB. Compliance with cardiac rehabilitation services. *J Cardiopulmonary Rehabil* 1991;11:115–127.
37. Oldridge NB, Spencer J. Exercise habits and perceptions before and after

graduating or dropout from supervised cardiac exercise rehabilitation. *J Cardiac Rehabil* 1985;5:313–319.

38. Ghali JK, Kadakia S, Cooper R, et al. Precipitating factors leading to decompensation of heart failure. Traits among urban blacks. *Arch Intern Med* 1988; 148:2013–2016.

39. Vinson JM, Rich MW, Sperry JC, et al. Early readmission of elderly patients with congestive heart failure. *J Am Geriatr Soc* 1990;38:1290–1295.

40. Luepker RV. Patient adherence: A 'risk factor' for cardiovascular disease. *Heart Dis Stroke* 1993;2:418–421.

41. Psaty BM, Koepsell TD, Wagner EH, et al. The relative risk of incident coronary heart disease associated with recently stopping the use of beta-blockers. *JAMA* 1990;263:1653–1657.

42. West of Scotland Coronary Prevention Study Group. Compliance and adverse event withdrawal: Their impact on the West of Scotland Coronary Prevention Study. *Eur Heart J* 1997;18:1718–1724.

43. Strandberg TE, Lehto S, Pyorala K, et al. Cholesterol lowering after participation in the Scandinavian Simvastatin Survival Study (4S) in Finland. *Eur Heart J* 1997;18:1725–1727.

44. Ornish D, Scherwitz LW, Billings JH, et al. Intensive lifestyle changes for reversal of coronary heart disease. *JAMA* 1998;280:2001–2007.

45. Cleary PD. Changing clinician behavior: Necessary path to improvement or impossible dream? *Ann Intern Med* 1999;131:859–860.

46. Davis D, O'Brien MA, Freemantle N, et al. Impact of formal continuing medical education: Do conferences, workshops, rounds, and other traditional continuing education activities change physician behavior or health care outcomes? *JAMA* 1999;282:867–874.

47. Oxman AD, Thomson MA, Davis DA, et al. No magic bullets: A systematic review of 102 trials of interventions to improve professional practice. *CMAJ* 1995;153:1423–1431.

48. Institute of Medicine. Clinical Practice Guidelines. Washington, DC: National Academy Press; 1990.

49. Langner NR, Rowe PC, Davies R. The next generation: Poor compliance with risk factor guidelines in the children of parents with premature coronary heart disease. *Am J Public Health* 1994;84:68–71.

50. AGS Clinical Practices Committee. American Geriatric Society. The use of oral anticoagulants (warfarin) in older people. *J Am Geriatr Soc* 2000;48: 224–227.

51. Bowker TJ, Clayton TC, Ingham J, et al. A British Cardiac Society survey of the potential for the secondary prevention of coronary disease: ASPIRE (Action on Secondary Prevention through Intervention to Reduce Events). *Heart* 1996;75:334–342.

52. Vogel RA. Risk factor intervention and coronary artery disease: Clinical strategies. *Coron Artery Dis* 1995;6:466–471.

53. McBride P, Schrott HG, Plane MB, et al. Primary care practice adherence to National Cholesterol Education Program guidelines for patients with coronary heart disease. *Arch Intern Med* 1998;158:1238–1244.

54. Sueta CA, Chowdhury M, Boccuzzi SJ, et al. Analysis of the degree of undertreatment of hyperlipidemia and congestive heart failure secondary to coronary artery disease. *Am J Cardiol* 1999;83:1303–1307.

55. Burt VL, Culter JA, Higgins M, et al. Trends in the prevalence, awareness, treatment, and control of hypertension in the adult US population. Data from the health examination surveys, 1960 to 1991. *Hypertension* 1995;26: 60–69.

56. Berlowitz DR, Ash AS, Hickey EC, et al. Inadequate management of blood pressure in a hypertensive population. *N Engl J Med* 1998;339:1957–1963.
57. Pilote L, Califf RM, Sapp S, et al. Regional variation across the United States in the management of acute myocardial infarction. GUSTO-1 Investigators. Global utilization of streptokinase and tissue plasminogen activator for occluded coronary arteries. *N Engl J Med* 1995;333:565–572.
58. Gottlieb SS, McCarter RJ, Vogel RA. Effect of beta-blockade on mortality among high-risk and low-risk patients after myocardial infarction. *N Engl J Med* 1998;339:489–497.
59. Wang TJ, Stafford RS. National patterns and predictors of beta-blocker use in patients with coronary artery disease. *Arch Intern Med* 1998;158:1901–1906.
60. Krumholz HM, Radford MJ, Wang Y, et al. Early beta-blocker therapy for acute myocardial infarction in elderly patients. *Ann Intern Med* 1999;131:648–654.
61. Mendelson G, Aronow WS. Underutilization of beta-blockers in older patients with prior myocardial infarction or coronary artery disease in an academic, hospital-based geriatrics practice. *J Am Geriatr Soc* 1997;45:1360–1361.
62. Aronow WS. Prevalence of use of beta blockers and of calcium channel blockers in older patients with prior myocardial infarction at the time of admission to a nursing home. *J Am Geriatr Soc* 1996;44:1075–1077.
63. Lau J, Antman EM, Jimenez-Silva J, et al. Cumulative meta-analysis of therapeutic trials for myocardial infarction. *N Engl J Med* 1992;327:248–254.
64. Stafford RS, Saglam D, Blumenthal D. National patterns of angiotensin-converting enzyme inhibitor use in congestive heart failure. *Arch Intern Med* 1997;157:2460–2464.
65. Nohria A, Chen YT, Morton DJ, et al. Quality of care for patients hospitalized with heart failure at academic medical centers. *Am Heart J* 1999;137:1028–1034.
66. Deedwania PC. Underutilization of evidence-based therapy in heart failure. An opportunity to deal a winning hand with ace up your sleeve. *Arch Intern Med* 1997;157:2409–2412.
67. Leon AS, Certo C, Comoss P, et al. Scientific evidence of the value of cardiac rehabilitation services with emphasis on patients following myocardial infarction—Section 1: Exercise conditioning component. *J Cardiopulmon Rehabil* 1990;10:79–87.
68. Mark DB, Naylor CD, Hlatky MA, et al. Use of medical resources and quality of life after acute myocardial infarction in Canada and the United States. *N Engl J Med* 1994;331:1130–1135.
69. Oldridge NB, Guyatt GH, Fischer M, et al. Cardiac rehabilitation after myocardial infarction: Combining data from randomized clinical trials. *JAMA* 1988;260:945–980.
70. Stahle A, Mattsson E, Ryden L, et al. Improved physical fitness and quality of life following training of elderly patients after acute coronary events. A 1 year follow-up randomized controlled study. *Eur Heart J* 1999;20:1475–1484.
71. Ades PA, Maloney A, Savage P, et al. Determinants of physical functioning in coronary patients: Response to cardiac rehabilitation. *Arch Intern Med* 1999;159:2357–2360.
72. Oldridge N, Guyatt G, Jones N, et al. Effects on quality of life with comprehensive rehabilitation after acute myocardial infarction. *Am J Cardiol* 1991;67:1084–1089.

73. Dorn J, Naughton J, Imamura D, et al. Results of a multicenter randomized clinical trial of exercise and long-term survival in myocardial infarction patients: The National Exercise and Heart Disease Project (NEHDP). *Circulation* 1999;100:1764–1769.

74. Lim LL-Y, Johnson NA, O'Connell RL, et al. Quality of life and later adverse health outcomes in patients with suspected heart attack. *Aust NZ J Pub Health* 1998;22:540–546.

75. Lewin RJ, Ingleton R, Newens AJ, et al. Adherence to cardiac rehabilitation guidelines: A survey of rehabilitation programmes in the United Kingdom. *BMJ* 1998;316:1354–1355.

76. Cook DJ, Greengold NL, Ellrodt AG, et al. The relation between systematic reviews and practice guidelines. *Ann Intern Med* 1997;127:210–216.

77. Pathman DE, Konrad TR, Freed GL, et al. The awareness-to-adherence model of the steps to clinical guideline compliance. The case of pediatric vaccine recommendations. *Med Care* 1996;34:873–889.

78. James PA, Cowan TM, Graham RP, et al. Family physicians' attitudes about and use of clinical practice guidelines. *J Fam Pract* 1997;45:341–347.

79. Cabana MD, Rand CS, Powe NR, et al. Why don't physicians follow clinical practice guidelines? A framework for improvement. *JAMA* 1999;282: 1458–1465.

80. Tunis SR, Hayward RS, Wilson MC, et al. Internists' attitudes about clinical practice guidelines. *Ann Intern Med* 1994;120:956–963.

81. Grol R. National standard setting for quality of care in general practice: Attitudes of general practitioners and response to a set of standards. *Br J Gen Pract* 1990;40:361–364.

82. Grimshaw JM, Russell IT. Effect of clinical guidelines on medical practice: A systematic review of rigorous evaluations. *Lancet* 1993;342:1317–1322.

83. Conroy M, Shannon W. Clinical guidelines: Their implementation in general practice. *Br J Gen Pract* 1995;45:371–375.

84. Davis DA, Taylor-Vaisey A. Translating guidelines into practice. A systematic review of theoretic concepts, practical experience and research evidence in the adoption of clinical practice guidelines. *CMAJ* 1997;157:408–416.

85. Worrall G, Chaulk P, Freake D. The effects of clinical practice guidelines on patient outcomes in primary care: A systematic review. *CMAJ* 1997;156: 1705–1712.

86. Department of Health. Methods to promote the implementation of research findings in the NHS—priorities for evaluation. Leeds: Research and Development Directorate, Department of Health; 1995.

Subject Index